The Pelvic Girdle

To memories of my mother;
may her spirit live forever in my memory

For Churchill Livingstone:

Publishing Director, Health Professions: Mary Law
Project Development Manager: Mairi McCubbin
Project Manager: Ailsa Laing
Designer: Judith Wright
Illustrations Manager: Bruce Hogarth

The Pelvic Girdle

An approach to the examination and treatment of the lumbopelvic–hip region

Diane Lee BSR MCPA FCAMT

Instructor/Examiner for the Orthopaedic Division of the Canadian Physiotherapy Association

Foreword by

Paul Hodges MD PhD BPhty

NHMRC Senior Research Fellow and Professor, Department of Physiotherapy,
The University of Queensland, Brisbane, Australia

THIRD EDITION

This book has been endorsed by the MACP

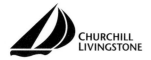

MANIPULATION
ASSOCIATION OF
CHARTERED
PHYSIOTHERAPISTS

CHURCHILL
LIVINGSTONE

EDINBURGH LONDON NEW YORK OXFORD PHILADELPHIA ST LOUIS SYDNEY TORONTO 2004

CHURCHILL LIVINGSTONE
An imprint of Elsevier Limited

First published 1989
Second edition 1999
Third edition 2004
    Reprinted 2005

ISBN 0 443 07373 2

British Library Cataloguing in Publication Data
A catalogue record for this book is available from the British Library

Library of Congress Cataloguing in Publication Data
A catalogue record for this book is available from the Library of Congress

Note
Knowledge and best practice in this field are constantly changing. As new research and experience broaden our knowledge, changes in practice, treatment and drug therapy may become necessary or appropriate. Readers are advised to check the most current information provided (i) on procedures featured or (ii) by the manufacturer of each product to be administered, to verify the recommended dose or formula, the method and duration of administration, and contraindications. It is the responsibility of the practitioner, relying on experience and knowledge of the patient, to make diagnoses, to determine dosages and the best treatment for each individual patient, and to take all appropriate safety precautions. To the fullest extent of the law, neither the publisher nor the authors assumes any liability for any injury and/or damage.

The Publisher

ELSEVIER   your source for books,
           journals and multimedia
           in the health sciences
www.elsevierhealth.com

Working together to grow
libraries in developing countries
www.elsevier.com | www.bookaid.org | www.sabre.org

ELSEVIER   BOOK AID   Sabre Foundation
           International

The
publisher's
policy is to use
**paper manufactured
from sustainable forests**

Printed in China

Contents

Foreword

Bridging the gap between science and clinical practice presents enormous challenges. Often we are faced with clinical techniques that develop with little consideration of biomechanical and neurophysiological findings or, conversely, basic science that contributes little to the progression of clinical practice. What Diane Lee and her colleagues have attempted and largely achieved here is a successful collaboration between science and practice. The result is an integrated clinical approach that incorporates a blend of concepts that are underpinned by research and clinical ideas that are based on observation of countless patients. Diane's clinical reasoning, based on observation of patterns of function and dysfunction, is attractive and thought-provoking.

A major feature that is obvious in the progression of each new edition of this book is how new advances in science and practice have been embraced, molded, challenged and refined into a working clinical model. It would appear that no new challenge or idea goes without notice. A great strength of the book is its open discussion of the evolution of ideas.

A multitude of people have developed and refined clinical techniques for the assessment and management of the pelvic girdle system. This book presents an amalgamation of these ideas into an integrated package. A strength of the book is how it flows from one approach to the next. The only weakness of this method is possible confusion regarding what comes from who and what has been adapted and progressed.

A major strength is the extrapolation and extension of established models. For instance, Diane has introduced a new level of complexity to the active straight leg raise test developed by Mens. Rather than simply use the test to evaluate load transfer through the pelvis Diane has taken the test to the next level, with multiple variants to establish the specific pattern of muscle activity that is problematic or beneficial. Another example is Diane's interpretation of the neutral zone hypothesis of Panjabi. Panjabi's model was specifically designed to explain the behaviour of motion segments and provide a model to explain changes in control of intervertebral motion that may contribute to the development of pain and disability. Diane has extended this model to include additional dysfunctions, such as intermittent loss of stability and subluxation.

A final example is the extrapolation of the concept of failed load transfer to urinary incontinence. Recent data from my group has defined the postural function of the pelvic floor muscles and has identified that incontinence is associated with increased risk of low back pain (Smith et al, unpublished data). The integration of this data and the concept of failed load transfer is likely to lead to improved management of incontinence. Although all of these developments require validation and support, they provide fuel for future research.

I have been fortunate for several years to collaborate clinically with Linda-Joy Lee. Her take on my group's approach to assessment and training of the muscle system has been faithfully described and integrated along with additional techniques to address specific issues of the pelvic girdle. Linda-Joy is currently taking the critical step to understand the 'other side' and is completing her PhD in my laboratory investigating motor control of the trunk and interaction of the lumbopelvic systems. If this book is any indication, I am convinced that this will lead to many new extrapolations into clinical practice.

In summary I commend Diane Lee and her collaborators for their intelligent summary of the field and their thoughtful clinical take on science and clinical practice. I am sure the developments will progress clinical practice and look forward to the next steps.

Brisbane 2004   Paul Hodges

Preface

When I was approached by the publishers about writing the third edition of this text I didn't think there was enough material to warrant a new edition at this time. After completing this update, I now realize that there have been significant advances in our understanding of the low back and pelvis over the past 5 years and a major revision to the second edition has occurred! As before, Chapters 1–4 review the history of interest in the pelvic girdle, its physical evolution through time both in the species and individually, and the relevant anatomy necessary to understand the subsequent material in the text. There are new anatomical figures in Chapters 4 and 9, which Frank Willard, Serge Gracovetsky, Carl DeRosa, Lance Twomey, and James Taylor have kindly allowed me to use. Thank you for sharing your beautiful work.

Chapter 5 is a brand new chapter for this text and presents in greater detail the integrated model of function that was developed in collaboration with Andry Vleeming through our many hours of discussion and teaching together. I am, as always, indebted to him for his confidence in me as I share this work with you. This model was originally derived from anatomical and biomechanical studies of the pelvis, as well as from the clinical experience of treating patients with lumbopelvic pain. This approach addresses why the lumbopelvic-hip region is painful and no longer able to sustain and transfer loads, as opposed to an approach that seeks to identify pain-generating structures. It has long been recognized that physical factors impact on joint function. The model suggests that joint mechanics can be influenced by multiple factors, some intrinsic to the joint itself, while others are produced by muscle action which is in turn influenced by the emotional state.

This text focuses on the assessment and treatment of the first three components of this model (form closure, force closure, and motor control) and its application to the lumbar spine, pelvic girdle, and hip.

The biomechanics of the lumbopelvic-hip region are updated in Chapter 6. Of significance is the recent PhD work of Barbara Hungerford, physiotherapist, from Sydney, Australia. Hungerford confirmed some of the biomechanics (both osteokinematics and arthrokinematics) proposed in the second edition; in particular, those that occur on the non-weight-bearing side of the pelvis during one-leg standing in healthy individuals. Her research also revealed that during one-leg standing a different arthrokinematic glide (previously unknown and unpredicted) occurs at the sacroiliac joint on the weight-bearing side when the force closure mechanism is effective. She went on to show that this 'locking-in' glide at the sacroiliac joint does not occur when there is insufficient compression (ineffective force closure) of the pelvis. This research has been clinically developed into specific tests (Ch. 8) for analyzing load transfer through the pelvis and hip.

The assessment of the lumbopelvic-hip region (Ch. 8) is co-written with Linda-Joy Lee. I have had the pleasure of working and teaching with Linda-Joy for the last 3 years and she continues to amaze me with her brilliance and clinical wisdom far beyond her graduate years. She gently challenges my long-held paradigms; she improves my writing and my PowerPoint presentations and, through the results she achieves with her patients, encourages me to explore areas of clinical practice that at times frighten me (dry needling). Together, we have learned how to teach others to achieve *mobile* stability through touch, imagery, and movement – a different way to exercise. Thank you Linda-Joy for sharing this part of your journey with me; I look forward to watching you fly.

The assessment presented in Chapter 8 follows the integrated model and includes tests for functional analysis (load transfer) as well as specific regional tests for analysis of form closure, force closure, and motor control. The work of Vleeming, Buyruk, and Damen has had a significant impact on our knowledge regarding the interpretation of joint play tests for form closure. Individually, their research has shown that we cannot predict how much mobility an individual's sacroiliac joint should have and therefore we cannot reliably diagnose 'hypomobility' or 'hypermobility' from joint play tests alone. Perhaps this is why intertester reliability has been so poor for motion analysis *in vivo*. What they have shown is that, in health, mobility of the left and right sacroiliac joint should be symmetric and that asymmetry is predictive of dysfunction and pain. The clinical significance of this research is expanded further in both Chapters 8 and 9. The active straight leg raise (ASLR) test is a validated clinical test for measuring effective load transfer between the trunk and lower limbs. It was originally introduced by Mens & Vleeming and has been further developed in this edition, based on clinical experience over the last 5 years. It is proposed that, by varying the location of manual compression during the ASLR, further information can be gained, which assists the clinician when prescribing manual therapy and/or exercises to improve mobility, stability, and motor control (Ch. 10).

A major change in this edition is the classification, assessment, and treatment of the muscles of the local and global systems. This is in response to the proliferation of research in this area, notably by Paul Hodges, Lorimer Moseley, Peter O'Sullivan, and others. We have been fortunate to learn directly from these leaders during their visits to our clinic (and ours to theirs) and by the opportunity of one of us (Linda-Joy Lee) to assist Paul Hodges on his courses in North America. We are indeed indebted to them for their trust and confidence that we will represent their material well in a clinical text such as this. The neuromuscular research pertaining to the local system has impressed upon us the sensitivity of the lumbar, sacroiliac, and hip joints to compression (or lack thereof) and the impact that variable compression can have on function of the low back, pelvis, and hip. We now understand that a diagnosis of 'stability' cannot be reached by one

test alone and the significance of Panjabi's interdependent concept of stability (1992b). It is indeed a complex concept, which we often attempt to simplify for study.

It has also become clear that the global system is essentially an integrated sling system, comprised of several muscles, which produces forces. A muscle may participate in more than one sling and the slings may overlap and interconnect depending on the task being demanded. It is proposed that the slings have no beginning or end but rather connect to assist in the transference of forces. It is possible that the slings are all part of one interconnected myofascial system and the particular sling that is identified during any motion is merely due to the activation of selective parts of the whole sling. This leads us to question the validity of 'specific' testing for muscle strength and whether this is indeed possible. A different way of analyzing effective force transfer through slings as well as analyzing the extensibility of a sling is presented in Chapter 8.

In 2002, Jackie Whittaker joined our team and has shared her clinical experience using real-time ultrasound imaging both for assessment and treatment of the muscles of the lumbopelvic local system. In Chapter 8, she presents her clinical interpretation of the research in this field; it has certainly opened my eyes and hands to another dimension for clinical assessment and treatment. Thank you, Jackie, for taking this on and tolerating my multiple edits. Your enthusiasm is contagious and I think I even understand it when I can slow you down just a bit. Which way does the green dot go again?

Chapter 9 considers the clinical findings from the subjective and objective examination for specific lumbar, pelvic girdle, and hip impairments according to the integrated model. The chapter concludes with a discussion of stress urinary incontinence, or ineffective force closure of the urethra. I believe that orthopedic manual therapists who focus on restoring function to the local system of the low back and pelvis and therapists who specialize in pelvic floor dysfunction are treating the same condition: failed load transfer through the lumbopelvic region, including the organs. The dysfunction is manifested either through a loss of effective force closure of the joints of the low back and pelvis (pain and loss of mobility/stability), or loss of effective force closure of the urethra (incontinence). The research clearly suggests that we are merging to a common understanding of both function and dysfunction of the whole pelvis and not just its parts.

Treatment for specific impairments of the lumbo-pelvic-hip region is the challenge of Chapter 10 and is also co-written with Linda-Joy Lee. Treatment for the impaired lumbopelvic-hip region must be pre-scriptive since every individual has a unique clin-ical presentation. Rarely will only one dysfunction be present (one stiff joint or one poorly controlled joint); more commonly, multiple problems coexist such that the most effective treatment consists of a unique combination of techniques and exercises specific for each patient. The effective management of lumbopelvic-hip pain and dysfunction requires attention to all four components: form closure, force closure, motor control, and emotions. Ultimately, function requires stability with mobility (not rigid-ity) of the joints and organs for any endeavor the individual chooses to do. This chapter presents spe-cific manual therapy techniques and exercises for restoring mobile stability for the lumbopelvic-hip region. The role of external supports and the indica-tions for prolotherapy are discussed.

In closing, I hope you enjoy the changes in this edition and feel, as I now do, that it was time to update the second edition.

Canada, 2004   Diane Lee

Acknowledgments

In addition to the contribution of the clinicians mentioned in the Preface, I would like to acknowledge the support of those who helped see this project to its completion. All of the clinical photographs are new thanks to Goran Basaric (photographer) and Melanie Coffey (model) and several of the anatomical and biomechanical line drawings are improved or new thanks, once again, to Frank Crymble. The anatomical figures in Chapter 9 are from Primal Pictures. Thank you, Sloan Hickman, for your generous corporate vision and for allowing me to use them here. The picture for the cover of this edition is provided courtesy of Roland Lorente, who is the official photographer for Les Grands Ballets Canadiens de Montréal. He holds the copyright for this photo and has kindly allowed me to use it here. The dancers captured in this wonderful pose clearly portray the goal of this book: restoring confident stability with mobility. Lisa Davies (the dancer on the right) is a principal soloist with Les Grands Ballets and Linda-Joy and I truly enjoyed the opportunity to work with her. Finally, I would also like to thank Mary Law and Churchill Livingstone for their patience and support while waiting for the completion of this edition.

As always, I am especially grateful for my family, Tom, Michael, and Chelsea, who allow me the time, and provide the encouragement, so necessary to complete a project such as this. This edition is dedicated to my mother, whose life's journey gave her the challenge of Alzheimer's disease, and my father, whose life's journey gave him the challenge of her care. The lesson for me has been to take the time to remember them both.

Abbreviations

ASIS	anterior superior iliac spine
ABLR	active bent leg raise
ASLR	active straight leg raise
CT	computed tomography
DISH	diffuse idiopathic skeletal hyperostosis
EMG	electromyogram
EO	external oblique
ERSL	extended, rotated/sideflexed left
ERSR	extended, rotated/sideflexed right
FRSL	flexed, rotated/sideflexed left
IAP	intraabdominal pressure
ILA	inferior lateral angle
IMS	intramuscular stimulation
IO	internal oblique
MUI	mixed urinary incontinence
PAVM	passive accessory vertebral motion
PICR	path of the instantaneous center of rotation
PIIS	posterior inferior iliac spine
PIVM	passive intervertebral motion
PNF	proprioceptive neuromuscular facilitation
PSIS	posterior superior iliac spine
RSA	roentgen stereophotogrammetric analysis
RTUS	real-time ultrasound
SIJ	sacroiliac joint
SUI	stress urinary incontinence
TA	transversus abdominis
UI	urinary incontinence
UUI	urge urinary incontinence

Chapter 1

A historical review

According to Weisl (1955) the first medical practitioners to express an interest in the pelvic girdle were Hippocrates (460–377 BC), Vesalius (AD 1543) and Pare (AD 1643). According to the historical records (reported by Weisl 1955), Hippocrates and Vesalius both felt that the sacroiliac joints were immobile, whereas Pare believed that motion of this joint could occur in women during pregnancy. Then in 1698 De Diemerbroeck demonstrated that mobility could occur apart from pregnancy. It appears that from the seventeenth century until today, a controversy has existed as to the classification and composition of the SIJ, the quantity, if any, of motion, and the specific biomechanics which accompany movement of the lower extremities and trunk.

The joint has been implicated as the cause of many symptoms including sciatica; in fact, at the turn of the twentieth century Albee (1909) and Goldthwait & Osgood (1905) proposed that sciatica developed from direct pressure on the lumbosacral plexus as it crossed the anterior aspect of the SIJ. This pressure was thought to be caused by "subluxed, relaxed or diseased sacroiliac joints" (Meisenbach 1911). Treatment consisted of manipulative reduction of the sacrum followed by immobilization, in plaster, in spinal hyperextension for 6 months. Following the classic paper by Mixter & Barr (1934) on prolapsed intervertebral disks and the clinical ramifications of pressure on the lumbosacral nerve roots intraspinally, the SIJ was felt to be less significant and lesions of this articulation were regarded as rare (Cyriax 1954).

Research over the last 50 years has revealed significant information pertaining to the anatomy and function of the pelvic girdle. In 1992, the first Interdisciplinary World Congress on Low Back and Pelvic Pain (Vleeming et al 1992b) exposed the current state of knowledge in this area; most was empirical. It was clear that more research was necessary to understand the biomechanics, to develop valid assessment tests and to determine the best way to treat lumbopelvic dysfunction. Three years later, the second World Congress (Vleeming et al 1995c) brought forth a wealth of information, validated through research, that has become part of the foundation for rehabilitation of the lumbopelvic region. Two more World Congresses (Vienna 1998, Montreal 2001) have occurred since the second edition of this text was published and each has helped to consolidate the scientific basis for the diagnosis and treatment of the impaired lumbopelvic region.

The integrated function of the low back, pelvic girdle, and lower extremity is becoming clear. The most reliable, sensitive, and specific diagnostic tests/procedures and treatment techniques/exercises are still open to debate; however, we now have evidence to support sound inclusion criteria for defining the impairment and thus investigating it independently from the pain it can produce. Once again, it is appropriate to record the current thoughts on the anatomy, biomechanics, assessment, and treatment of the lumbopelvic-hip complex. The integrated model of function (Lee & Vleeming 1998, 2003) continues to be the foundation for this work. Some parts of this model are firmly supported by research while others remain to be validated. With each passing year, today's ideas become historical reviews – this edition attempts to bridge the historical gap from 1998 to 2004.

Chapter 2

Evolution and comparative anatomy

In collaboration with

James Meadows MCPA MCSP FCAMT

Instructor for the Orthopaedic Division of the Canadian Physiotherapy Association and the North American Institute of Orthopedic Manipulative Therapy. Founder and director of Swodeam Consulting

INTRODUCTION

The human lumbopelvic-hip region, while in many respects unique in the animal world for its evolutionary adaptation to orthograde bipedalism, is based on a design originating almost half a billion years ago. The absence of fossils of human pelves older than five million years supports the assumption that the adaptation to bipedalism is recent. This chapter will briefly outline the evolutionary steps which have facilitated human gait. Subsequently, the changes in human structure and posture as a result of bipedalism will be described.

EVOLUTION OF THE PELVIC GIRDLE

The pelvic girdle first appeared as a pair of small cartilaginous elements lying in the abdomen of primitive fish (Romer 1959, *Encyclopedia Britannica* 1981, Young 1981, Stein & Rowe 1982, Nelson & Jurmain 1985, Gracovetsky & Farfan 1986). The "fin fold" theory maintains that lateral folds formed in ancient fish to prevent rolling and buckling of the undulating body. As the folds contributed to propulsion and steering, they gradually began to fragment. From this fragmentation, two paired lateral fins were formed, the pectoral and pelvic fins. The pectoral fin was the primary propeller and was the largest and the most stable of the two. Since stability was not a functional requirement of the pelvic girdle, there was no need for axial attachment nor attachment between the two sides.

With migration on to land, the pelvic fin rapidly developed into the powerhouse of locomotion and consequently increased stability of the pelvic girdle was required. The pectoral fin (and its later development, the forelimb) was relegated to the role of steering – a reversal of the original roles.

STABILIZATION OF THE PELVIC GIRDLE

The pelvic girdle has evolved towards increased stability both at the pubic symphysis and at the sacroiliac joints. The original innominate bone contained two elements which together formed the puboischium. During the stabilization process, the puboischium enlarged and united with the opposite side via the puboischial symphysis. Intrapelvic stability was subsequently increased; however, stability between the primitive innominate bone and the axial skeleton was also required. A dorsal projection developed on the puboischium (ultimately forming the ilium) directed towards the axial skeleton.

Simultaneously, the costal element of the axial skeleton enlarged and fused with one (or more) preanal vertebra to form the sacrum. The iliac projection of the primitive innominate bone and the enlarged costal process of the primitive sacrum formed the first sacroiliac joint. The initial union was ligamentous. Thus, direct articulation between the axial and appendicular skeletons occurred. At this stage, the pelvic girdle had a full inventory of the elements present today in all tetrapods.

The number of vertebrae which contribute to the sacrum varies from species to species and depends on the degree of stability or mobility required at the sacroiliac joint. Many amphibians and reptiles have only one or two sacral vertebrae whereas higher mammals have five. The extreme of sacral development is found in the bird where the synsacrum includes the fusion of the sacral, lumbar, and caudal thoracic vertebrae. This, together with the huge sternum, provides the stability necessary to anchor the muscles which move the wings.

As the locomotive pattern of vertebrates progressed from crawling to the linear-limb quadripedal and bipedal gait of advanced mammals, the role of the ilium became more significant. The bone provided the major pelvic attachment for the limb musculature as well as the articular surface for the sacroiliac joint.

COMPARATIVE ANATOMY

The structure of the human pelvic girdle reflects the adaptation required for bipedal gait (Keagy &

Brumlik 1966, Tuttle 1975, Farfan 1978, Goodall 1979, Rodman & McHenry 1980, Stein & Rowe 1982, Swindler & Wood 1982, Basmajian & Deluca 1985, Nelson & Jurmain 1985, Williams 1995) (Fig. 2.1). The surface area of the ilia has increased whereas the length of the ischium and the pubis has decreased. The posterior muscles have lost some bulk secondary to the increased stability of the sacroiliac joint. Sufficient mobility of the sacroiliac joint has been maintained for bipedalism.

SACRUM

The sacrum has increased in size, thus accommodating the increased osseous attachment of the gluteus maximus muscle. The articular surface of the sacroiliac joint has also increased in size and facilitates the increased compression produced in bipedal stance. The surface itself has become more incongruous (Ch. 3) and facilitates intrapelvic stability.

INNOMINATE

The ilia have undergone dramatic changes in response to bipedalism. The bone has twisted (Fig. 2.1) such that the lateral aspect is now directed anteriorly. The gluteus medius and minimus muscles have migrated anteriorly and their function has subsequently changed. In the ape, the gluteus medius and minimus muscles are femoral extensors, while in humans they act as femoral abductors (Fig. 2.2) and thus prevent a Trendelenburg gait.

In addition to the reorientation of the ilium, a fossa has developed (the iliac fossa) which increases the surface area available for the attachment of the gluteal and iliacus muscles. The reduction in extensor power caused by the anterior migration of the gluteus medius and minimus muscles is therefore compensated for. The iliac fossa also facilitates the enlargement of the iliacus muscle, which plays a significant role in the maintenance of erect human posture.

The anatomical changes apparent in the ischium reflect the alteration in function of the hamstring muscle group (see below). Although these muscles have continued to be involved in femoral extension, constant activity is not a requirement of bipedal stance in humans. Subsequently, the ischial body and tuberosity have become reduced in both length and width (Fig. 2.1). The vertical dimension of the pubic symphysis has also decreased with the evolution of efficient bipedal gait.

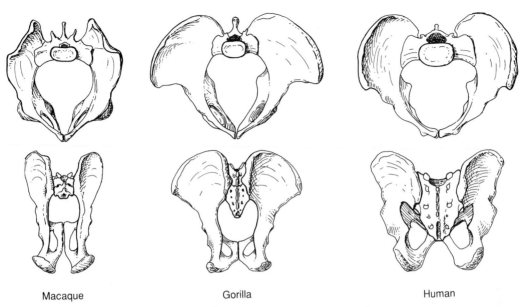

Figure 2.1 Comparative anatomy of the pelvic girdle. (Redrawn from Stein & Rowe 1982.)

Macaque   Gorilla   Human

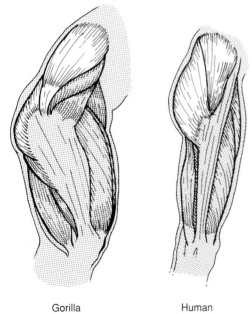

Gorilla   Human

Figure 2.2 The gluteus medius and minimus muscles in the gorilla function as femoral extensors while in humans they act as femoral abductors.

ACETABULUM

The acetabulum has become deeper as well as reoriented in an anterolateral direction. This reorientation projects the femoral neck anteriorly and, together with

the angle of inclination, ensures that the leg adducts at heel strike to place the foot beneath the acetabulum. The ligaments of the hip joint (Figs 4.23 and 4.24) are extensive in comparison to those of the ape, where they are almost non-existent.

POSTURE

The human vertebral column, in comparison to other primates, differs primarily in its posture. The human vertebral column and innominates have rotated posteriorly through 90° to bring the head above the feet (Fig. 2.3). The sacral base is no longer horizontal as it is in non-human mammals, but neither has it rotated through 90° (Abitbol 1995, 1997). The angle of the sacral promontory with the fifth lumbar vertebra is acute. Consequently, the spine organized into a vertical column even though the orientation of the sacrum facilitated a more horizontal row. Caudally, the lumbosacral angle and lumbar lordosis developed. This curve was compensated for by the development of a thoracic kyphosis.

In all non-human primates, the lumbar spine is kyphotic. However, it is possible for a non-human primate to achieve a lumbar lordosis, as was witnessed by Goodall (1979) in her Gombe Stream Reserve study. One ape in this study contracted poliomyelitis as an infant, which affected the function of one arm. Since the characteristic "knuckle walk"

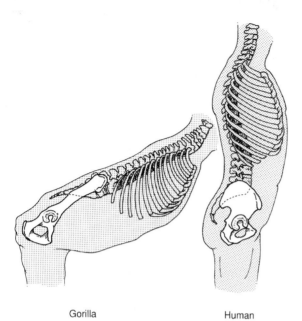

Gorilla   Human

Figure 2.3 Posterior rotation of the vertebral column and the innominates has led to the development of the lumbosacral lordosis and the thoracic kyphosis.

was not possible, the animal had developed a bipedal gait for locomotion. To facilitate this, a marked lumbar lordosis had developed. However, the attachment of the gluteal muscles in the ape prevents simultaneous extension of the lumbar spine and the femur and since neither the osseous nor the myofascial structure had changed, an increase in both hip and knee flexion had to occur in order to maintain the line of gravity within the base of support.

The bipedal posture of the ape depends on the massive gluteal and hamstring muscles whose major role is to stabilize the pelvic girdle and the trunk on the flexed hips. Constant activity in both muscle groups is required since the line of gravity of the bipedal ape falls considerably anterior to the coronal axis of the hip joint. Consequently, the

attachments of the posterior muscles in the ape are widespread and the ischial body and tuberosity are massive. Conversely, in humans, the line of gravity falls slightly posterior to the coronal axis of the hip joint (Fig. 8.1) and therefore the requirements for postural balance are both reduced and reversed. According to Abitbol (1997), erect posture can be effortless when the center of the sacroiliac joint (biauricular line) and the center of the acetabulum (biacetabular line) form a vertical line when the sagittal plane of the pelvis is viewed laterally. The body weight is more efficiently balanced and tends to extend the pelvic girdle on the femora. To prevent this, slight recruitment of the psoas major muscle is required to maintain the optimal bipedal posture. Only intermittent activity is required from the hamstring muscle group and consequently the ischial body and tuberosity have become considerably reduced in size.

Summary

The human lumbopelvic-hip complex has developed from the primate pelvic girdle which evolved for an arboreal lifestyle. The current vertebral curvatures are relatively recent; the early hominids and even Neanderthals had different vertebral curvatures. The curves are interdependent and any factor which causes a change in one results in a compensatory change in all others. The major structural changes in *Homo sapiens* appear to have evolved to facilitate the most bioenergetically efficient gait among terrestrial tetrapods.

ACKNOWLEDGMENT

For this contribution, I am indebted to Jim Meadows.

Chapter 3

The pelvis – its anatomy through time

CHAPTER CONTENTS

EMBRYOLOGY AND DEVELOPMENT

DEVELOPMENT OF BONES

Sacrum

The sacrum derives its name from the Latin word *sacer*, meaning sacred. It is thought that the sacrum was the only bone to be preserved following the burning of a witch and as such must have been sacred. Fryette credits the "ancient Phallic Worshipers [for naming] the base of the spine the Sacred Bone" (Fryette 1954). The bone is derived from the fusion of five mesodermal somites. During the 4th embryonic week, 42–44 pairs of somites arise from the paraxial mesoderm. Although not consistently, the sacrum evolves from the 31st to the 35th somites, each of which divides into three components – the sclerotome, myotome, and dermatome (Fig. 3.1). The sclerotome multiplies and migrates both ventrally and dorsally to surround the notochord and the evolving spinal cord. Subsequently, each sclerotome divides into equal cranial and caudal components

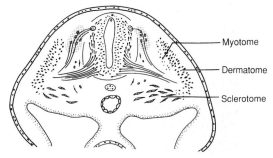

Figure 3.1   Differentiation of the mesodermal somite into sclerotome, myotome, and dermatome. (Redrawn from Williams 1995.)

separated by a sclerotomic fissure which in the sacrum progresses to develop a rudimentary intervertebral disk composed of fibrocartilage. The adjacent sclerotomic segments then fuse to form the centrum of the sacral vertebral body. The dorsal aspect of the sclerotome, which has migrated posteriorly, forms the vertebral arch (the neural arch is part of this), while the ventrolateral aspect becomes the costal process (ala of the sacrum) (Fig. 3.2). This process appears only in the upper two or three sacral segments and is responsible for forming the auricular sacral surface.

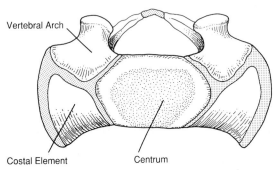

Figure 3.2 The sclerotome of the future sacrum differentiates into three parts: the centrum, the vertebral arch, and the costal element or process.

Chondrification of the sacrum precedes ossification and begins during the 6th embryonic week (Rothman & Simeone 1975). The primary ossification centers for the centrum and each half of the vertebral arch appear between the 10th and the 20th week, while the primary centers for the costal elements appear later, between the 6th and the 8th month.

The three components of the sacral segment (Fig. 3.2) – the costal element, the vertebral arch, and the centrum – remain separated by hyaline cartilage up until 2–5 years of age when the costal element (ala of the sacrum) unites with the vertebral arch. This unit then fuses to the centrum and to the other vertebral arch in the 8th year.

The conjoined costal element, vertebral arch, and centrum of each sacral segment remain separated from those above and below by hyaline cartilage laterally and by fibrocartilage medially (Fig. 3.3). A cartilaginous epiphysis extends the entire length of the lateral aspect of the sacrum. Fusion of the sacral segments occurs after puberty in a caudocranial direction with the simultaneous appearance of secondary ossification centers for the centrum, spinous process, transverse processes, and costal elements. The adjacent margins of the sacral vertebrae ossify after the 20th year; however, the central portion of the intervertebral disk can remain unossified even after middle life.

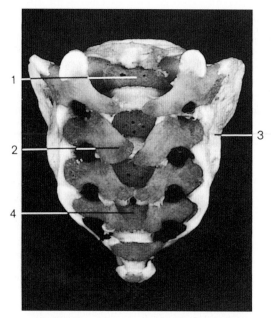

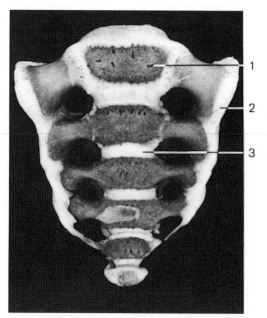

Figure 3.3 Ossification of the sacrum. **Left: Posterior aspect:** note the centrum (1), the vertebral arch (2), the lateral epiphysis (3), and the sacral canal (4). **Right: Anterior aspect:** note the centrum (1), the lateral epiphysis (2), and the intervertebral disk (3). (Reproduced with permission from Rohen & Yokochi 1983.)

Innominate

The innominate has a Latin derivation, *innominatus*, meaning having no name. It appears during the 7th embryonic week as three bones – the ilium, the ischium, and the pubis – which are derived from a small proliferating mass of mesenchyme from the somatopleure in the developing limb bud. Three primary ossification centers appear before birth, one for the ilium above the sciatic notch during the 8th intrauterine week, one for the ischium in the body of the bone during the 4th month, and one for the pubis in the superior ramus between the 4th and 5th months. At birth, the iliac crest, the acetabular fossa, and the inferior ischiopubic ramus are cartilaginous (Fig. 3.4). The inferior ischiopubic ramus ossifies during the 7th to 8th year. The iliac crest and the acetabular fossa develop secondary ossification centers during puberty but can remain unossified until 25 years of age. When treating adolescents, it is pertinent to recall the stage of development before applying vigorous mobilization or manipulation techniques.

DEVELOPMENT OF JOINTS

Sacroiliac joint

According to Bellamy et al (1983), the development of the sacroiliac joint (SIJ) commences during the 8th week of intrauterine life. As in other synovial joints, a trilayer structure initially appears in the mesenchyme between the ilium and the costal element of the sacrum. Cavitation begins both peripherally and centrally by the 10th week and by the 13th week the enlarged cavities are separated by fibrous septa. These findings are not consistent with Walker's (1984, 1986) study of 36 fetuses in which she noted that cavitation did not begin until the 32nd week (Fig. 3.5). The stage at which cavitation is complete and the fibrous bands disappear is controversial. Bellamy et al (1983) state that the cavity is fully developed by the 8th month and that the fibrous septa soon disappear whilst Walker (1986) notes that, unlike most synovial joints which show complete cavitation by the 12th week, the SIJ remains separated by fibrous bands at birth and she questions their persistence in some joints into adulthood. Bowen & Cassidy (1981) report that the 10 specimens studied in this age group did not contain the fibrous septa previously noted in late fetal life. Schunke (1938) was the first to describe these intraarticular bands and felt that they disappeared in the first year of life.

The synovium of the joint develops from the mesenchyme at the edges of the primordial cavity, as does the articular capsule which is thin and pliable at this stage (Bowen & Cassidy 1981). All investigators

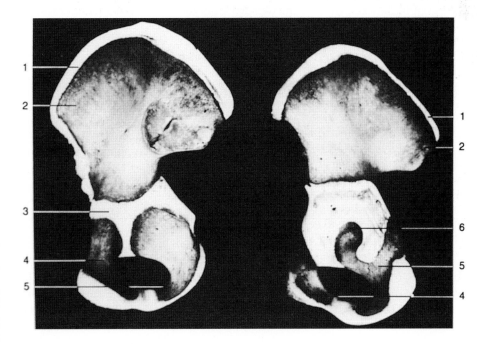

Figure 3.4 The medial (left) and lateral (right) aspect of the left innominate bone and the ossification process. Note the cartilage of the iliac crest (1), the ilium (2), the cartilage separating the ilium, pubis and ischium (3), the pubis (4), the ischium (5) and the acetabulum (6). (Reproduced with permission from Rohen & Yokochi 1983.)

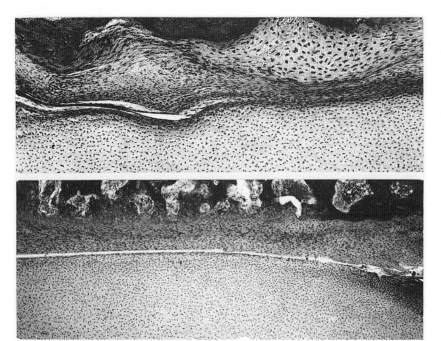

Figure 3.5 Cavitation of the sacroiliac joint. **Top:** Sacroiliac joint of a fetus at 16 weeks of gestation. Note the proximity of the iliac bone to the joint surface, the partial cavitation of the joint, and the presence of a fibrous band connecting the two surfaces. **Bottom:** Sacroiliac joint of a fetus at 34 weeks of gestation. Note that cavitation is almost complete except for a few loose fibrous bands. (Reproduced with permission from Walker 1986.)

note (Schunke 1938, Bowen & Cassidy 1981, Walker 1986, Kampen & Tillmann 1998) the macroscopic and microscopic differences between the cartilage which lines the articular surfaces of the ilium and the sacrum.

The ilium is lined with a type of fibrocartilage which is bluer, duller and more striated than the hyaline cartilage which lines the sacrum (Plates 1 and 2) and this difference is noted right from birth (Kampen & Tillmann 1998). The depth of the cartilage is also different. According to Bowen & Cassidy (1981), the sacral hyaline cartilage is three to five times thicker than the iliac fibrocartilage. This is consistent with the findings of Schunke (1938), MacDonald & Hunt (1951) and Kampen & Tillmann (1998), but differs from the studies of Walker (1986), who found that the sacral hyaline cartilage was 1.7 times thicker than the iliac fibrocartilage, although this finding may vary depending upon which aspect of the joint was being studied. All agree that the corresponding articular surfaces were smooth and flat at this stage, although Walker (1984) found elevations and depressions on her full-term infants as well. Bowen & Cassidy (1981) note that during handling of the fetal pelves, the joint was capable of gliding in a multitude of directions.

Pubic symphysis and hip joint

The pubic symphysis is a non-synovial joint which contains a thick fibrocartilaginous disk between thin layers of hyaline cartilage. The symphysis is present by the end of the second month of gestation (Gamble et al 1986) with thick cartilaginous end-plates at birth (9–10 mm) that become thin (200–400 µm) with skeletal maturity. The secondary ossification centers appear in early puberty and, by mid-adolescence, the joint has reached its mature size. It is beyond the scope of this text to describe the detailed embryology of the hip joint; however, several references are included for the interested reader (Strayer 1971, Watanabe 1974, Siffert & Feldman 1980, Walker 1980a, b, 1981).

THE SACROILIAC JOINT AND AGING

At birth, the pelvic girdle is far from complete developmentally. A major part of the unit is cartilaginous and the articular anatomy contributes little to intrapelvic stability. The changes which occur within the SIJs over the next seven decades are significant for the biomechanics, assessment, and treatment of the pelvic girdle in the varying age groups.

THE FIRST DECADE (0–10 YEARS)

Bowen & Cassidy (1981) studied seven pelves in this age group and report that the surfaces of the SIJ remain primarily flat (Plate 2), with the major restraint to passive motion being provided by the

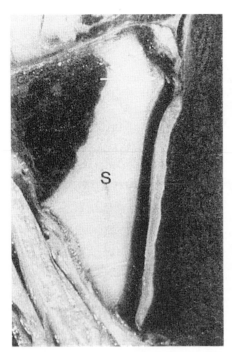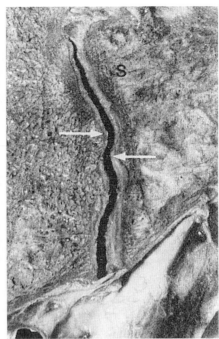

Figure 3.6   A coronal section through two embalmed male specimens: the left aged 12 years and the right over 60 years. Note the planar nature of the sacroiliac joint in the young and the presence of ridges and grooves (arrows) in the old. S, sacrum. (Reproduced with permission from Vleeming et al 1990a.)

very strong interosseous ligaments. The articular cartilage remains as noted prenatally.

THE SECOND AND THIRD DECADES (11–30 YEARS)

The availability of cadavers for investigation in this age group is limited; the data obtained is, therefore, based on few specimens. Sashin's (1930) investigation of age-related intraarticular changes is perhaps the most extensive; 42 specimens in his study belonged to this age group. The study of Resnick et al (1975) included only two specimens, MacDonald & Hunt's (1951) seven, Bowen & Cassidy's (1981) seven, and Walker's (1986) none.

Early in the second decade the SIJ appears planar; however, by the beginning of the third decade all specimens manifest a convex ridge which runs along the entire length of the articular surface of the ilium apposed to a corresponding sacral groove (Bowen & Cassidy 1981, Vleeming et al 1990a) (Fig. 3.6). The iliac fibrocartilaginous surface is duller, rougher, and intermittently coated with fibrous plaques (Plate 3). The deep articular cartilage is microscopically normal, but the superficial layers are fibrillated

and some crevice formation and erosion occurs by the end of the third decade. The sacral hyaline cartilage takes on a yellowish hue, although macroscopic changes are not evident at this stage. The collagen content of the fibrous capsule increases, thus reducing its extensibility. Passive articular motion is limited to a small angular motion coupled with a few millimeters of translation. Shibata et al (2002) investigated age-related changes (joint space narrowing, sclerosis, osteophytes, cysts, and erosion) of the SIJ via computed tomography (CT) and found changes beginning in the third decade.

THE FOURTH AND FIFTH DECADES (31–50 YEARS)

Several investigators (Schunke 1938, Bowen & Cassidy 1981, Walker 1984, 1986, Faflia et al 1998, Shibata et al 2002) feel that the changes noted in the articular surfaces during this stage represent a degenerative process. The changes occur earlier in males (fourth decade) than females (fifth decade). Vleeming et al (1990a, b) feel that since these changes are asymptomatic in most, they reflect a functional adaptation secondary to an increase in body weight

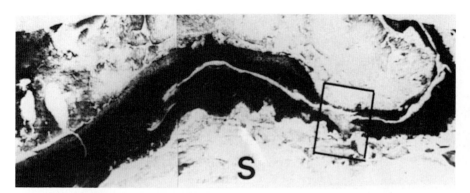

Figure 3.7 Sacroiliac joint of a male, 60 years of age. Note the variability in the depth of both the sacral (S) and the iliac cartilage at different sites. (Reproduced with permission from Walker 1986.)

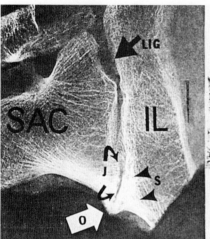

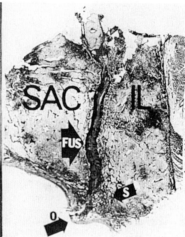

Figure 3.8 **Left:** This radiograph of a coronal section through the sacroiliac joint of a cadaver over 70 years of age illustrates narrowing of the joint space (J), sclerosis of the bone (S) and osteophyte formation (O) secondary to the degenerative process. Note the space for the interosseous ligament (LIG). SAC indicates the sacrum and IL the ilium. **Right:** This photomicrograph reveals the thickened trabeculae in the sclerotic region (S), an area of fibrous intraarticular fusion (FUS) and the previously noted osteophyte (O). (Reproduced with permission from Resnick et al (1975) and the publishers J. B. Lippincott.)

during puberty and not a degenerative process. They studied the effects of the cartilage texture on the friction coefficient of the joint (Vleeming et al 1990b) and found that, together with the development of ridges and grooves, the fibrillated surface increased friction and thus stability of the SIJ. This was felt to reflect an adaptation to bipedalism.

The articular surfaces increase in irregularity, with marked fibrillation occurring on the iliac side by the end of the fourth decade (Plate 4). Plaque formation and peripheral erosion of cartilage progress to subchondral sclerosis of bone on the iliac side. The joint space contains flaky, amorphous debris. The articular capsule thickens but still permits the translatory motion noted in the second and third decades (Bowen & Cassidy 1981). Bony hypertrophy with some lipping of the sacral articular margins was noted in some specimens in the fifth decade. Shibata et al (2002) found degeneration to be more frequent in this age group and found sclerosis to be common on the upper and middle anterior of the articular surface of the ilium whereas osteophytes were common on the anterior surface of the sacrum. Women showed more advanced signs of degeneration and parous women tended to progress faster than nulliparous women.

THE SIXTH AND SEVENTH DECADES (51–70 YEARS)

At this stage (Figs 3.7 and 3.8), the articular surfaces become totally irregular with deep erosions occasionally exposing the subchondral bone. Peripheral osteophytes enlarge and often bridge the anterior margin and inferior lip of the joint. Fibrous interconnections between the articular surfaces are commonplace; however, "when stressed, all specimens maintained some degree of mobility, although this was restricted when compared with the younger specimens" (Bowen & Cassidy 1981). Vleeming et al (1992a) found that even in old age small movements of the SIJ are possible and ankylosis of this joint is not normal. Faflia et al (1998) also note that ankylosis of the SIJ was rare and, like Shibata et al

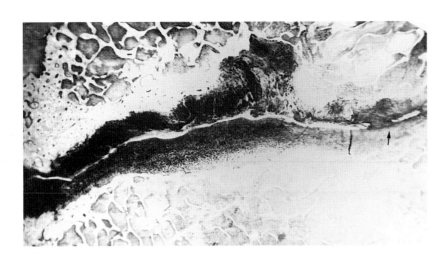

Figure 3.9   Sacroiliac joint of a female, 81 years of age. Note the erosion of the articular cartilage and the intraarticular fibrous connection (arrow). (Reproduced with permission from Walker 1986.)

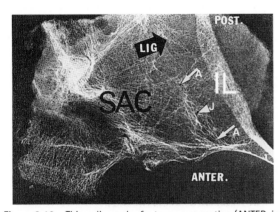

Figure 3.10   This radiograph of a transverse section (ANTER. is the anterior aspect of the pelvis and POST. is the posterior aspect) through the sacroiliac joint (J) illustrates the intra-articular ankylosis (A) of ankylosing spondylitis. Note the ossification of the interosseous ligament (LIG). SAC indicates the sacrum and IL the ilium. (Reproduced with permission from Resnick et al (1975) and the publishers J. B. Lippincott.)

(2002), found joint changes in all subjects imaged in this age group. Interestingly, Faflia et al (1998) found a higher prevalence of asymmetric non-uniform SIJ narrowing and extensive subchondral sclerosis in obese and multiparous women when age-matched to men, normal-weight women, and non-multiparous women.

THE EIGHTH DECADE (OVER 70 YEARS)

Intraarticular fibrous connections are more often the rule, with some periarticular osteophytosis present (Plate 5, Fig. 3.9). Cartilaginous erosion and plaque formation is extensive and universal, filling the joint space with debris. Consequently, the joint space is markedly reduced. Intraarticular bony

ankylosis is rarely reported and usually thought to be associated with ankylosing spondylitis (Fig. 3.10). Schunke (1938) reports that the average age of the specimens with bony ankylosis is considerably less than those without fusion, confirming a probable pathological cause.

In Walker's study (1986), 15 adult cadavers between 49 and 84 years of age were investigated for age-related changes. "Changes observed in adult specimens were similar to those of previous reports, but from examination of the entire joint, this report emphasizes the inherent variability of the SIJ, both within and between joints, at any of the ages studied."

THE PUBIC SYMPHYSIS AND AGING

In the fourth decade, smooth undulations appear along the margins of the joint and the bone begins to compact. This process continues and in the sixth decade the superior and inferior edges of the symphysis are clearly demarcated on X-ray and a dense sclerotic streak is present. This sclerosis continues and marginal osteophytes may appear (Gamble et al 1986).

Summary

That the SIJ degenerates with time is not unique to this articulation. The significance of this degeneration for function is unknown. Clinically, it appears that advancing age does not mean the loss of mobility. Current evidence supports the view that the presence or absence of SIJ mobility and its significance to the patient's presenting complaints are best judged by clinical evaluation.

Chapter 4

Anatomy

CHAPTER CONTENTS

HISTORY

The following historical data comes from Lynch (1920). The earliest record of anatomical data pertaining to the pelvic girdle is credited to Bernhard Siegfried Albinus (1697–1770) and William Hunter (1718–1783). According to Lynch (1920), these anatomists were the first to demonstrate that the sacroiliac joint (SIJ) was a true synovial joint, a finding apparently confirmed by Meckel in 1816. Von Luschka, in 1854, was the first to classify the joint as diarthrodial (Lynch 1920). Further anatomical studies conducted by Albee in 1909 on 50 postmortem specimens confirmed that the joint was lined with a synovial membrane and contained by a well-formed articular capsule. His findings were confirmed by Brooke in 1924. It wasn't until 1938 (Schunke 1938) that the variations in the articular cartilage lining the iliac surface were noted. In 1957, Solonen conducted a comprehensive study of the osteology and arthrology of the pelvic girdle, from which some findings will be reported later in this chapter.

The pelvic girdle as a unit supports the abdomen and the organs of the lower pelvis and also provides a dynamic link between the vertebral column and the lower limbs. It is a closed osteoarticular ring composed of six or seven bones which include the two innominates, the sacrum, the one or two bones which together form the coccyx and the two femora, as well as six or seven joints which include the two sacroiliac, the sacrococcygeal, often an intercoccygeal, the pubic symphysis, and the two hip joints.

OSTEOLOGY: THE BONES

SACRUM

Little wonder that the ancient Phallic Worshipers named the base of the spine the sacred bone. It is the seat of the transverse center of gravity, the keystone of the pelvis, the foundation of the spine. It is closely associated with our greatest abilities and disabilities, with our greatest romances and tragedies, our greatest pleasure and pains (Fryette 1954).

The sacrum is a large triangular bone situated at the base of the spine wedged between the two innominates. It is formed by the fusion of five sacral vertebrae (see Fig. 3.3), and the vertebral equivalents are easily recognized. The sacrum is highly variable both between individuals and between the left and right sides of the same bone. In spite of this, certain anatomical features are consistent and only those

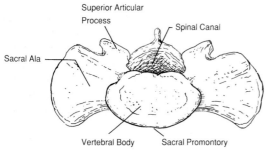

Figure 4.1 The cranial aspect of the first sacral vertebra – the sacral base.

which are essential to the description and evaluation of function will be described here.

The cranial aspect of the first sacral vertebra (Fig. 4.1), the sacral base, consists of the vertebral body anteriorly (the anterior projecting edge being the sacral promontory) and the vertebral arch posteriorly. Laterally, the transverse processes of the first sacral vertebra are fused with the costal elements (see Fig. 3.2) to form the alae of the sacrum. Variations have been noted (Grieve 1981) in the height of the sacral alae as well as the body of the S1 vertebra. The orientation of the superior articular processes of the S1 vertebra is also variable (see below).

The posterior surface of the sacrum (Fig. 4.2) is convex in both the sagittal and the transverse planes. The spinous processes of the S1–S4 vertebrae are fused in the midline to form the median sacral crest. Lateral to the median sacral crest, the intermediate sacral crest is formed by the fused laminae of the S1–S5 vertebrae. The laminae and inferior articular processes of the S5 (and occasionally the S4) vertebra remain unfused in the midline. They project caudally to form the sacral cornua, and together with the posterior aspect of the vertebral body of the S5 vertebra, form the sacral hiatus. The lateral sacral crest represents the fused transverse processes of the S1–S5 vertebrae. Between this crest and the intermediate sacral crest lie the dorsal sacral foramina which transmit the dorsal sacral ramus of each sacral spinal nerve. There are three deep depressions in the lateral sacral crest at the levels of the S1, S2, and S3 vertebrae. These depressions contain the strong

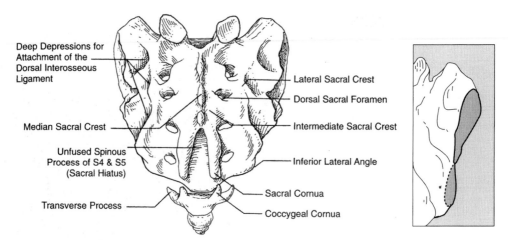

Figure 4.2 The posterior aspect of the sacrum and coccyx. **Inset:** the orientation of the three components of the auricular surface are shaped like a propeller. (Redrawn from Vleeming et al 1997.)

attachments of the interosseous sacroiliac ligament (Fig. 4.2 and see Fig. 4.13).

The lateral sacral crest fuses with the costal element to form the lateral aspect of the sacrum (Fig. 4.3). Superiorly, the lateral aspect of the sacrum is wide, while inferiorly the anteroposterior dimension narrows to a thin border which curves medially to join the S5 vertebral body. This angle is called the inferior lateral angle of the sacrum (Figs 4.2 and 4.4). The articular surface of the sacrum is auricular in shape (L-shaped) and is contained entirely by the costal elements of the first three sacral segments.

The short arm of the L-shaped surface (Fig. 4.3) lies in the vertical plane and is contained within the first sacral segment. The long arm lies in the antero-posterior plane within the second and third sacral segments. The contours of the articular surface are

reported (Weisl 1954, 1995, Solonen 1957, Kapandji 1970, Vleeming et al 1990a) to be highly variable and depend on the age of the individual studied (see Ch. 3). Investigators have reported (Kapandji 1974) the presence of a curved furrow bordered by two longitudinal crests corresponding to a convex longitudinal crest on the articular surface of the ilium. However, Solonen (1957) in his study of 30 skeletons concluded that there were "numerous depressions, elevations and other irregularities … In no case was there a distinct ridge-furrow or eminence-depression formation. On the contrary, the impression was gained that great irregularity prevails in respect to the surface formations" (Solonen 1957). His study; however, did not consider the age-related changes which may have been present in his specimens.

The anterior surface of the sacrum (Fig. 4.4) is concave in both the sagittal and the transverse planes. In the midline, four interbody ridges represent the sclerotomic fissures which are not always completely fused. Lateral to the fused vertebral bodies are four ventral sacral foramina which transmit the ventral ramus of each sacral spinal nerve as well as the segmental ventral sacral artery. The costal elements project laterally from the middle of each vertebral body between the ventral sacral foramina and fuse with those above and below as well as with the transverse processes posteriorly to form the lateral aspect of the sacrum.

The orientation of the articular surface of the sacrum in both the coronal and the transverse planes has been studied by Solonen (1957) and a summary of his findings is presented in Table 4.1. These observations represent the common findings but variations

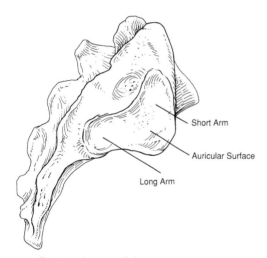

Figure 4.3   The lateral aspect of the sacrum.

Short Arm

Auricular Surface

Long Arm

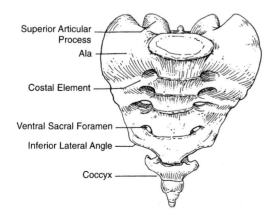

Superior Articular Process

Ala

Costal Element

Ventral Sacral Foramen

Inferior Lateral Angle

Coccyx

Figure 4.4   The anterior aspect of the sacrum and coccyx.

Table 4.1   Orientation of the articular surface of the sacrum in the coronal and transverse planes as described by Solonen (1957) and as shown graphically in Figure 4.5

Coronal plane	
90% of the specimens narrowed inferiorly at S1	Fig. 4.5A and B
85% of the specimens examined narrowed inferiorly at S2	Fig. 4.5B
80% of the specimens examined narrowed superiorly at S3	Fig. 4.5A
Transverse plane	
S1 and S2 narrow posteriorly	
S3 narrows anteriorly	

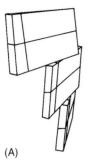
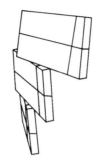
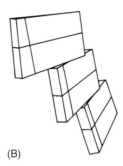
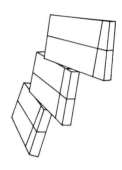

(A)   (B)

Figure 4.5   Stereometric drawings of two pelves studied by Solonen (1957) illustrating the variation found in the orientation of the sacral articular surface. (Redrawn with permission from Solonen 1957.)

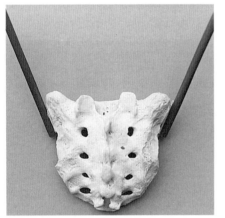
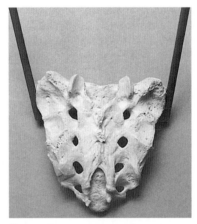
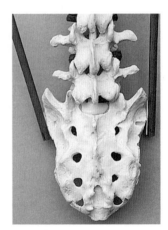

Figure 4.6   Figure 4.7   Figure 4.8

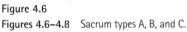
Figures 4.6–4.8   Sacrum types A, B, and C.

were noted. The stereometric drawings of two pelves studied by Solonen are illustrated in Figure 4.5. Vleeming et al (1997) describe the orientation of the three components of the auricular surface as resembling those of a propeller (Fig. 4.2 inset).

Fryette (1954) examined 23 sacra and subsequently classified the bone into three types: A, B, and C (Figs 4.6–4.8). This classification depends on the orientation of the sacral articular surface in the coronal plane, which he found to correlate with the orientation of the superior articular processes of the S1 vertebra. The type A sacrum narrows inferiorly at S1 and S2 and superiorly at S3. The orientation of the superior articular processes in this group is in the coronal plane. The type B sacrum narrows superiorly at S1 and the orientation of the superior articular processes in this group is in the sagittal plane. The type C sacrum narrows inferiorly at S1 on one side (type A) and superiorly at S1 on the other (type B). The orientation of the superior articular processes is in the

coronal plane on the type A side and in the sagittal plane on the type B.

In conclusion, there is a high incidence of variability in the plane of the SIJ, in both the coronal and the transverse planes as well as in the shape of the articulating surfaces. Grieve (1981) has noted that "Each joint exhibits at least two planes slightly angulated to one another and often three – their disposition and area are not always similar when sides are compared in the same individual." As clinicians, we are never relieved of the necessity for accurate clinical evaluation given the anatomical uncertainty of the individual being assessed.

COCCYX

The coccyx (Figs 4.2 and 4.4) is represented by four fused coccygeal segments although the first is commonly separate. The bone is roughly triangular;

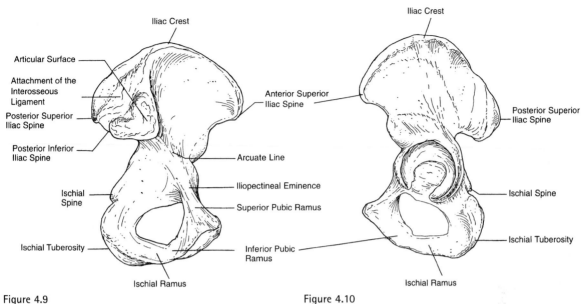

Figure 4.9

Figure 4.10

Figures 4.9 and 4.10   The medial and lateral aspects of the innominate.

the base bears an oval facet which articulates with the inferior aspect of the S5 vertebral body. The first coccygeal segment contains two rudimentary transverse processes as well as two coccygeal cornua which project superiorly to articulate with the sacral cornua.

INNOMINATE

There are three parts to the innominate, the ilium, the ischium and the pubis, which in the adult are fused to form one bone, the innominate (Figs 4.9 and 4.10 and see Fig. 3.4). Only the anatomical features pertinent to the description and evaluation of function will be described here.

Ilium

The ilium is a fan-like structure forming the superior aspect of the innominate and contributing to the superior portion of the acetabulum. The iliac crest is convex in the sagittal plane and sinusoidal in the transverse plane such that the anterior portion is concave medially while the posterior portion is convex medially. The curve reversal occurs in the same coronal plane as the short arm of the L-shaped articular surface. The anterior superior iliac spine (ASIS)

and the posterior superior iliac spine (PSIS) are at either end of the iliac crest. Inferior to the PSIS, the ilium curves irregularly to end at the posterior inferior iliac spine (PIIS). This is often the site of an accessory SIJ (Trotter 1937, Solonen 1957).

Several anatomical points are worthy of note on the medial aspect of the ilium. The articular surface lies on the posterosuperior aspect of the medial surface. Like the sacrum, the articular surface is L-shaped with the axis of the short arm in the craniocaudal plane, while the long arm has an anteroposterior axis. A variety of elevations, depressions, ridges, and furrows have been reported and develop with age (see Ch. 3). Superior to the articular surface, the medial aspect of the ilium is very rough and affords attachment to the strong interosseous sacroiliac ligament which has been noted (Colachis et al 1963) to remain intact when the sacrum and the innominate are forced apart in cadavers. The SIJ cannot be palpated given the depth of the articulation and this point should be noted when studying the anatomy.

Anteriorly, the arcuate line of the ilium appears at the angle between the short and the long arms of the articular surface and projects anteroinferiorly to reach the iliopectineal eminence, a point at which the ilium and the pubis unite. This line between the SIJ and the iliopectineal eminence represents a line of force transmission from the vertebral column to the lower limb and is reinforced by subperiosteal trabeculae (Kapandji 1974).

Pubis

The inferomedial aspect of the innominate is formed by the pubis which articulates with the pubis of the opposite side via the pubic symphysis. It joins the ilium superiorly via the superior pubic ramus which constitutes the anterior one-fifth of the acetabulum. Inferiorly, the inferior pubic ramus projects postero-laterally to join the ischium on the medial aspect of the obturator foramen. The lateral surface of the pubis is directed towards the lower limb and affords attachment for many of the medial muscles of the thigh. The pubic tubercle is located at the lateral aspect of the pubic crest approximately 1 cm lateral to the mid symphyseal line.

Ischium

The inferolateral one-third of the innominate is formed by the ischium. The upper part of the body of the ischium forms the floor of the acetabulum as well as the posterior two-fifths of the articular surface of the hip joint. From the lower part of the body, the ischial ramus projects anteromedially to join the inferior ramus of the pubis. The ischial tuberos-ity is a roughened area on the posterior and inferior aspect of the ischial body and is the site of strong muscular and ligamentous attachments. Superior to the tuberosity, the ischial spine projects medially. This process is also the site of ligamentous and muscular attachments (see Figs 4.12 and 4.18).

Acetabulum

The acetabulum (see Figs 4.10 and 4.22) is formed from the fusion of the three bones which make up the innominate (see Fig. 3.4). It is roughly the shape of a hemisphere and projects in an anterolateral and inferior direction. The lunate surface represents the articular portion of the acetabulum while the non-articular portion constitutes the floor, or the acetabu-lar fossa. This fossa is continuous with the acetabular notch located between the two ends of the lunate surface.

FEMORA

Clinically, it is important to note that the angle of inclination of the femoral neck to the shaft of the

femur, as well as the angle of anteversion between the femoral neck and the coronal plane, are highly variable. This variability will be reflected in both the pattern and the range of motion available at the hip joint (Kapandji 1970).

ARTHROLOGY: THE JOINTS

SACROILIAC JOINT

The SIJ (Fig. 4.11) is classified as a synovial joint or diarthrosis (Bowen & Cassidy 1981). According to Bowen & Cassidy (1981), Albinus and Hunter were the first to note the presence of a synovial mem-brane within the joint. In 1850, Koelcher identified synovial fluid within the joint on dissection (Bowen & Cassidy 1981).

The shape, as well as the articular cartilage, have been previously described (see Ch. 3). To summar-ize, the sacral surface is covered with hyaline cartil-age while the iliac surface is covered with a type of fibrocartilage (see Ch. 3, Plates 1–4). The depth of the articular cartilage differs both within the same

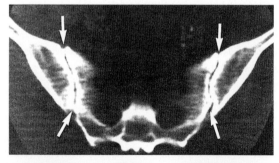

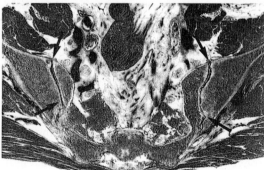

Figure 4.11 A computed tomography scan (top) with a photograph of the corresponding anatomical section (bottom) through the synovial portion of a cadaveric sacroiliac joint (arrows). (Reproduced with permission from Lawson et al (1982) and the publishers Raven Press.)

articular surface and on apposing sides (see Fig. 3.7). Most investigators report (MacDonald & Hunt 1951, Solonen 1957, Bowen & Cassidy 1981) a ratio of 1:3 between the iliac and sacral surfaces.

The joint capsule is composed of two layers, an external fibrous layer which contains abundant fibroblasts, blood vessels, and collagen fibers, and an inner synovial layer. The chronological changes in the articular capsule have been described (Ch. 3). Anteriorly, the capsule is clearly distinguished from the overlying ventral sacroiliac ligament, while posteriorly the fibers of the capsule and the deep interosseous ligament are intimately blended. Inferiorly, the capsule blends with the periosteum of the contiguous sacrum and innominates.

Like other synovial joints, the SIJ capsule is supported by overlying ligaments and fascia, some of which are the strongest in the body. They include the ventral sacroiliac, interosseous sacroiliac, long dorsal sacroiliac, sacrotuberous, sacrospinous, and iliolumbar ligaments.

Ventral sacroiliac ligament

The ventral sacroiliac ligament (Fig. 4.12) is the weakest of the group and is little more than a thickening of the anterior and inferior parts of the joint capsule (Bowen & Cassidy 1981, Williams 1995).

Interosseous sacroiliac ligament

The interosseous sacroiliac ligament is the strongest of the group and completely fills the space between the lateral sacral crest and the iliac tuberosity (Figs 3.8 and 4.13). The fibers are multidirectional and can be divided into a deep and a superficial group. The deep layer attaches medially to three fossae on the lateral aspect of the dorsal sacral surface (Fig. 4.2) and laterally to the adjacent iliac tuberosity. The superficial layer of this ligament is a fibrous sheet which attaches to the lateral sacral crest at S1 and S2 and to the medial aspect of the iliac crest. This structure is the primary barrier to direct palpation of the SIJ in its superior part and its density makes intraarticular injections extremely difficult.

Long dorsal sacroiliac ligament

The dorsal sacroiliac ligament (Fig. 4.14) attaches medially to the lateral sacral crest at S3 and S4 and laterally to the PSIS and the inner lip of the iliac crest. It lies posterior to the interosseous ligament and is separated from it by the emerging dorsal branches of the sacral spinal nerves and blood vessels. It can be palpated directly caudal to the PSIS as a thick band and at this point it is covered by the fascia of the gluteus maximus muscle. Medially, fibers of this ligament attach to the deep lamina of the posterior layer

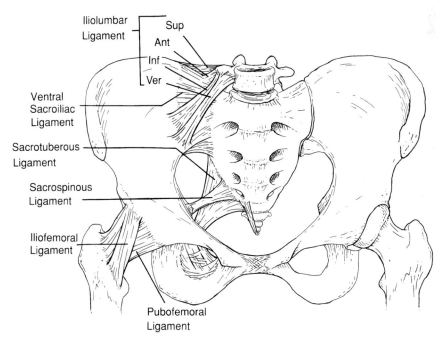

Figure 4.12   The ligaments of the pelvic girdle viewed from the anterior aspect.

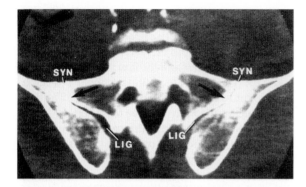

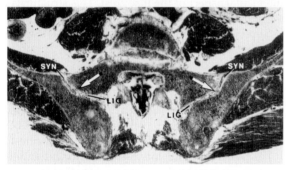

Figure 4.13 A computed tomography scan (top) with a photograph of the corresponding anatomical section (bottom) through the sacroiliac joint. Note the depth of the synovial portion (SYN) of the joint and the interosseous ligament (LIG). (Reproduced with permission from Lawson et al (1982) and the publishers Raven Press.)

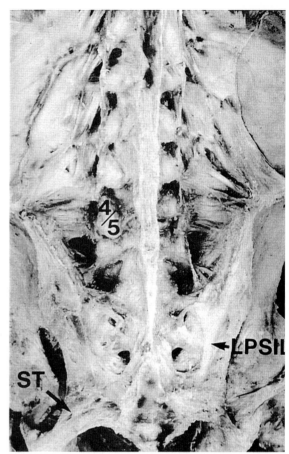

Figure 4.14 A dorsal view of the female pelvic girdle. LPSIL, the long dorsal sacroiliac ligament, 4/5, the zygapophyseal joint between L4 and L5; ST, the sacrotuberous ligament. (Reproduced with permission from Willard (1997) and the publishers Churchill Livingstone.)

of the thoracodorsal fascia and the aponeurosis of the erector spinae muscle (Vleeming et al 1996). At a deeper level, connections have been noted between the long dorsal ligament and the multifidus muscle (Willard 1997). Laterally, fibers blend with the superior band of the sacrotuberous ligament.

Tension can be increased in this ligament during motion of the sacrum and contraction of the muscles which blend with it. During counternutation of the sacrum, the ligament tightens (Fig. 4.15) (Vleeming et al 1996). During nutation of the sacrum, the ligament slackens. Contraction of the erector spinae muscle as well as loading of the sacrotuberous ligament will also increase tension in this ligament, whereas contraction of the latissimus dorsi and the gluteus maximus muscles has been found to reduce the tension (Vleeming et al 1997). The skin overlying the ligament is a frequent area of pain in patients with lumbosacral and pelvic girdle dysfunction (Fortin et al 1994a, b, 1997, 1999). Tenderness on palpation of the long dorsal sacroiliac ligament does not necessarily incriminate this tissue, given the nature of

pain referral from both the lumbar spine and the SIJ. Chapter 8 outlines specific stress tests for this structure.

Sacrotuberous ligament

This ligament is composed of three large fibrous bands, the lateral, medial, and superior (Fig. 4.16) (Willard 1997). The lateral band connects the ischial tuberosity and the PIIS and spans the piriformis muscle, from which it receives some fibers. The medial band (inferior arcuate band) attaches to the transverse tubercles of S3, S4, and S5 and the lateral margin of the lower sacrum and coccyx. These fibers run anteroinferolaterally to reach the ischial tuberosity. The fibers of this band spiral, such that those

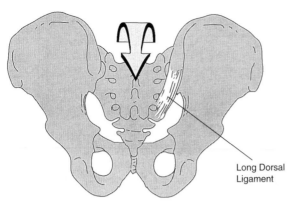

Figure 4.15   Counternutation of the sacrum tightens the long dorsal ligament. This increase in tension can be palpated just inferior to the posterior superior iliac spine. (Redrawn from Vleeming et al 1996.)

arising from the lateral aspect of the ischial tuberosity insert into the caudal part of the sacrum while those from the medial aspect of the ischial tuberosity attach cranially (Vleeming et al 1996). The superior band runs superficial to the interosseous ligament and connects the coccyx with the PSIS. The gluteus maximus also attaches to the sacrotuberous ligament and its contraction can increase the tension in the sacrotuberous ligament (Vleeming et al 1989a, b).

Phylogenetically, the sacrotuberous ligament represents the tendinous insertion of the biceps femoris muscle in lower vertebrates (Williams 1995). In some humans, this ligament still receives some fibers from the biceps femoris muscle (Fig. 4.17) (Vleeming et al 1989a, 1995b). The fibers of the biceps femoris muscle can bridge the ischial tuberosity completely to attach directly into the sacrotuberous ligament.

The tendons of the deep laminae of the multifidus muscle can also blend into the superior surface of the sacrotuberous ligament (Fig. 4.16) (Willard 1997). The ligament is pierced by the perforating cutaneous nerve (S2, S3) which subsequently winds around the inferior border of the gluteus maximus muscle to supply the skin covering the medial and inferior part of the buttock, perhaps a source of paresthesia when entrapped.

Sacrospinous ligament

The sacrospinous ligament (Figs 4.12 and 4.18) attaches medially to the lower, lateral aspect of the sacrum and the coccyx. Laterally, the apex of this triangular ligament attaches to the ischial spine of the

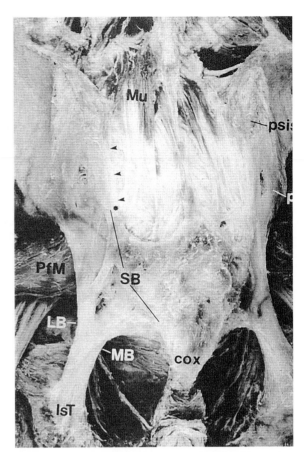

Figure 4.16   A dorsal view of the male pelvic girdle, ligaments intact and all but the deepest laminae of multifidus (Mu) removed. The arrowheads mark the long dorsal ligament beneath the lateral band (LB) of the sacrotuberous ligament. The medial band (MB) of the sacrotuberous ligament traverses the ischial tuberosity (IsT) and the coccyx. The superior band of the sacrotuberous ligament (SB) runs superficial to the long dorsal ligament to connect the coccyx with the posterior superior iliac spine. Tendons of the multifidus (Mu) pass between the superior band and the long dorsal ligament to insert into the body of the sacrotuberous ligament. (Reproduced with permission from Willard (1997) and the publishers Churchill Livingstone.)

innominate. Proximally, fibers blend with the capsule of the SIJ (Willard 1997). It is closely connected to the coccygeus muscle, of which it may represent a degenerated part (Williams 1995).

Iliolumbar ligament

Bogduk (1997) describes five bands of the iliolumbar ligament: anterior, superior, inferior, vertical (Fig. 4.12), and posterior (Fig. 4.19). The anterior

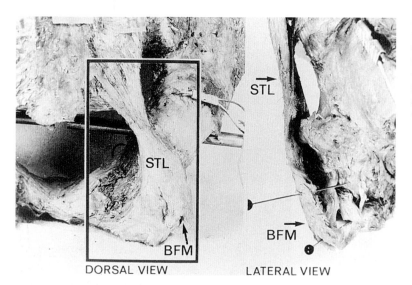

DORSAL VIEW   LATERAL VIEW

Figure 4.17 The biceps femoris muscle (BFM) has been found to alter tension in the sacrotuberous ligament (STL) through its indirect (attaching to the ischial tuberosity first), and in some, direct (bypassing the ischial tuberosity) connection to the ligament. (Reproduced with permission from Vleeming et al 1995b.)

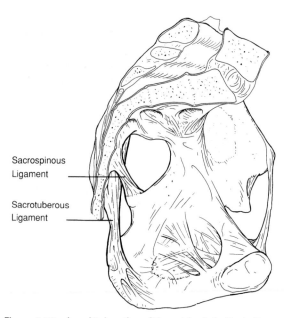

Figure 4.18 A sagittal section of the pelvic girdle illustrating the anchoring effect of the sacrotuberous ligament on the sacral base.

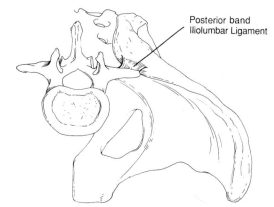

Figure 4.19 A transverse section of the lumbosacral junction illustrating the attachment of the posterior band of the iliolumbar ligament.

band attaches to the anteroinferior aspect of the entire length of the transverse process of the L5 vertebra. It blends with the superior band anterior to the quadratus lumborum muscle to attach to the anterior margin of the iliac crest. The superior band arises from the tip of the transverse process of the L5 vertebra. Laterally, the band divides to envelop the quadratus lumborum muscle before inserting on to the iliac crest. The posterior band also arises from the tip

of the transverse process of the L5 vertebra. Laterally, it inserts on to the iliac tuberosity posteroinferiorly to the superior band. The inferior band arises both from the body and the inferior border of the transverse process of the L5 vertebra. Inferiorly, the fibers cross the ventral sacroiliac ligament obliquely to attach to the iliac fossa. The vertical band arises from the anteroinferior border of the transverse process of the L5 vertebra. These fibers descend vertically to attach to the posterior aspect of the arcuate line.

Willard (1997) reports that the individual bands of the iliolumbar ligament are highly variable in number and form, but consistently arise from the transverse processes of the L4 and L5 vertebrae, blending inferiorly with the sacroiliac ligaments and laterally with the iliac crest. Previous descriptions of the evolution of this ligament from the quadratus lumborum muscle in the second decade of life (Luk et al 1986) have been refuted with the discovery of this ligament in the fetus (Uhtoff 1993, Hanson & Sonesson 1994). Both Bogduk (1997) and Willard (1997) speculate that these ligaments are responsible for maintaining the stability of the lumbosacral junction in both the coronal and the sagittal planes.

SACROCOCCYGEAL JOINT

The sacrococcygeal joint is classified as a symphysis although synovial joints have been found at this articulation. Maigne (1997) examined nine specimens and found one fibrocartilaginous disk, four synovial joints, and four mixed (part synovial and part fibrocartilaginous). All of the specimens were older and it is not known if the sacrococcygeal joint can change from one form to another during a lifetime. The supporting ligaments include the ventral sacrococcygeal ligament, dorsal sacrococcygeal ligament, and the lateral sacrococcygeal ligament.

The ventral sacrococcygeal ligament represents the continuation of the anterior longitudinal ligament of the vertebral column. The dorsal sacrococcygeal ligament has two layers. The deep layer attaches to the posterior aspect of the body of the S5 vertebra and the coccyx (analogous to the posterior longitudinal ligament), whereas the superficial layer bridges the margins of the sacral hiatus and the posterior aspect of the coccyx, thus completing the sacral canal. Laterally, the intercornual ligaments, or the lateral sacrococcygeal ligaments, connect the sacral and coccygeal cornua.

INTERCOCCYGEAL JOINT

The intercoccygeal joint is classified as a symphysis in the young since the first two segments are separated via a fibrocartilaginous disk. With time, the joint usually ossifies; however, it occasionally remains synovial.

PUBIC SYMPHYSIS

This joint contains a fibrocartilaginous disk (Fig. 4.20a), has no synovial tissue or fluid, and therefore is classified as a symphysis – a Greek term for "growing together" (Gamble et al 1986). The osseous surfaces are covered by a thin layer of hyaline cartilage; however, they are separated by the fibrocartilaginous disk. The posterosuperior aspect of the disk often contains a cavity which is not seen before the age of 10 years (Williams 1995). This is a nonsynovial cavity and may represent a chronological degenerative change. The supporting ligaments of this articulation (Fig. 4.20a–c) include the superior pubic ligament, inferior arcuate ligament, posterior pubic ligament, and the anterior pubic ligament.

The superior pubic ligament is a thick fibrous band which runs transversely between the pubic tubercles of the pubic bones. Inferiorly, the arcuate ligament blends with the fibrocartilaginous disk to attach to the inferior pubic rami bilaterally. According to Gamble et al (1986), this ligament provides most of the joint's stability. The posterior pubic ligament (Fig. 4.20b) is membranous and blends with the adjacent periosteum while the anterior ligament of the pubic symphysis is very thick and contains both transverse and oblique fibers (Kapandji 1974). It receives fibers from the aponeurotic expansion of the abdominal musculature as well as the adductor longus muscle which decussates across the joint (Fig. 4.20c).

HIP JOINT

The hip joint (Fig. 4.21a) is classified as an unmodified ovoid synovial joint (MacConaill & Basmajian 1977). The head of the femur forms roughly two-thirds of a sphere, and except for a small fovea it is covered by hyaline cartilage which decreases in depth toward the periphery of the surface (Fig. 4.21b). The acetabulum has been described (see Osteology: The Bones section, above). The lunate surface of the acetabulum (Fig. 4.22) is lined with hyaline cartilage while the non-articular portion, the acetabular fossa, is filled with loose areolar tissue and covered with synovium. The acetabulum is deepened by a fibrocartilaginous labrum which on cross-section is triangular in shape. The base of the labrum attaches to the rim of the acetabulum except inferiorly where it is deficient at the acetabular–notch, which is bridged by the transverse acetabular ligament. The apex of the labrum is lined with articular cartilage and lies inside the hip joint as a free border; the capsule of the joint attaches to the labrum at its peripheral base, thus creating a circular recess.

The articular capsule encloses the joint and most of the femoral neck. Medially, it attaches to the base

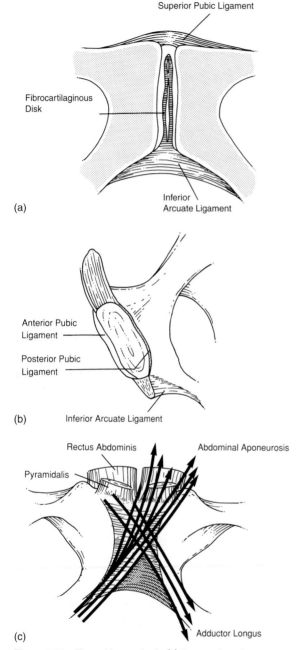

(a)

(b)

(c)

Figure 4.20 The pubic symphysis. (a) A coronal section. (b) A sagittal section through the fibrocartilaginous disk. (c) The anterior aspect. (Redrawn from Kapandji 1974.)

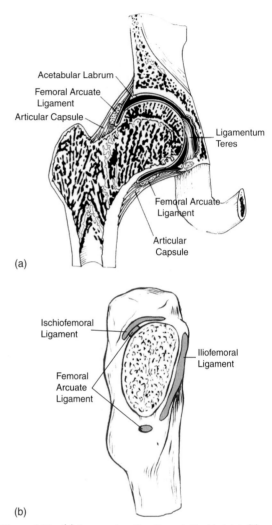

(a)

(b)

Figure 4.21 (a) A coronal section through the hip joint. (b) Medial view of the proximal femur. (Redrawn from Hewitt et al 2002.)

of the acetabular labrum and extends 5–6 cm beyond this point on to the innominate. Inferiorly, the medial attachment is to the transverse acetabular ligament. Laterally, the capsule inserts on to the femur anteriorly along the entire extent of the trochanteric line, posteriorly to the femoral neck above the trochanteric crest, superiorly to the base of the femoral neck, and inferiorly to the femoral neck above the lesser trochanter. The superficial bands of the capsular fibers are predominantly longitudinal while the deep bands are circular (Hewitt et al 2002). The ligaments which are intimately blended with, and support, the capsule include the iliofemoral ligament, pubofemoral ligament, the ischiofemoral ligament, and the femoral arcuate ligament. There are two intraarticular ligaments, the ligamentum teres and the transverse acetabular ligament. Hewitt et al (2002) tested some of these ligaments to failure in tension and also

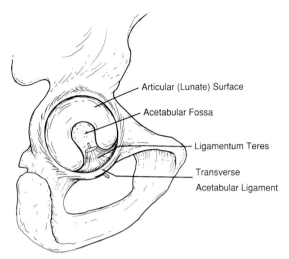

Articular (Lunate) Surface

Acetabular Fossa

Ligamentum Teres

Transverse
Acetabular Ligament

Figure 4.22   The acetabulum.

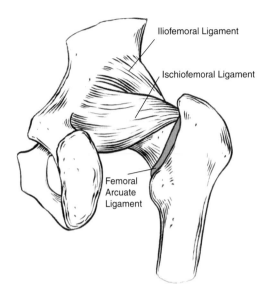

Iliofemoral Ligament

Ischiofemoral Ligament

Femoral
Arcuate
Ligament

Figure 4.24   The ligaments of the posterior aspect of the hip joint.

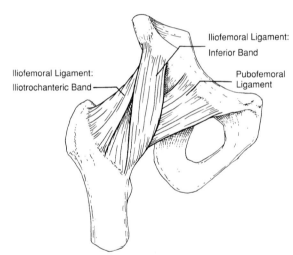

Iliofemoral Ligament:
Inferior Band

Iliofemoral Ligament:
Iliotrochanteric Band

Pubofemoral
Ligament

Figure 4.23   The ligaments of the anterior aspect of the hip joint.

noted the stiffness value (force/displacement) at the point of failure.

Iliofemoral ligament

The iliofemoral ligament (Figs 4.12, 4.23, and 4.24) is extremely strong and reinforces the anterior aspect of the hip joint. It is triangular in shape and attaches to the anterior inferior iliac spine at its apex. Inferolaterally, it diverges into two bands, the lateral iliotrochanteric band which inserts on to the superior aspect of the trochanteric line and the medial inferior band which inserts on to the inferior aspect of the trochanteric line. Together, these two bands

form an inverted Y, the center of which is filled with weaker ligamentous tissue. Hewitt et al (2002) noted that both bands of the iliofemoral ligament resisted a greater tensile force than the ischiofemoral and femoral arcuate ligaments and failed with the least amount of displacement. This ligament exhibited the greatest stiffness. The iliofemoral ligament restricts extension of the hip.

Pubofemoral ligament

The pubofemoral ligament (Figs 4.12 and 4.23) attaches medially to the iliopectineal eminence and the superior pubic ramus as well as to the obturator crest and membrane. Laterally, it attaches to the anterior surface of the trochanteric line. The capsule of the hip joint is unsupported by any ligament between the pubofemoral ligament and the inferior band of the iliofemoral ligament; however, the tendon of the psoas major muscle crosses the joint at this point, contributing to its dynamic support. A bursa is located here between the tendon of the psoas muscle and the capsule and occasionally will communicate directly with the synovial cavity of the hip joint. Hewitt et al (2002) did not test this ligament in their study.

Ischiofemoral ligament

The ischiofemoral ligament (Fig. 4.24) arises medially from the ischial rim of the acetabulum and its labrum. Laterally, the fibers spiral superoanteriorly over the back of the femoral neck to insert anterior to the trochanteric fossa deep to the iliofemoral ligament. Some fibers from this ligament also run transversely to blend with those forming the femoral arcuate ligament, formerly called the zona orbicularis (Hewitt et al 2002). The ischiofemoral ligament primarily restricts internal rotation of the hip as well as adduction of the flexed hip. This ligament failed under lower tensile loads than the iliofemoral ligament and exhibited greater displacement at the point of failure (less stiff) (Hewitt et al 2002).

Femoral arcuate ligament

This ligament was previously called the zona orbicularis and some changes in its anatomy have been noted (Hewitt et al 2002). The fibers are circular and located in the deep posterior capsule (Figs 4.21 and 4.24). It originates at the greater trochanter and passes deep to the ischiofemoral liagment posteriorly to insert inferiorly at the lesser trochanter. It does not cross the hip joint; however, it functions to tense the capsule at the limits of extension and flexion. In tension studies (Hewitt et al 2002), this ligament exhibited the least amount of stiffness and failed at the lowest force.

Ligamentum teres

The ligamentum teres (Figs 4.21a and 4.22) attaches laterally to the anterosuperior part of the fovea of the femoral head and medially via three bands to either end of the lunate surface of the acetabulum inferiorly and to the upper border of the transverse acetabular ligament.

Transverse acetabular ligament

This ligament is a continuation of the acetabular labrum inferiorly and converts the acetabular notch into a foramen through which the intraarticular vessels pass to supply the head of the femur (Fig. 4.22). In addition to the ligamentous support, the hip joint is dynamically stabilized by numerous muscles, including the iliacus, rectus femoris, pectineus, gluteus minimus, piriformis, obturator externus, obturator internus, superior and inferior gemellus muscles, as well as the fascia latae of the thigh, all of which partially insert into the articular capsule.

MYOLOGY: THE MUSCLES

There are 35 muscles which attach directly to the sacrum and/or innominate and function with the ligaments and fascia to produce synchronous motion and stability of the trunk and extemities. It is not the intent of this text to describe the anatomy of each of these muscles but rather to highlight certain muscles which will be discussed in greater depth in later chapters of this text.

TRANSVERSUS ABDOMINIS

The transversus abdominis (Fig. 4.25) is the deepest abdominal muscle and arises from the lateral one-third of the inguinal ligament, the anterior two-thirds of the inner lip of the iliac crest, the lateral raphe of the thoracodorsal fascia, and the internal aspect of the lower six costal cartilages interdigitating with the costal fibers of the diaphragm. From this broad

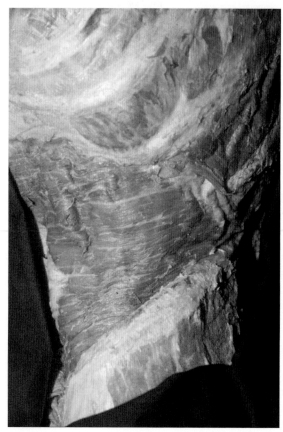

Figure 4.25   A lateral view of the transversus abdominis. (Reproduced with permission from DeRosa 2001.)

attachment, the muscle runs transversely around the trunk where its upper and middle fibers blend with the fascial envelope of the rectus abdominis, reaching the linea alba in the midline through a complex and variable bilaminar aponeurosis (Fig. 4.26). Superior to the umbilicus, the aponeurotic fibers of transversus abdominis pass *posterior* to rectus abdominis in either a superior or inferior direction to blend with the aponeurotic fibers of the contralateral transversus abdominis and internal oblique (Fig. 4.26b top). Below the umbilicus, all of the aponeurotic fibers run inferiorly with the anterior lamina passing *anterior* to the rectus abdominis and the posterior lamina passing *posterior* to the rectus abdominis. Caudally, the posterior laminar fibers gradually pass anterior to the rectus abdominis along with the anterior laminar fibers (Rizk 1980) (Fig. 4.26b bottom). Inferiorly, the inguinal fibers of transversus abdominis blend with the insertion of the internal oblique muscle to form the conjoint tendon to attach to the pubic crest posterior to the superficial inguinal ring. Urquhart et al (2001) have noted differences in the fiber orientation of the upper, middle, and lower regions of transversus abdominis. The upper fibers were oriented superomedially, middle region inferomedially, and the lower region inferomedially (more so than the middle region). The transversus abdominis is innervated by the anterior primary rami of T7–T12 and L1.

MULTIFIDUS

The deepest fibers of the multifidus muscle in the lumbar spine (the laminar fibers) arise from the posteroinferior aspect of the lamina and articular capsule of the zygapophyseal joint and insert on to the mammillary process two levels below (Bogduk 1997) (Fig. 4.27 and see Fig. 4.33). The remainder of the muscle arises medially from the spinous process, blending laterally with the laminar fibers. Inferiorly, the superficial fascicles of multifidus insert *three* levels below, such that those arising from the L1 vertebra insert on to the mammillary processes of the L4, L5, and S1 vertebrae as well as the medial aspect of the iliac crest. Inferiorly, the fibers from the spinous

(a)

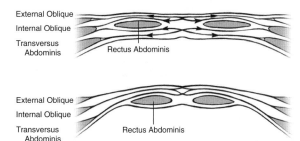

(b)

Figure 4.26   (a) The anterior fascia of transversus abdominis is bilaminar. Above the umbilicus the decussating fibers pass either superomedially or inferomedially and create a cross-hatched pattern, whereas below the umbilicus all the fibers travel inferomedially. (Redrawn from Richardson et al 1999.) (b) The pattern of decussation of the anterior fascia of the external oblique, internal oblique, and transversus abdominis above (top) and below the umbilicus (bottom). (Redrawn from Williams 1995.)

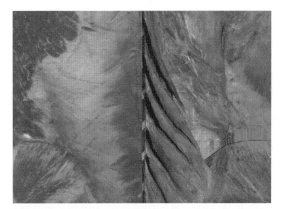

Figure 4.27   **Right**: superficial fibers of the lumbar multifidus. **Left**: thoracodorsal fascia. Courtesy of Gracovetsky (personal library).

process of the L2 vertebra (superficial multifidus) insert on to the mammillary processes of the L5 and S1 vertebrae and the PSIS of the innominate. The fibers from the spinous process of the L3 vertebra insert on to the S1 articular process, the superolateral aspect (costal element) of the S1 and S2 segments, and the iliac crest. The fibers from the spinous process of the L4 vertebra insert on to the lateral sacral crest and the area of bone between this crest and the dorsal sacral foramina, while those from the L5 vertebra insert on to the intermediate sacral crest inferiorly to S3. Within the pelvis, the multifidus muscle also attaches to the deep laminae of the posterior thoracodorsal fascia at a raphe which separates it from the gluteus maximus muscle (Willard 1997). Here, fibers from the multifidus pass beneath the posterior sacroiliac ligaments to blend with the sacrotuberous ligament (Fig. 4.16). At the lumbosacral junction, the multifidus is the largest muscle. In the lumbar spine, the superficial (and more lateral) multisegmental fibers are known (Moseley et al 2002) to be phasic in function (responsible for angular motion) whereas the deep fibers have a more tonic function (are non-direction-specific and responsible for stabilization).

The fascicles are innervated by the medial branch of the dorsal ramus such that all of the fascicles which arise from the same spinous process are innervated by the same nerve regardless of the inferior extent of their insertion (Bogduk 1983, 1997).

THE DEEP BACK WALL AND FLOOR OF THE PELVIS

The deep back wall of the pelvis is comprised of the ischiococcygeus muscle which lies in the same plane as the piriformis, another muscle of the deep back wall. The pelvic floor is comprised of the levator ani muscle (puborectalis, pubococcygeus, and iliococcygeus) and the fascia from which it arises (Figs 4.28 and 4.29), also known collectively as the "levator plate."

The pelvic fascia

The pelvic floor takes origin from the osseus perimeter of the internal pelvis as well as from certain fascial structures. The arcus tendineus fascia (Fig. 4.28) is a thick fascial band (often called the white line) which is suspended between its anterior and posterior attachments. It is located medial to the fascia overlying the obturator internus muscle. Anteriorly,

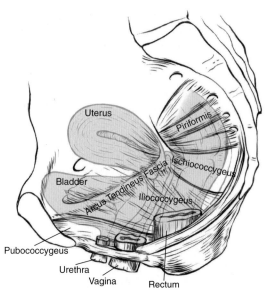

Figure 4.28   The relationship between the muscles, fascia, and organs (transparent) of the pelvic floor.

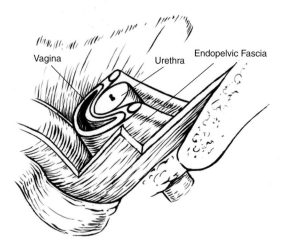

Figure 4.29   The "functional hammock." Downward pressure compresses the urethra against the endopelvic fascia, effectively force-closing this structure. Attenuation of the fascial support system is one cause of lost urethral force closure and stress urinary incontinence. (Redrawn from DeLancey 1994.)

the arcus tendineus fascia is a well-defined tendon which attaches 1 cm above and 1 cm lateral to the midline of the inferior border of the pubic symphysis (DeLancey 1994). The posterior attachment of the arcus is to the ischial spine. As the arcus proceeds posteriorly from its tendinous attachment to the pubic bone, it fuses with surrounding structures and becomes a broad aponeurotic band blending with the endopelvic fascia. The endopelvic fascia is a dense horizontal fascial aponeurosis which lies between the anterior vaginal wall and the urethra (Fig. 4.29) and provides support to these structures. Laterally, the endopelvic fascia attaches to the arcus tendineus fascia bilaterally, providing a hammock-like support for the urethra and vagina (Fig. 4.29) (DeLancey 1994). Posteriorly, the endopelvic fascia blends with the internal surface of the pubococcygeus, puborectalis, and iliococcygeus muscles. These muscles support the endopelvic fascia and thus the urethra and vagina by stiffening the functional "hammock."

Ischiococcygeus

The ischiococcygeus arises from the ventral aspect of the sacrospinous ligament and the ischial spine and inserts into the apex of the sacrum between S4 and S5. Together with the piriformis, ischiococcygeus forms the deep back wall of the pelvis. This muscle is supplied by ventral rami of the sacral plexus, S3 and S4.

Piriformis

The piriformis muscle arises from the anterior aspect of the S2, S3, and S4 segments of the sacrum as well as the ventral capsule of the SIJ, the anterior aspect of the PIIS of the ilium, and often the upper part of the sacrotuberous ligament. Its exit from the pelvis is through the greater sciatic foramen and it attaches to the greater trochanter of the femur. The nerve supply is from the ventral rami of L5 and S1.

Levator ani

The levator ani is part of the pelvic floor and is comprised of three muscles, the pubococcygeus, puborectalis, and iliococcygeus. The pubococcygeus and puborectalis arise from the inner surface of the pubic bone 2.5–4 cm above the arcus tendineus fascia (Fig. 4.28). Posterior fibers of the pubococcygeus arise from the anterior half of the arcus tendineus fascia. Pubococcygeus passes posteriorly, inferior to the puborectalis, and attaches to a midline raphe posterior to the rectum. Through this raphe, fibers unite and continue posteriorly from the anorectal flexure to attach to the anterior aspect of the last two coccygeal segments. The puborectalis passes posteriorly

lateral to the urethra, vagina (females), and rectum to unite with its counterpart to form a muscular sling at the anorectal flexure; there is no posterior osseus attachment. The iliococcygeus originates from the medial aspect of the ischial spine and the posterior part of the arcus tendineus fascia. Fibers from this muscle attach to the anterior aspect of the coccyx. The anteromedial portion of the levator ani is supplied by branches of the pudendal nerve while the posterolateral region is supplied directly from the sacral plexus S3 and S4 (Williams 1995).

DIAPHRAGM

The diaphragm is a modified half-dome which separates the thorax from the abdominal cavity (Fig. 4.30). It has an extensive attachment to the xyphoid, internal surface of the lower six ribs (interdigitates with the transversus abodminis), and lumbar spine. The crura of the diaphragm arise from the anterolateral aspect of the bodies and intervertebral disks of L1–L3 on the right and L1–L2 on the left. Laterally, fibers arise from the medial and lateral arcuate ligaments, which are thick bands of fascia which arch over the psoas major and quadratus lumborum. From this circumferential origin, fibers converge on to a central tendon – a thin, strong aponeurosis of collagen fibers. The motor fibers to the diaphragm are from the phrenic nerve (C3 and C4) while the sensory supply comes from the lower six or seven intercostal nerves (T6–T12).

EXTERNAL OBLIQUE

The external oblique is the largest abdominal muscle with eight digitations arising from the external surfaces and inferior borders of the lower eight ribs. This origin interdigitates with fibers of serratus anterior and latissimus dorsi. The upper attachments of the external oblique arise close to the costochondral joints, the middle attachments to the body of the ribs, and the lowest to the tip of the cartilage of the 12th rib. Inferiorly, the posterior fibers descend vertically to attach to the outer lip of the anterior half of the iliac crest. The upper and middle fibers end in the anterior abdominal aponeurosis (Fig. 4.31). Rizk (1980) investigated this structure in 41 specimens and discovered that the aponeurosis of the external oblique was bilaminar (Fig. 4.26b). The two layers cross the midline to blend with the fascia of the opposite side with the deep layer being continuous

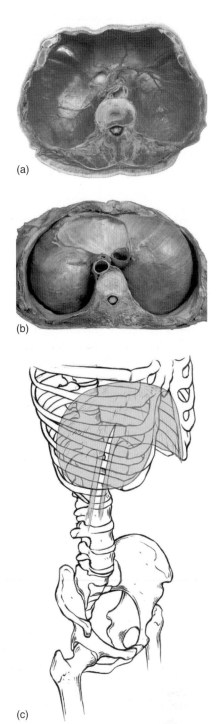

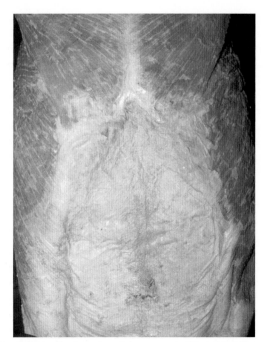

Figure 4.31 The insertion of the external oblique into the anterior abdominal aponeurosis. (Reproduced with permission from DeRosa 2001.)

Figure 4.30 (a) An anatomical dissection of the diaphragm viewed from below. (Reproduced with permission from Primal Pictures.) (b) An anatomical dissection of the diaphragm viewed from above. (Reproduced with permission from Primal Pictures.) (c) A three-dimensional graphic representation of the respiratory diaphragm.

with the contralateral internal oblique. The superficial layer merges with the superficial layer of the contralateral side. The deep and superficial layers produce a cross-hatched appearance as their orientation is 90° to one another. The external oblique muscle is innervated by the ventral rami of the T7–T12 spinal nerves.

INTERNAL OBLIQUE

The internal oblique lies between the external oblique and the transversus abdominis and arises from the lateral two-thirds of the inguinal ligament, anterior two-thirds of the intermediate line of the iliac crest, and the lateral raphe of the thoracodorsal fascia. The posterior fibers ascend laterally to reach the tips of the 11th and 12th ribs and the 10th rib near the costochondral junction. The anterior fibers arising from the inguinal ligament arch inferomedially to blend with the aponeurosis of transversus abdominis and attach to the pubic crest. The intermediate fibers pass superomedially to insert into a bilaminar aponeurosis (Rizk 1980), blending with the aponeurosis of the external oblique and transversus abdominis, forming a decussating network of fascia across the midline of the body (Fig. 4.26b). The internal

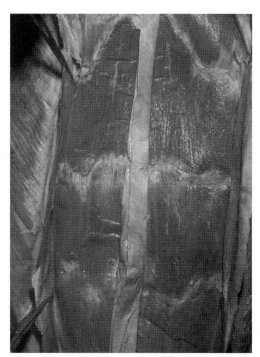

Figure 4.32 Rectus abdominis. Note the three horizontal tendinous bands which receive attachment from the external oblique muscle. (Reproduced with permission from DeRosa 2001.)

oblique muscle is innervated by the ventral rami of the T7–T12 and L1 spinal nerves.

RECTUS ABDOMINIS

The rectus abdominis muscle is a long muscular strap and is just lateral to the anterior midline of the abdomen. It arises from the pubic crest and tubercle as well as the ligaments of the symphysis pubis. The aponeurotic expansions of this muscle, along with those of the transversus abdominis, internal oblique, pyramidalis, and adductor longus muscles, interdigitate anterior to the symphysis to form a dense network of fibers and thus contribute to the stability of this articulation (see Fig. 4.20c) (Kapandji 1974, Williams 1995). The muscle inserts into the fifth to seventh costal cartilages (sometimes as high as the third costal cartilage) and xyphoid process. Rectus abdominis is separated by three horizontal tendinous bands (Fig. 4.32) which receive attachment from the external oblique muscle (DeRosa 2001). The rectus abdominis is enclosed in a fascial sheath formed by the decussating aponeurosis of the external and internal oblique muscles as well as the bilaminar

aponeurosis of the transversus abdominis. The medial borders of the rectus abdominis connect through this bilaminar aponeurosis, collectively known as the linea alba. The nerve supply is through the ventral rami of the lower six or seven thoracic spinal nerves.

PYRAMIDALIS

This triangular muscle is located anterior to the inferior aspect of the rectus abdominis muscle and is enclosed within its sheath (Fig. 4.20c). The base attaches to the os pubis as well as to the symphysis while the apex blends with the linea alba midway between the umbilicus and the pubis. This muscle is innervated by the subcostal nerve which is the ventral ramus of the T12 spinal nerve.

ERECTOR SPINAE

Longissimus thoracis pars lumborum

This muscle arises from five muscle fascicles, the deepest of which is from the L5 vertebra overlapped by those from L4, then L3, then L2, and finally L1 (Bogduk 1997). Medially, these laminae arise from the accessory and the medial end of the dorsal surface of the transverse processes. The fibers from the L1–L4 vertebrae insert via a common tendon into the medial aspect of the lumbar intermuscular aponeurosis which attaches inferiorly to the medial aspect of the PSIS just lateral to the fascicle from L5.

Longissimus thoracis pars thoracis

The thoracic component of longissimus thoracis is the largest part of the erector spinae group in the thoracic spine and forms the bulk of the paravertebral muscle mass adjacent to the spine. It arises from the ribs and transverse processes of T1–T12 and descends to attach via the aponeurosis of the erector spinae to the spinous processes of the lumbar spine and sacrum (Fig. 4.33). Each fascicle descends a variable length with those from the upper thorax reaching to L3 while the lower fascicles bridge the lumbar spine completely.

Iliocostalis lumborum pars lumborum

This muscle arises as four overlapping fascicles from the tips of the transverse processes of the L1–L4 vertebrae (lateral to the lumbar longissimus) and

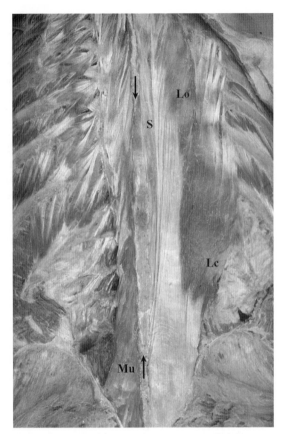

Figure 4.33 Longissimus thoracis pars thoracis (Lo), iliocostalis lumborum pars thoracis (Lc) and superficial fibers of multifidus (Mu) can be clearly seen in this beautiful dissection of Willard. S, spinalis. (Reproduced with permission from Willard (1997) and the publishers Churchill Livingstone.)

from the middle layer of the thoracodorsal fascia. Inferiorly, the muscle inserts on to the iliac crest lateral to the PSIS.

Iliocostalis lumborum pars thoracis

The thoracic component of iliocostalis lumborum is large and the most lateral part of the erector spinae muscle group. Fascicles from the inferior borders of the angles of the lower seven to eight ribs originate lateral to the attachment of iliocostalis thoracis and descend to attach to the ilium and sacrum with the thoracic component of the longissimus thoracis to form the aponeurosis of erector spinae (Fig. 4.33). These thoracic fascicles have no attachment to the lumbar vertebra bridging the gap between the thorax and the pelvis.

The erector spinae aponeurosis is derived from the tendons of the longissimus thoracis pars thoracis and iliocostalis lumborum pars thoracis. This muscle is innervated from the lateral and intermediate branches of the segmental dorsal spinal rami.

THORACODORSAL FASCIA

The thoracodorsal fascia is a critical structure when considering transference of load from the trunk to the lower extremity (Vleeming et al 1995a). Several muscles, important in providing stability to the pelvic girdle, attach to this fascia and can affect tension within it. They include the transversus abdominis, internal oblique, gluteus maximus, latissimus dorsi, erector spinae, multifidus, and biceps femoris.

Its anatomy is complex (Vleeming et al 1995a, Bogduk 1997, Barker & Briggs 1999). There are three layers to the fascia: the anterior, middle, and posterior. The anterior layer is thin and covers the anterior aspect of the quadratus lumborum muscles. It attaches medially to the transverse processes and blends with the intertransverse ligaments. The middle layer is posterior to the quadratus lumborum. It arises medially from the tips of the transverse processes and provides origin to the aponeurosis of the transversus abdominis.

There are two laminae which comprise the posterior layer of the thoracodorsal fascia. The superficial lamina is predominantly derived from the aponeurosis of the latissimus dorsi muscle (Fig. 4.34) and contains oblique fibers which run caudomedially. In the midline, strong connections exist to attach the fascia to the supraspinal ligaments and the spinous processes of the lumbar vertebrae cranial to L4. According to Willard (1997), the posterior border of the ligamentum flavum becomes the supraspinous ligament, which in turn is anchored to the thoracodorsal fascia (Figs 4.35 and 4.36). Through these attachments, tension of the thoracodorsal fascia is transmitted to the ligamentum flavum and, according to Willard (1997), assists in the alignment of the lumbar vertebrae. The superficial laminae also receives some fibers from the external oblique and the lower trapezius muscles (Vleeming et al 1995a).

Caudal to L4, midline connections are very loose and actually cross the midline to reach the opposite iliac crest and sacrum. Over the sacrum, the superficial lamina blends with the fascia of the gluteus maximus. These fibers run in a caudolateral direction from a medial attachment to the median sacral crest and occasionally as far cranial as the L4 spinous process (Fig. 4.37).

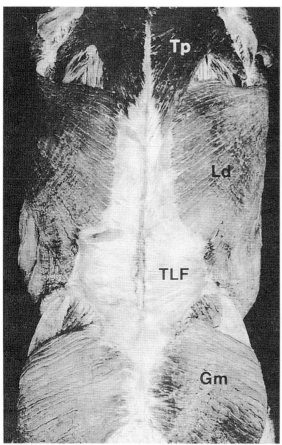

Figure 4.34   A posterior view of the thoracolumbar fascia (TLF) illustrates the attachments of latissimus dorsi (Ld) and gluteus maximus (Gm) into the superficial lamina of the posterior layer. Note the small attachment of the lower fibers of the trapezius muscle (Tp). (Reproduced from Willard (1997) with permission of Churchill Livingstone.)

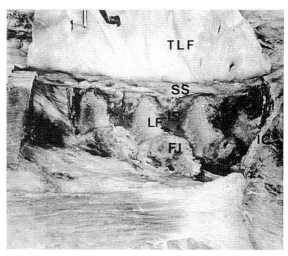

Figure 4.35   Dorsolateral view of the lumbar spine. The thoracolumbar fascia (TLF) blends with the supraspinous ligament (SS) and interspinous ligament (IS), ligamentum flavum (LF) and the facet joint (FJ) capsule. IC is the iliac crest. (Reproduced from Willard (1997) with permission of Churchill Livingstone.)

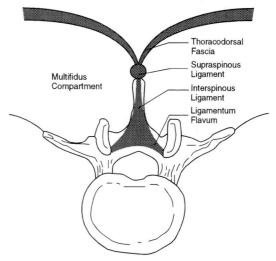

Figure 4.36   Horizontal view of the lumbar region illustrating the ligamentum flavum/interspinous ligament/supraspinous ligament/thoracodorsal fascia connections. This mechanism plays a significant role in stabilization training of the lumbo-pelvic-hip region. (Redrawn from Willard (1997) with permission of the publishers Churchill Livingstone.)

The deep lamina of the posterior layer of the thoracodorsal fascia is also complex with several muscular connections (Fig. 4.38). The fibers run in a caudolateral direction attaching medially to the interspinous ligaments and caudally to the PSIS, iliac crest, and posterior sacroiliac ligaments. Above the pelvis, the deep lamina attaches to the lateral raphe and blends with the middle layer of the thoracodorsal fascia. The internal oblique and the transversus abdominis muscles attach to this lateral raphe. Over the pelvis, some fibers blend with the deep fascia of the erector spinae muscle (forming the roof over the sacral multifidus: see Fig. 7.1) and the sacro-tuberous ligament.

Tension of the thoracodorsal fascia can be increased through motion of the arms, trunk, and lower extremity. Contraction or lengthening of the many muscles which attach into the fascia can influence its tension. Coupled with the anterior musculature and the anterior abdominal fascia (Fig. 4.39), a "circle of integrity is created." In this manner, stability of the pelvic girdle and low back is enhanced

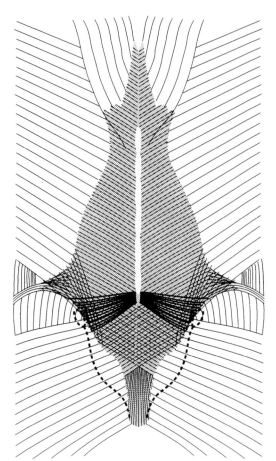

Figure 4.37 The superficial lamina of the thoracodorsal fascia. (Redrawn from Vleeming et al (1997) with permission of the publishers Churchill Livingstone.)

and load is effectively transferred from the trunk to the lower extremity.

THE FASCIA OF THE LEG

The fascia of the lower extremity envelops the muscles and via its extensive attachments to the pelvic girdle can influence its function and subsequently become symptomatic in dysfunction. The fascia encircles the pelvic girdle by attaching to the sacrum, coccyx, iliac crest, inguinal ligament, superior pubic ramus, inferior pubic ramus, ischial ramus, ischial tuberosity, and sacrotuberous ligament. Superiorly, it blends with the thoracodorsal and abdominal fascia of the trunk. From the iliac crest, the fascia descends over the gluteus medius muscle before splitting to envelop the gluteus maximus muscle. The two bands meet at the lower border of this muscle

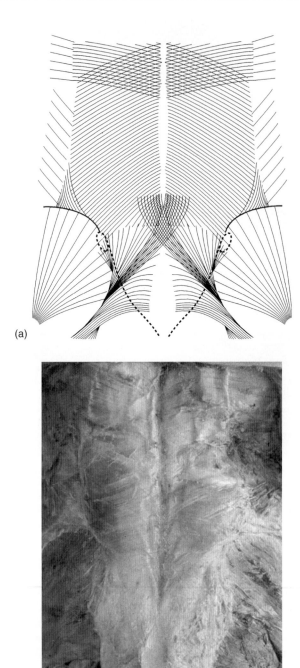

(a)

(b)

Figure 4.38 (a) The deep lamina of the thoracodorsal fascia. (Redrawn from Vleeming et al (1997) with permission of the publishers Churchill Livingstone.) (b) The deep lamina of the thoracodorsal fascia forms the roof of multifidus and blends with the sacrotuberous ligament. (Courtesy of A. Vleeming.)

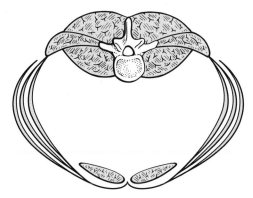

Figure 4.39 A graphic representation of the components of the circle of integrity.

and facilitate its insertion into the iliotibial tract which represents a lateral thickening of the fascia.

The iliotibial tract attaches inferiorly to the condyles of the femur and the tibia, and to the head of the fibula, blending with the crural fascia and aponeurotic extensions of the quadriceps muscle. The fascia is continuous in the thigh with two intermuscular septa which attach to the linea aspera.

The tensor fascia latae muscle inserts into the iliotibial tract anterior to the attachment of the gluteus maximus muscle. This muscle is also enveloped by two layers of the fascia. The superficial layer reaches the iliac crest lateral to the muscle while the deep layer blends medially with the capsule of the hip joint.

NEUROLOGY: THE NERVES

Understanding the neurology of the lumbopelvic-hip region is essential since rehabilitation involves the restoration of optimal neurological function. Muscle control in posture and locomotion depends directly on both the central and peripheral nervous systems. Janda (1986) notes that "It is almost impossible clinically to differentiate the primary changes in muscle from their secondary reaction due to an altered or impaired central nervous regulation, as the quality of muscle function depends directly on the central nervous system activity." In addition, emotional states are known to influence basic muscle tone and patterning (Holstege et al 1996). Wyke (1981, 1985) has shown that articular neurology has both direct and reflex influences on muscle tone locally and globally. In addition, afferent input from articular structures contributes to perception of posture and motion.

Altered afferent input from the articular mechanoreceptors can have profound influences on both static and dynamic pelvic girdle function. Several studies (Mattila et al 1986, Bullock-Saxton et al 1994, Uhlig et al 1995, Hides et al 1996, Hodges & Richardson 1996, Dangaria & Naesh 1998, Hodges & Moseley 2003) have shown that changes in muscle fiber type, muscle bulk, and recruitment patterns occur with pain and pathology. However, simply relieving pain does not necessarily restore optimum function; these changes can remain even when pain subsides (Bullock-Saxton et al 1994, Hides et al 1996). Changes in the proprioceptive and motor control systems alter movement patterns and strategies of load transfer. The result is less efficient movement, suboptimal function, a higher risk for recurrence of pain and injury (Hides et al 2001), and altered joint forces (due to altered axes of joint rotation) that may lead to earlier degenerative changes and pain.

MACROSCOPIC ARTICULAR NEUROLOGY

The most extensive study of the macroscopic innervation of the SIJ was done in 1957 by Solonen. He examined 18 joints in nine cadavers and found that posteriorly all of the joints were innervated from branches of the posterior rami of the S1 and S2 spinal nerves. Bradlay (1985) reported that the dorsal sacroiliac ligaments receive supply from the lateral divisions of the dorsal rami of the L5, S1, S2, and S3 spinal nerves. This was later confirmed by Grob et al (1995). According to Willard et al (1998), the dorsal sacral plexus (S1, S2, S3) forms in the sacral gutter inferior to the sacral attachment of multifidus and superficial to the sacrotuberous ligament and divides into medial and lateral divisions. The medial divisions supply multifidus while the lateral divisions pass either through or under the long dorsal ligament where they are flattened to a very thin layer. These branches innervate the posterior aspect of the SIJ. Anteriorly, Solonen (1957) found that the articular innervation was not always consistent nor necessarily symmetrical. Of the 18 specimens examined, all of the joints were innervated by branches from the ventral rami of the L5 spinal nerve, 17 from L4, 11 from S1, four from S2, one from L3, and 15 received innervation from the superior gluteal nerve. Grob et al (1995) were unable to confirm any innervation from the ventral rami. Fortin et al (1999) concur with Grob et al and feel that the SIJ is only innervated from the dorsal rami S1–S4. They suggest that the investigators who have reported innervation of the joint from ventral rami have mistaken blood vessels for nerves since both are imaged with the same staining technique. The wide distribution of innervation is reflected clinically in the variety of pain patterns reported by patients with SIJ dysfunction (Fortin et al 1994a).

The pubic symphysis is innervated from branches from the pudendal and genitofemoral nerves (Gamble et al 1986).

The hip joint is innervated by branches from the obturator nerve (L2, L3, L4), the nerve to the quadratus femoris (L2, L3, L4), and the superior gluteal nerve (L5, S1) (Grieve 1986). As well, the joint receives branches from the nerves which supply the muscles crossing the joint. The hip joint is principally derived from the L3 segment of mesoderm with contributions from L2 to S1, hence the potential for a variety of patterns of pain referral.

The outer one-third of the lumbar intervertebral disk is innervated posteriorly by the sinuvertebral nerve (Bogduk 1983, 1997) and laterally by the ventral rami and gray rami communicantes of the spinal nerve. Nociceptors (see below) have been located here, thus the anatomical potential for primary disk pain. The zygapophyseal joints of the L5 and S1 vertebrae are innervated via the medial branch of the dorsal ramus of the L4, L5, and S1 spinal nerves.

MICROSCOPIC ARTICULAR NEUROLOGY

Accurate information from mechanoreceptors in the joint is required by the central nervous system so that the activity of the motor units essential for position, motion, and stability of the joint is coordinated (Hodges & Moseley 2003). This mechanism protects the joint from excessive motion and coordinates the timing of motor recruitment such that habitual movements are produced in an efficient and biomechanically safe manner.

There is more than one classification of joint receptors (Wyke 1981, Rowinski 1985). Essentially, there are receptors in all layers of the capsule, in all ligaments and fascia, and within all parts of the muscles. Some have a low threshold for discharge and are slow in adapting. They report on static position of the joint, muscle length and tone, and intraarticular pressure. Others have a low threshold for discharge and adapt very quickly. These receptors report dynamic changes in the environment, including changes in joint position (direction, quantity, and

velocity). The receptors which have a high threshold for discharge adapt very slowly and are protective. The effect of these receptors is reflexively to inhibit further muscle contraction and prevent further stretch of the joint capsule. Both myelinated and non-myelineated axons are found in the ventral portion of the SIJ capsule (Fortin et al 1999).

Nociceptors are located throughout the articular and myofascial system. They respond to extremes of mechanical deformation and/or chemical irritation (potassium ions, lactic acid, polypeptide kinins, 5-hydroxytryptamine, acetylcholine, norepinephrine (noradrenaline), prostaglandins, histamine) and are high-threshold, non-adapting receptors. These receptors contribute to the perception of pain (nociception); however, the afferent input can be significantly altered both peripherally and centrally.

According to Wyke (1981) the central effects of articular mechanoreceptor activity are threefold: reflex, perceptual, and pain suppression.

REFLEX EFFECTS

Depolarization of the afferent fibers from the low-threshold articular mechanoreceptors reaches the fusimotor neurons polysynaptically, thus contributing to the gamma feedback loop from the muscle spindle both at rest and during joint motion. "By this means the articular mechanoreceptors exert reciprocally coordinated reflexogenic influences on muscle tone and on the excitability of stretch reflexes in all the striated muscles" (Wyke 1981). When this capsular reflex is activated, the discharging receptors facilitate the muscles antagonistic to the occurring movement. When the high-threshold articular mechanoreceptors are discharged, the reflex effect is projected polysynaptically to the alphamotoneurons and this results in local muscular inhibition. Nociceptors affect the discharge from the alpha-motoneuron pool and can distort the normal, coordinated, mechanoreceptor reflex system (Gandevia 1992).

Perceptual effects

Afferent input from the articular mechanoreceptors travels polysynaptically via the posterior and dorsal spinal columns to reach the paracentral and parietal regions of the cerebral cortex, thus contributing significantly, though not solely, to both postural and kinesthetic awareness.

The observation that capsulectomy of the hip joint performed in the course of hip replacement surgery does not result in total loss of postural sensation at the hip leaves no doubt that while joint capsule mechanoreceptors contribute to awareness of static joint position, they are not the sole source of perceptual experience, and other recent studies suggest that their contribution in this regard is supplementary to and coordinated with that provided by the inputs from cutaneous and myotactic [muscle spindle] mechanoreceptors!

(Wyke 1981)

Pain

According to Grieve (1981):

No matter where it is felt in the body, and no matter from what cause, pain – which is the commonest of all clinical symptoms encountered in medical practice – represents a disturbance of neurological function.

Unlike taste, touch, or smell, pain is not a primary neurological sensation but rather a complex neurological phenomenon influenced by patterns of activity in specific afferent systems as well as by past and present experiences.

Impulses subserving pain are not transmitted centrally by small-diameter fibers only. The entire spectrum of afferent fibers may be stimulated by peripheral noxious stimuli, depending upon the intensity of the stimulus. The experience of pain depends upon mechanisms of convergence, summation, and modulation both peripherally in the spinal cord and centrally in the brainstem and cortex.

The theory of peripheral modulation, or spinal gating, was originally proposed by Melzak & Wall (1965). Briefly, the gate-control mechanism depends on large-fiber activity (mechanoreceptor) which presynaptically inhibits the transmission of impulses from the small-fiber nociceptors at the substantia gelatinosa. Thus "by rhythmic movement of the body, or a body part, and by cutaneous contact and soft tissue compression, i.e. stroking, holding and by rhythmic manual or mechanical mobilization techniques, the large-diameter (6–12 and 13–17 μm) mechanoreceptors are stimulated" (Grieve 1981) and subsequently modulate the transmission of nociceptor activity.

Centrally, the perception of pain can be influenced by psychological factors, including past experience, anxiety, and culture, and drugs such as caffeine, alcohol, and barbiturates, all of which increase the experience of pain (Butler 2000, Butler & Moseley 2003). The presence of pain and the fear of pain are known to impact motor control (Hodges & Moseley 2003).

ANGIOLOGY: THE BLOOD SUPPLY

The hip joint is supplied by the obturator, the medial and lateral femoral circumflex, and the superior and inferior gluteal arteries and veins (Singleton & LeVeau 1975, Crock 1980, Grieve 1981). The acetabular fossa, its contents as well as the head of the femur, receive supply from the acetabular branch of the obturator and medial femoral circumflex vessels via the ligamentum teres. The vascular anatomy is inconsistent and rarely sufficient to sustain the viability of the head of the femur following interruption of other sources of supply.

Experimental findings (Astrom 1975) point to a connection between aching pain, elevation of intraosseous pressure and impaired [venous] drainage of spongiosa. Rhythmic mobilizations of this articulation are extremely effective in relieving persistent aches associated with osteoarthritis. Together with the effects of mechanoreceptor discharge during these techniques perhaps improved circulation plays a role in pain suppression. (Grieve 1981)

The nutrient arteries and veins for the sacrum arise from the lateral and median sacral system. The lateral sacral vessels arise from the posterior trunk of the internal iliac and descend over the anterolateral aspect of the sacrum. The two longitudinal arteries give off anterior central branches which course medially to anastomose with the median sacral artery. The anterior central branches send feeder vessels into the centrum of the sacrum. At the level of the ventral sacral foramina, spinal branches supply the cauda equina as well as the contents of the sacral canal. The foraminal branch, after passing through the dorsal sacral foramina, supplies the posterior aspect of the medial and intermediate sacral crests as well as the posterior musculature. Venous drainage is via vessels which accompany the arteries and subsequently drain into the common iliac system.

The nutrient supply for the innominate is derived from the iliac branches of the obturator and iliolumbar vessels as well as the superior gluteal vessels (Williams 1995).

Chapter 5

Principles of the integrated model of function and its application to the lumbopelvic–hip region

CHAPTER CONTENTS

INTRODUCTION

This chapter introduces the principles of an integrated model for managing impaired function. This model comes from anatomical and biomechanical studies of the pelvis, as well as from the clinical experience of treating patients with lumbopelvic pain (Lee 2001b, Lee & Vleeming 2003). This approach addresses why the pelvis is painful and no longer able to sustain and transfer loads as opposed to one which seeks to identify pain-generating structures. Several studies have sought to understand pelvic function. The anatomical research on the sacroiliac joint (SIJ) and the connections between it and the lumbopelvic muscles (Vleeming et al 1990a, b, 1995b, 1996, Snijders et al 1993a) led to conclusions regarding the role the passive and active elements play in stabilization of the pelvis (form and force closure of joints). The timing of specific muscle activation (Hodges 1997, 2003, Hodges & Richardson 1997, Hodges et al 1999, 2001a, 2003b, Hungerford 2002) and the pattern of muscular co-contraction (or lack thereof) in patients with low back pain (Hides et al 1994, 1996, Hodges & Richardson 1996, O'Sullivan 2000, Hungerford 2002, O'Sullivan et al 2002, Hodges 2003, Hodges & Moseley 2003) further enhanced the force closure theory and suggested a crucial role for motor control. Based on this knowledge, functional tests for the pelvis were developed (Buyruk et al 1995a, b, 1999, Lee 1999, Mens et al 1999, 2001) and treatment protocols were established (Lee 1999, Richardson et al 1999, O'Sullivan 2000). Clinically, it was soon apparent that the patient's emotional state could significantly influence the outcome. Over time, the integrated model of function was developed (Lee & Vleeming 1998, 2003).

THE INTEGRATED MODEL OF FUNCTION

The integrated model of function (Fig. 5.1) has four components – three that are physical:

1. form closure (structure)
2. force closure (forces produced by myofascial action)
3. motor control (specific timing of muscle action/inaction during loading) and one that is psychological:
4. emotions.

The proposal is that joint mechanics can be influenced by multiple factors (articular, neuromuscular, and emotional) and that management requires attention to all.

Managing dysfunction requires an understanding of function. A primary function of the lumbo-pelvic-hip region is to transfer the loads generated by body weight and gravity during standing, walking, and sitting (Snijders et al 1993a, b) (Fig. 5.2). How well this load is managed dictates how efficient function will be. According to Panjabi (1992a, b), stability (effective load transfer) is achieved when the passive, active, and control systems work together (Fig. 5.3). Snijders et al (1993a, b) believe that the passive, active, and control systems produce approximation of the joint surfaces, which is essential if stability is to be insured. The amount of approximation required is variable and difficult to quantify since it is essentially dependent on an individual's structure (form closure) and the forces they need to control (force closure). The term "adequate" has been used (Lee & Vleeming 1998, 2003) to describe how much approximation is necessary and reflects the non-quantitative aspect of this measure. Essentially, it means "not too much" and "not too little"; in other words, just enough to suit the existing situation. Consequently, the ability to transfer load through the pelvis effectively is dynamic and depends on:

1. optimal function of the bones, joints, and ligaments (form closure or joint congruency) (Vleeming et al 1990a, b)

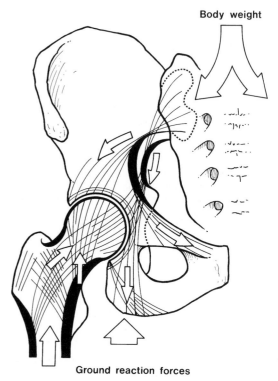

Figure 5.2 The orientation of the bony trabeculae within the pelvic girdle corresponds to the lines of force met during load transfer through the pelvic girdle. (Redrawn from Kapandji 1970.)

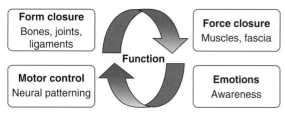

Figure 5.1 The integrated model of function (Lee & Vleeming 1998).

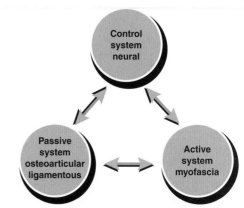

Figure 5.3 Conceptual model from Panjabi (1992b), illustrating the components which provide stability.

2. optimal function of the muscles and fascia (force closure) (Vleeming et al 1995b, Richardson et al 1999, 2002, O'Sullivan 2000, Hungerford 2002)

3. appropriate neural function (motor control, emotional state) (Bo & Stein 1994, Holstege et al 1996, Hodges 1997, 2003, Hodges et al 1999, 2001c, 2003b, Hodges & Gandevia 2000b, Hungerford 2002).

FORM CLOSURE

The term "form closure" was coined by Vleeming & Snijders (Vleeming et al 1990a, b, Snijders et al 1993a, b) and is used to describe how the joint's structure, orientation, and shape contribute to stability and potential mobility (Fig. 5.4). All joints have a variable amount of form closure and the individual's inherent anatomy will dictate how much additional force (force closure) is needed to ensure stabilization when loads are increased. The "form" of the lumbar spine, pelvic girdle, and hip (the bones, joints, and ligaments) has been described in detail in Chapter 4. The potential mobility (biomechanics) for each region will be discussed in Chapter 6.

THE LUMBAR SPINE

The "form" of the lumbar spine contributes to its ability to resist compression, torsion, and posteroanterior shear, forces encountered during activities of daily living, in the following ways.

Compression

Compression of an object results when two forces act towards each other. The main restraint to compression in the lumbar spine is the vertebral body/annulus-nucleus unit, although the zygapophyseal joints have been noted (Farfan 1973, Kirkaldy-Willis 1983, Gracovetsky et al 1985, Gracovetsky & Farfan 1986, Bogduk 1997) to support up to 20% of the axial compression load (Fig. 5.5). Both the annulus and the nucleus transmit the load equally to the end-plate of the vertebral body. The thin cortical shell of the vertebral body provides the bulk of the compression strength, being simultaneously supported by a hydraulic mechanism within the cancellous core, the contribution of which is dependent upon the rate of loading. When compression is applied slowly (static loading), the nuclear pressure rises, distributing its force on to the annulus and the end-plates. The annulus bulges circumferentially and the end-plates bow towards the vertebral bodies. Fluid is squeezed out of the cancellous core via the veins; however, when the rate of compression is increased, the small vessel size may retard the rate of outflow such that the internal pressure of the vertebral body rises, thus increasing the compressive strength of the unit. In this manner, the vertebral body supports and protects the intervertebral disk against compression overload (McGill 2002). The anatomical structure which initially yields to high loads of compression is the hyaline cartilage of the end-plate, suggesting that this structure is weaker than the peripheral parts of the end-plate (Bogduk 1997).

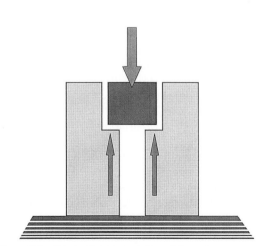

Figure 5.4 Schematic representation of form closure (Vleeming et al 1990a, b, Snijders et al 1993a).

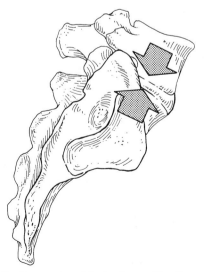

Figure 5.5 Compression of the lumbosacral junction.

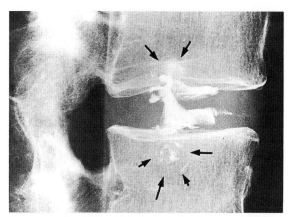

Figure 5.6 Superior and inferior end-plate fractures (Schmorl's nodes) detected via a diskogram. Note the penetration of the dye into both the superior and inferior vertebral bodies through the end-plate (arrows). (Reproduced with permission from Farfan 1973.)

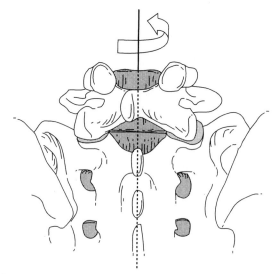

Figure 5.7 Right axial torsion of the L5 vertebra is resisted by osseous impaction of the left zygapophyseal joint and capsular distraction of the right zygapophyseal joint as well as the segmental ligaments, the intervertebral disk, and the myofascia.

The fracture appears radiographically as a Schmorl's node (Fig. 5.6) (Kirkaldy-Willis et al 1978, Kirkaldy-Willis 1983). This lesion is commonly seen at the higher lumbar levels. McGill states that the vertebral bony elements fail at the higher load rates whereas the end-plate (no specification as to which part) fails first at low rates (McGill 2002). The zygapophyseal joints do not contribute to weight-bearing when in the neutral position, given that their sagittal and coronal components are oriented vertically. When the segment is extended, the inferior articular process of the superior vertebra glides inferiorly and impacts the pars interarticularis. When axial compression is applied in this lordotic position, load can be transferred through the inferior articular process to the lamina (Bogduk 1997).

Torsion or rotation

When a force is applied to an object at any location other than the center of rotation, it will cause the object to rotate about an axis through this pivot point. The magnitude of the torque force can be calculated by multiplying the quantity of the force by the distance the force acts from the pivot. Axial rotation of the lumbar vertebra occurs when the bone rotates about a vertical axis through the center of the body (Fig. 5.7) and is resisted by anatomical factors located within the vertebral arch (65%) as well as by the structures of the vertebral body/intervertebral disk unit (35%) (Gracovetsky & Farfan 1986, Bogduk 1997).

At the lumbosacral junction, the superior articular process of the sacrum (see Fig. 4.2) is squat and strong in comparison to the inferior articular process of the L5 vertebra which is much longer and receives less support from the pedicle. Consequently, the inferior process is more easily deflected when the zygapophyseal joint is loaded at 90° to its articular surface. This process can deflect 8–9° medially during axial torsion beyond which trabecular fractures and residual strain deformation will occur (Farfan 1973, Bogduk 1997).

The structure and orientation of the annular fibers are critical to the ability of the intervertebral disk to resist torsion. "The concentric arrangement of the collagenous layers of the annulus ensures that when the disk is placed in tension, shear or rotation, the individual fibers are always in tension" (Kirkaldy-Willis 1983). Under static loading conditions, injuries occur with as little as 2° and certainly by 3.5° of axial rotation (Gracovetsky & Farfan 1986). The iliolumbar ligament (see Figs 4.12 and 4.19) plays an important role in minimizing torque forces at the lumbosacral junction. The longer the transverse process of the L5 vertebra and consequently the shorter the iliolumbar ligament, the stronger is the resistance of the segment to torsion (Farfan 1973).

Axial compression also increases the segmental torque strength by 35% (Gracovetsky & Farfan 1986). During forward flexion of the lumbar spine,

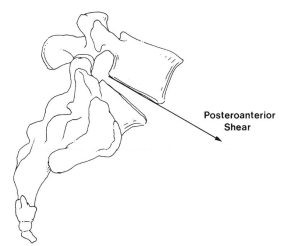

Figure 5.8 Posteroanterior shear of the L5 vertebra on the sacrum.

the instantaneous center of rotation moves forward (see Fig. 6.3), thus increasing the compressive load and consequently the ability of the joint to resist torsion (Farfan 1973, Gracovetsky & Farfan 1986).

Posteroanterior translation

Translation occurs when an applied force produces sliding between two planes. Posteroanterior translation occurs in the lumbar spine when a force attempts to displace a superior vertebra anterior to the one below (Fig. 5.8). The anatomical factors which resist posteroanterior shear at the lumbosacral junction are primarily the impaction of the inferior articular processes of L5 against the superior articular processes of the sacrum and the iliolumbar ligaments (Bogduk 1997). Secondary factors include the intervertebral disk, the anterior longitudinal ligament, the posterior longitudinal ligament, and the midline posterior ligamentous system (Twomey & Taylor 1985).

Dynamically, the posterior midline ligaments, the thoracodorsal fascia, and the muscles which generate tension within this system are important in balancing the anterior shear forces which occur when large loads are lifted (force closure) (Gracovetsky & Farfan 1986, Vleeming et al 1990a, b, 1995a, 1997, Hides et al 1994, 1996, Richardson & Jull 1995, Hodges & Richardson 1996, Adams & Dolan 1997, Bogduk 1997, Hodges et al 2003b). The optimal method of loading the spine should balance both compression and translation such that the magnitude of the resultant force does not exceed the strength of the joint. Consequently, both the articular (form closure) and

the myofascial components (force closure) are required to balance the moment of a large external load.

THE PELVIC GIRDLE

How does the "form" of the pelvic girdle contribute to stability of the SIJs? The SIJs transfer large loads and their shape is adapted to this task. The articular surfaces are relatively flat and this helps to transfer compression forces and bending moments (Vleeming et al 1990a, b, Snijders et al 1993a, b). However, a relatively flat joint is theoretically more vulnerable to shear forces. The SIJ is anatomically protected from shear in three ways. First, the sacrum is wedge-shaped in both the anteroposterior and vertical planes (Figs 4.1 and 4.2) and thus is stabilized by the innominates. The articular surface of the SIJ is comprised of two to three sacral segments and each is oriented differently (Fig. 4.5) (Solonen 1957). Second, in contrast to other synovial joints, the articular cartilage is not smooth but irregular, especially on the ilium (Sashin 1930, Bowen & Cassidy 1981) (Plates 1–5, Ch. 3). Third, a frontal dissection through the SIJ reveals cartilage-covered bony extensions protruding into the joint (Vleeming et al 1990a), ridges, and grooves (Fig. 3.6). They seem irregular, but are in fact complementary. All three factors enhance stabilization of the SIJ when compression (force closure) is applied to the pelvis. Again, both the articular (form closure) and the myofascial components (force closure) are required to balance the moment of a large external load.

The pubic symphysis has less form closure than the SIJ in that the joint surfaces are relatively flat. The joint surfaces are bound by a fibrocartilatinous disk which is supported externally by superior, inferior, anterior, and posterior ligaments. The pubic symphysis is vulnerable to shear forces in both the vertical and horizontal plane and relies on dynamic elements (myofascia), in addition to the passive structures, for stability.

THE HIP

The hip is subjected to forces equal to multiples of the body weight and requires osseous, articular, and myofascial integrity for stability. The form closure factors which contribute to stability at the hip include the anatomical configuration of the joint as well as the orientation of the trabeculae and the orientation of the capsule and the ligaments during habitual movements.

During erect standing, the superincumbent body weight is distributed equally through the pelvic girdle to the femoral heads and necks. Each hip joint supports approximately 33% of the body weight which subsequently produces a bending moment between the neck of the femur and its shaft (Singleton & LeVeau 1975). A complex system of bony trabeculae exists within the femoral head and neck to prevent superoinferior shearing of the femoral head during erect standing (Fig. 5.2) (Kapandji 1970). The hip joint is an unmodified ovoid joint, a deep ball and socket, and its shape precludes significant shearing in any direction yet facilitates motion (Ch. 6).

FORCE CLOSURE

If the articular surfaces of the lumbar spine, pelvic girdle, and hip were constantly and completely compressed, mobility would not be possible. However, compression during loading is variable and therefore motion is possible (Ch. 6) and stabilization required. This is achieved by increasing compression across the joint surface at the moment of loading (force closure – Fig. 5.9). The amount of force closure required depends on the individual's form closure and the magnitude of the load. The anatomical structures responsible for force closure are the ligaments, muscles, and fascia.

For every joint, there is a position called the close-packed, or self-locked, position in which there is maximum congruence of the articular surfaces and maximum tension of the major ligaments. In this position, the joint is under significant compression and the ability to resist shear forces is enhanced by the tension of the passive structures and increased

friction between the articular surfaces (Vleeming et al 1990b, Snijders et al 1993a, b). For the zygapophyseal joints of the lumbar spine this position is end-range extension, for the sacroiliac joints full nutation of the sacrum or posterior rotation of the innominate (Vleeming et al 1989a, b, van Wingerden et al 1993), and for the hip joint extension combined with abduction and internal rotation.

Studies have shown (Egund et al 1978, Lavignolle et al 1983, Sturesson et al 2000, Hungerford 2002) that nutation of the sacrum occurs bilaterally whenever the lumbopelvic spine is loaded. The amount of sacral nutation varies with the magnitude of the load. Full sacral nutation (self-locking or close-packing) occurs during forward and backward bending of the trunk (Sturesson et al 2000). Counternutation of the sacrum, or anterior rotation of the innominate, is thought to be a relatively less stable position for the SIJ. The long dorsal ligament becomes taut during this motion (Fig. 4.15); however, the other major ligaments (sacrotuberous, sacrospinous, and interosseus) are less tensed (Vleeming et al 1996).

The orientation of the capsule and the articular ligaments of the hip joint (see Figs 4.23 and 4.24) contribute to force closure of the hip during functional motions (Table 5.1). Extension of the femur winds all of the extraarticular ligaments around the femoral

Table 5.1   Force closure secondary to tension of the ligaments of the hip joint during motion of the femur

Femoral motion	Ligament	Tension
Extension	All extraarticular ligaments	Taut
Flexion/adduction	All ligaments	Slack
Lateral rotation	Iliotrochanteric	Taut
	Pubofemoral	Taut
	Ischiofemoral	Slack
Medial rotation	Iliofemoral	Slack
	Pubofemoral	Slack
	Ischiofemoral	Taut
Abduction	Pubofemoral	Taut
	Inferior band[a]	Taut
	Ischiofemoral	Taut
	Iliotrochanteric	Slack
Adduction	Iliotrochanteric	Taut
	Inferior band[a]	Slack
	Ischiofemoral	Slack
	Pubofemoral	Slack

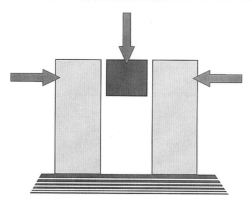

Figure 5.9   Schematic representation of force closure (Vleeming et al 1990a, b, Snijders et al 1993a).

[a]Inferior band of iliofemoral ligament.

neck and renders them taut. The inferior band of the iliofemoral ligament is under the greatest tension in extension. Flexion of the femur unwinds the ligaments, and when combined with slight adduction, predisposes the femoral head to posterior dislocation if sufficient force is applied to the distal end of the femur (e.g., dashboard impact).

During lateral rotation of the femur, the iliotrochanteric band of the iliofemoral ligament and the pubofemoral ligament become taut while the ischiofemoral ligament becomes slack. Conversely, during medial rotation of the femur, the anterior ligaments become slack while the ischiofemoral ligament becomes taut (Hewitt et al 2002).

Abduction of the femur tenses the pubofemoral ligament and the inferior band of the iliofemoral ligament as well as the ischiofemoral ligament. At the end of abduction, the neck of the femur impacts on to the acetabular rim, thus distorting and everting the labrum (Kapandji 1970). In this manner, the acetabular labrum deepens the articular cavity (improving form closure), thus increasing stability without limiting mobility. Adduction results in tension of the iliotrochanteric band of the iliofemoral ligament while the others remain relatively slack. Adduction of the flexed hip tightens the ischiofemoral ligament (Hewitt et al 2002). The ligamentum teres is under moderate tension in erect standing as well as during medial and lateral rotation of the femur.

Function would be significantly compromised if joints could only be stable in the close-packed position. In the neutral spinal position, an osteoligamentous spine (T1 to sacrum with no muscles attached) will buckle under approximately 20 N (about 4.4 lb) of compression load (Lucas & Bresler 1961, Panjabi et al 1989, Panjabi 1992a, b). Stability for load transfer is required throughout the entire range of motion and this is provided by the active, or neuromyofascial, system. In 1989, Bergmark proposed that muscles could be classified into two systems – a local and a global system. The local system pertains to those muscles essential for segmental or intrapelvic stabilization while the global system appears to be more responsible for regional stabilization (between the thorax and pelvis or pelvis and legs) and motion (Bergmark 1989, Richardson et al 1999, Comerford & Mottram 2001). There is a significant neurophysiological difference in the timing of contraction of these two muscle systems. When loads are predictable, the local system contracts prior to the perturbation (in anticipation) regardless of the direction of movement (Hodges 1997, 2003, Hodges & Richardson

1997, Hodges et al 1999, Moseley et al 2002, 2003) whereas the global system contracts later and is direction-dependent (Radebold et al 2000, 2001, Hodges 2003). While some researchers have embraced this classification (Richardson et al 1999, Comerford & Mottram 2001), others have not (McGill 2002).

The research is still lacking which enables classification of all muscles according to this system and clinically it appears that parts of some muscles may belong to both systems. With respect to the lumbopelvic region, the following muscles fit the criteria for classification as local stabilizers – the muscles of the pelvic floor (Constantinou & Govan 1982, Bo & Stein 1994, Sapsford et al 2001, Hodges 2003), the transversus abdominis (Hodges & Richardson 1997, Hodges 2003), the diaphragm (Hodges & Gandevia 2000a, b, Hodges 2003), and the deep fibers of multifidus (Moseley et al 2002, 2003) (Fig. 5.10). As research continues, more muscles will likely be added to this list. The deep (medial) fibers of psoas (Gibbons et al 2002), the medial fibers of quadratus lumborum (Bergmark 1989, McGill 2002), the lumbar parts of the lumbar iliocostalis and longissimus (Bergmark 1989), and the posterior fibers of the internal oblique (Bergmark 1989, O'Sullivan 2000) are some likely candidates. This text will focus on those in which the research clearly indicates that they are local stabilizers; however, it is not the intent to state that they are the only muscles that fit this role.

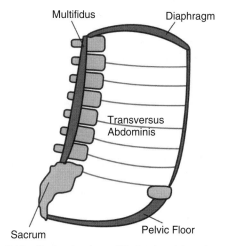

Figure 5.10 The local system of the lumbopelvic region consists of the muscles of the pelvic floor, the transversus abdominis, the diaphragm, and the deep fibers of multifidus. (Reproduced with permission from © Diane G. Lee Physiotherapist Corp.)

THE ROLE OF THE LOCAL MUSCLE SYSTEM

The function of the lumbopelvic local system is to stabilize the joints of the spine and pelvic girdle in preparation for (or in response to) the addition of external loads. This is achieved through several mechanisms, some of which include:

- increasing the intraabdominal pressure (McGill & Norman 1987, Cresswell 1993, Hodges & Gandevia 2000a, b, Hodges et al 2001a, 2003b, Hodges 2003)
- increasing the tension of the thoracodorsal fascia (Cresswell 1993, Vleeming et al 1995a, Willard 1997, Hodges 2003, Hodges et al 2003b) and/or
- increasing the articular stiffness (Hodges et al 1997a, Richardson et al 2002, Hodges 2003).

Research has shown (Constantinou & Govan 1982, Bo & Stein 1994, Hodges 1997, 2003, Hodges & Gandevia 2000a, b, Sapsford et al 2001, Hungerford 2002, Moseley et al 2002, 2003) that when the central nervous system can predict the timing of the load, the local system is anticipatory when functioning optimally. In other words, these muscles should work at low levels at all times and increase their action *before* any further loading or motion occurs.

Transversus abdominis

Dr. Paul Hodges' first PhD focused on the role of transversus abdominis in healthy individuals and the response of this muscle in patients with low back pain (Hodges & Richardson 1996, 1997). He was able to show that transversus abdominis is an anticipatory muscle for stabilization of the low back and is recruited prior to the initiation of any movement of the upper or lower extremity. He also showed that this anticipatory recruitment of transversus abdominis is absent or delayed in patients with low back pain. Dr. Paul Hodges has just completed his second PhD (2003: Neuromechanical control of the spine). This series of studies provides further information on *how* lumbopelvic stability is achieved. According to Hodges (2003), a key finding from this research is that:

> When the upper limbs were moved rapidly in response to a light, the anticipatory postural adjustment did not stiffen the trunk, but rather there was a consistent pattern of trunk motion that was specific to the direction of limb movement.

Stability is achieved through motion, not rigidity. Small angular displacements of the vertebra preceded the limb movement and occurred in the opposite direction (preparatory movement) to the predicted movements of the segment (resultant movement). In other words, during rapid bilateral flexion of the upper limbs, a small amount of segmental extension occurred in the lumbar spine (preparatory movement) before the arms moved (flexed). After the arms flexed, the lumbar segments flexed (resultant movement) a small amount. The opposite preparatory and resultant movements were noted during bilateral extension of the upper limbs. Transversus abdominis was the first trunk muscle recruited in all of these experiments yet did not render the trunk rigid. Hodges (2003) proposes that movement is used to dissipate or dampen the imposed internal and external forces which occur as a result of the perturbation. Therefore optimal stability requires mobility and a finely tuned motion control system. The clinical application of this research (Ch. 10) supports exercise programs which foster mobile stability (movements with control) as opposed to rigidity and bracing.

As part of a very interesting study with pigs, Hodges et al (2003b) differentiated the role of first, the intraabdominal pressure (IAP); second, the vertebral attachments of the crura of the diaphragm; and third, the fascial attachments of the middle layer of the thoracolumbar fascia on stability (resistance to flexion and extension) at L3–L4. The pigs were anesthetized and pins inserted into the spinous processes of L3 and L4. The resistance to segmental flexion and extension of L3–L4 was measured under different conditions.

1. The phrenic nerve was stimulated and the impact of an isolated contraction of the diaphragm on IAP and consequential stiffness (resistance to flexion/extension) at L3–L4 was noted. The IAP increased approximately 5 cm H_2O and the resistance to flexion at L3–L4 increased approximately 10%. There was no difference in the resistance to extension at L3–L4.

2. Transversus abdominis was electrically stimulated bilaterally. The intensity of the stimulus was set such that the IAP increased to similar levels as those in the phrenic nerve stimulation trials (#1: see below). The impact of this stimulation on stiffness (resistance to flexion/extension) at L3–L4 was noted. Again, resistance increased to flexion at L3–L4 but not statistically to extension (although a trend was noted). When transversus abdominis was stimulated

unilaterally there was no change in the resistance to either flexion or extension at L3–L4. Therefore a *bilateral* contraction of transversus abdominis is required for stiffness at L3–L4 to be increased.

3. To differentiate the role of IAP from the mechanical role of the crura of the diaphragm and the fascial attachments of transversus abdominis three further experiments were done:

a. A small incision was made in the abdominal wall and the phrenic nerve was stimulated to produce an isolated contraction of the diaphragm. It was noted that the IAP decreased to 17% of the IAP that occurred when the abdomen was closed. Subsequently, the resistance to flexion and extension was measured at L3–L4 (the diaphragm was stimulated through the phrenic nerve) and no change was noted. Therefore, the IAP is a significant contributor to resisting flexion at L3–L4 (contraction of the diaphragm increased the IAP which in turn produces an extensor moment).

b. The crura of the diaphragm were then cut and the abdomen closed. When a contraction of the diaphragm occurred through stimulation via the phrenic nerve, the IAP had returned to 87% of the previous measures (#1 above). Subsequently, the resistance to flexion and extension was measured at L3–L4 and, as previously observed, there was an increase in the resistance to flexion. However, in addition, the resistance to extension was significantly *decreased*, suggesting that the crura of the diaphragm provide some mechanical control for extension at L3–L4.

c. The middle layer of the thoracolumbar fascia was cut from the transverse processes at L2–L5 first unilaterally and then bilaterally. In both trials, the resistance to flexion and extension was measured at L3–L4 following bilateral stimulation of transversus abdominis. Although the IAP increased with the contraction of transversus abdominis, there was no difference in the stiffening effect in flexion and there was a *reduction* in the stiffness of extension. Transversus abdominis appears to play a mechanical role (along with the crura of the diaphragm) through its fascial attachments in resisting extension at L3–L4.

In conclusion, the IAP, the fascial attachments of transversus abdominis, and the crura of the diaphragm play a significant role in controlling flexion and extension in the lumbar spine (measured only at L3–L4). The IAP is increased through contraction of both the diaphragm and transversus abdominis and produces an extension moment (resistance to flexion). Extension is resisted by the fascial attachments of transversus abdominis and the crural attachments of the diaphragm.

Although it does not cross the SIJ directly, the transversus abdominis has an impact on stiffness of the SIJ (Richardson et al 2002) through, in part, its direct pull on the large attachment to the middle layer and the deep lamina of the posterior layer of the thoracodorsal fascia (Barker & Briggs 1999) (Figs 4.37 and 4.38). Richardson et al (2002) propose that contraction of the transversus abdominis produces a force which acts on the ilia perpendicular to the sagittal plane (i.e., approximates the ilia anteriorly) (Fig. 5.11). They also propose that the "mechanical action of a pelvic belt in front of the abdominal wall at the level of the transversus abdominis corresponds with the action of this muscle." At this time, the specific direction of force produced by an isolated contraction of transversus abdominis (i.e., without co-activation of multifidus) has not been validated through research but this hypothesis has been developed clinically as a means for diagnosis and exercise prescription (see active straight leg raise, Ch. 8).

In a study of patients with chronic low back pain, a timing delay or absence was found in which transversus abdominis failed to anticipate the initiation of arm and/or leg motion (Hodges & Richardson 1997a, 1999, Hodges 2001, 2003). Delayed activation of transversus abdominis means that the thoracodorsal fascia is not pretensed and the joints of the low

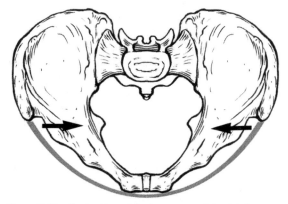

Figure 5.11 Contraction of the transversus abdominis is proposed to produce a force which acts on the ilia perpendicular to the sagittal plane (i.e., approximates the ilia anteriorly: arrows). (Reproduced with permission from © Diane G. Lee Physiotherapist Corp.)

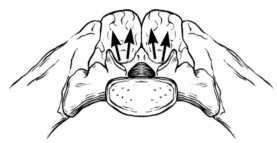

Figure 5.12 When the deep fibers of the multifidus contract, the muscle can be felt to broaden or swell (represented by the arrows in the deep layers of the muscle). This hydraulic amplifying mechanism (proposed by Gracovetsky 1990) "pumps up" the thoracodorsal fascia much like blowing air into a balloon (Vleeming et al 1995a). (Reproduced with permission from © Diane G. Lee Physiotherapist Corp.)

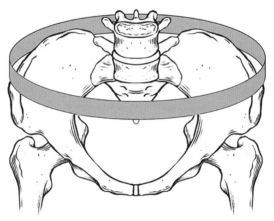

Figure 5.13 Together, multifidus and transversus abdominis form a corset of support for the lumbopelvic region, collectively called the "circle of integrity." (Reproduced with permission from © Diane G. Lee Physiotherapist Corp.)

back and pelvis are therefore not stiffened (compressed) in preparation for external loading and are potentially vulnerable to losing intrinsic stability.

Deep fibers of multifidus

Moseley et al (2002) have shown that the deep fibers of the multifidus muscle are also anticipatory for stabilization of the lumbar region and are recruited prior to the initiation of any movement of the upper extremity when the timing of the load is predictable (Moseley et al 2002). In contrast, the superficial and lateral fibers of the multifidus muscle were shown to be direction-dependent. In the pelvis, this muscle is contained between the dorsal aspect of the sacrum and the deep layers of the thoracodorsal fascia (Figs 4.16 and 4.27). When the deep fibers of the multifidus contract, the muscle can be felt to broaden or swell (Fig. 5.12). As the deep fibers of multifidus broaden, they "pump up" the thoracodorsal fascia much like blowing air into a balloon (Gracovetsky 1990, Vleeming et al 1995a). Using the Doppler imaging system, Richardson et al (2002) noted that a co-contraction of multifidus and transversus abdominis increased the stiffness of the SIJ. These authors state that "Under gravitational load, it is the transversely oriented muscles that must act to compress the sacrum between the ilia and maintain stability of the SIJ." Although multifidus is not oriented transversely, its contraction tenses the thoracodorsal fascia and it is likely this structure which imparts compression to the posterior pelvis. This has yet to be scientifically verified; however, this hypothesis has been developed clinically as a means for diagnosis and exercise prescription (Lee 2002) (see active straight leg raise, Ch. 8).

Several investigators (Hides et al 1994, Danneels et al 2000, O'Sullivan 2000, Hungerford 2002, Moseley et al 2002) have studied the response of multifidus in low back and pelvic pain patients and note that multifidus becomes inhibited and reduced in size in these individuals. The normal "pump-up" effect of multifidus on the thoracodorsal fascia, and therefore its ability to compress the pelvis, is lost when the size or function of this muscle is impaired. Rehabilitation requires both retraining (Hides et al 1996, O'Sullivan et al 1997) and hypertrophy of the muscle (Danneels et al 2001) for the restoration of proper force closure of the lumbopelvic region. Together, multifidus and transversus abdominis (along with their fascia) form a corset of support for the lumbopelvic region (Fig. 5.13) – the "circle of integrity."

The pelvic floor

The "roof and floor" of this local system (Fig. 5.10) are supported by the muscles of the pelvic floor and the respiratory diaphragm. The muscles of the pelvic floor (Figs 4.28 and 4.29) play a critical role in both stabilization of the pelvic girdle and in the maintenance of urinary and fecal continence (Constantinou & Govan 1982, Bo & Stein 1994, Ashton-Miller et al 2001, Peschers et al 2001a, Sapsford et al 2001, Dietz et al 2003). Constantinou & Govan (1982) measured the intraurethral and intrabladder pressures in healthy continent women during coughing and Valsalva (bearing down) and found that during a cough the intraurethral pressure increases approximately 250 ms before any pressure increase is detected in the bladder. This suggests that the urethra anticipates the impending load during coughing.

The increase in urethral pressure occurred simultaneously with the increase in bladder pressure during a Valsalva (no urethral anticipation). Constantinou & Govan suggest that the timing difference in pressure generation within the urethra and bladder during a cough versus a Valsalva may be due to the contraction of the pelvic floor during a cough and relaxation of the pelvic floor during a Valsalva.

Sapsford et al (2001) investigated the co-activation pattern of the pelvic floor and the abdominals via needle electromyogram (EMG) for the abdominals and surface EMG for the pelvic floor. In two subjects, fine-wire needle EMG was used to detect activation of the right pubococcygeus through the lateral vaginal wall. They found that the abdominals contract in response to a pelvic floor contraction command and that the pelvic floor contracts in response to both a "hollowing" and "bracing" abdominal command. The results from this research suggest that the pelvic floor can be facilitated by co-activating the abdominals and vice versa. Constantinou & Govan's suggestion that there may be a reflex connection between the pelvic floor and the urethra is supported by this research.

The diaphragm

The diaphragm is traditionally considered to be a respiratory muscle. Hodges (2003; Hodges et al 1997a, b; Hodges & Gandevia 2000a, b) investigated the role of the diaphragm as a stabilizer of the trunk during perturbation studies involving rapid, single (Hodges et al 1997b, 2001c) and rapid, repetitive (Hodges & Gandevia 2000b, Hodges et al 2001c) shoulder flexion. They found that EMG activity in both the costal and crural portions of the diaphragm occurred simultaneously with the transversus abdominis and approximately 20 ms prior to any EMG activity noted in the deltoid. They also noted that the anticipatory activity of the diaphragm depends on the magnitude of the perturbation and occurred regardless of the phase of respiration in which the shoulder was rapidly moved (Hodges et al 1997b). This research supports the classification of the diaphragm acting as a local stabilizer of the trunk in addition to its respiratory responsibilities.

Hodges & Gandevia (2000a, b) also noted that when loads to the trunk are sustained, the diaphragm responds tonically throughout the respiratory cycle for postural support of the trunk and simultaneously modulates this tonic activation to control the intrathoracic pressure necessary for breathing. An interesting pattern between the amplitude of activation of the

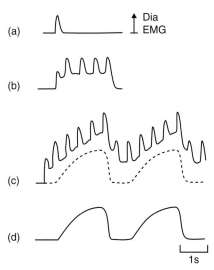

Figure 5.14 Electromyogram (EMG) activity of the diaphragm during single and repetitive trunk loading via upper-limb flexion with and without respiration. (a) Single-limb movement (shoulder flexion) without breathing. (b) Repetitive upper-limb movement without breathing. This tracing shows an increase in the tonic activation of the diaphragm along with the repetitive phasic bursts in response to the repetitive arm movements. (c) Combined tonic and phasic EMG modulation of the diaphragm during repetitive arm movement while breathing. The dashed line represents the inspiratory diaphragm EMG without limb movement and the line above is the phasic modulation which occurs when repetitive arm movement is added. (d) EMG activity of the diaphragm during respiration without any limb movement. (Redrawn from Hodges & Gandevia 2000b.)

diaphragm and the transversus abdominis was noted in the initial study (Hodges & Gandevia 2000a).

The amplitude of diaphragm EMG was higher in inspiration than expiration. The opposite pattern of activity modulation was found for both the right and left TrA [transversus abdominis]. Similar to the diaphragm, TrA was active throughout the respiratory cycle and was modulated with respiration, but the amplitude of TrA EMG was higher during expiration.
(Hodges & Gandevia 2000a)

When repetitive and sustained (10 s) perturbation of the trunk was added to the experiment (Hodges & Gandevia 2000b), another modulation of diaphragm activity was seen. There was a phasic modulation of activity which occurred at the frequency of the limb movement superimposed on the respiratory and tonic/postural activation (Fig. 5.14)!

Our data suggest that diaphragm EMG has three components: increased tonic activity, phasic modulation with respiration and phasic modulation with movement.
(Hodges & Gandevia 2000b)

In a subsequent study (Hodges et al 2001c), the authors noted that the tonic function (as well as the phasic modulation associated with arm movement) of both the diaphragm and transversus abdominis was reduced or absent after only 60 s of hypercapnea.

Blaney & Sawyer (1997) measured the amplitude of descent of the diaphragm from functional residual capacity to maximal inspiration in subjects who were about to undergo upper abdominal surgery and found the average displacement of the crural portion to be 5.5 ± 1.1 cm preoperatively. No significant difference was noted between abdominal versus lateral costal expansion breathing patterns. Postoperatively, the amplitude of the diaphragm descent decreased to 2.0 ± 1.0 cm (58% decrease) and again no significant difference was noted between the two breathing patterns. However, the authors did note that when the subject was instructed just to take a deep breath, the amplitude of descent was much less and they concluded that the proprioceptive input from the therapist's hands can play a significant role in the excursion of the diaphragm. Blaney et al (1999) subsequently measured diaphragmatic displacement during tidal breathing maneuvers (quiet breathing – not forced, not full) and noted that the excursion of the diaphragm varied with the pattern of breathing. They measured diaphragm displacement during upper chest, abdominal, and lateral costal breathing and found the mean amplitude to be 2.2, 3.1, and 2.4 cm respectively. Optimally, DeTroyer (1989) has found that quiet breathing should consist of 60% lateral costal expansion and 40% upper abdominal motion.

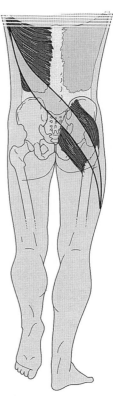

Figure 5.15 The posterior oblique sling of the global system includes the latissimus dorsi, gluteus maximus, and the intervening thoracodorsal fascia. (Redrawn from Vleeming et al 1995a.)

THE ROLE OF THE GLOBAL MUSCLE SYSTEM

In the past, four slings of muscle systems which stabilize the pelvis regionally (between the thorax and legs) have been described (Vleeming et al 1995a, b, Snijders et al 1993a). The posterior oblique sling (Fig. 5.15) contains connections between the latissimus dorsi and the gluteus maximus through the thoracodorsal fascia. The anterior oblique sling (Fig. 5.16) contains connections between the external oblique, the anterior abdominal fascia, and the contralateral internal oblique abdominal muscle and adductors of the thigh. The longitudinal sling (Fig. 5.17) connects the peroneii, the biceps femoris, the sacrotuberous ligament, the deep lamina of the thoracodorsal fascia, and the erector spinae. The lateral sling contains the primary stabilizers for the hip joint, namely the gluteus medius/minimus and tensor fascia latae and the lateral stabilizers of the thoracopelvic region.

These muscle slings were initially classified to gain a better understanding of how local and global

Summary

In conclusion, when the local system is functioning optimally, it provides anticipatory intersegmental stiffness of the joints of the lumbar spine (Hodges et al 2003b) and pelvis (Richardson et al 2002). This external force (force closure) augments the form closure (shape of the joint) and helps to prevent excessive shearing at the time of loading. This stiffness/compression occurs prior to the onset of any movement and prepares the low back and pelvis for additional loading from the global system. Simultaneously, the diaphragm maintains respiration while the pelvic floor assists in maintaining the position of the pelvic organs (continence) as load is transferred through the pelvis.

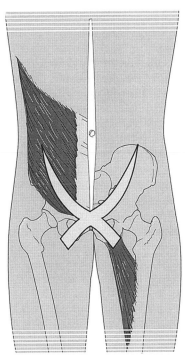

Figure 5.16 The anterior oblique sling of the global system includes the external oblique, the contralateral internal oblique, the adductors of the thigh, and the intervening anterior abdominal fascia.

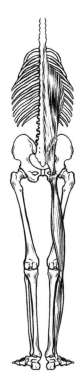

Figure 5.17 The longitudinal sling connects the peroneii, the biceps femoris, the sacrotuberous ligament, the deep lamina of the thoracodorsal fascia, and the erector spinae. (Reproduced with permission from © Diane G. Lee Physiotherapist Corp.)

stability of the pelvis could be achieved by specific muscles. It is now recognized that, although individual muscles are important for regional stabilization as well as for mobility, it is critical to understand how they connect and function together. A muscle contraction produces a force that spreads beyond the origin and insertion of the active muscle. This force is transmitted to other muscles, tendons, fasciae, ligaments, capsules, and bones that lie both in series and in parallel to the active muscle. In this manner, forces are produced quite distant from the origin of the initial muscle contraction. These integrated muscle systems produce slings of forces that assist in the transfer of load. Van Wingerden et al (2001, submitted) used the Doppler imaging system to analyze the effect of contraction of the biceps femoris, erector spinae, gluteus maximus, and latissiumus dorsi on compression of the SIJ. None of these muscles directly crosses the SIJ yet each was found to effect compression (increase stiffness) of the SIJ.

The global system of muscles is essentially an integrated sling system, comprised of several muscles, which produces forces. A muscle may participate in more than one sling and the slings may overlap

and interconnect depending on the task being demanded. The hypothesis is that the slings have no beginning or end but rather connect to assist in the transference of forces. It is possible that the slings are all part of one interconnected myofascial system and the particular sling (anterior oblique, posterior oblique, lateral, longitudinal), which is identified during any motion, is merely due to the activation of selective parts of the whole sling.

The identification and treatment of a specific muscle dysfunction (weakness, inappropriate recruitment, tightness) is important when restoring global stabilization and mobility (between the thorax and pelvis or between the pelvis and legs) and for understanding why parts of a sling may be inextensible (tight) or too flexible (lacking in support).

MOTOR CONTROL

Motor control pertains to patterning of muscle activation (Hodges & Richardson 1996, Hodges 2000, O'Sullivan et al 1997, Richardson et al 1999, O'Sullivan 2000, Comerford & Mottram 2001, Danneels et al 2001,

Moseley et al 2002, Hodges 2003), in other words, the timing of specific muscle action and inaction. Efficient movement requires coordinated muscle action, such that stability is ensured while motion is controlled and not restrained (Hodges et al 2001b, Hodges 2003). With respect to the lumbopelvic region, it is the coordinated action between the local and global systems that ensures stability without rigidity of posture and without episodes of collapse. Exercises that focus on sequencing muscle activation are necessary for restoring motor control (Richardson et al 1999, Lee 2001a, Lee DG 2003). The exercises in Chapter 10 focus on balancing tension and releasing compression within the slings of muscle systems and involve an extensive use of imagery. Imagery has been shown (Yue & Cole 1992, Franklin 1996, Gandevia 1999) to be effective in restoring neural patterning and increasing strength. Using imagery and specific sequencing of muscle activation, individual muscles are strengthened, lengthened, and appropriately timed/patterned during functional tasks.

EMOTIONS

Dr. Andry Vleeming (from Lee & Vleeming 2003)

Emotional states can play a significant role in human function, including the function of the neuromusculoskeletal system. Many chronic pelvic pain patients present with traumatized life experiences in addition to their functional complaints. Several of these patients adopt motor patterns indicative of defensive posturing which suggest a negative past experience. A negative emotional state leads to further stress. Stress is a normal response intended to energize our system for quick flight and fight reactions. When this response is sustained, high levels of epinephrine (adrenaline) and cortisol remain in the system (Holstege et al 1996), in part due to circulating stress-related neuropeptides (Sapolsky & Spencer 1997, Sapolsky et al 1997) which are released in anticipation of defensive or offensive behavior.

Emotional states (fight, flight, or freeze reactions) are physically expressed through muscle action and, when sustained, influence basic muscle tone and patterning (Holstege et al 1996). If the muscles of the pelvis become hypertonic, this state will increase compression of the SIJs (van Wingerden et al 2001, Richardson et al 2002). It is important to understand the patient's emotional state since the detrimental motor pattern can often only be changed by affecting the emotional state. Sometimes, it can be as simple as restoring hope through education and awareness of the underlying mechanical problem (Butler & Moseley 2003, Hodges & Moseley 2003). Other times, professional cognitive-behavioral therapy is required to retrain more positive thought patterns. A basic requirement for cognitive and physical learning is focused, or attentive, training – in other words, not being absent-minded. Teaching individuals to be "mindful" or aware of what is happening in their body during times of physical and/or emotional loading can reduce sustained, unnecessary muscle tone and therefore joint compression (Murphy 1992).

CONCLUSION

It has long been recognized that physical factors impact joint function. The model presented here suggests that joint mechanics can be influenced by multiple factors, some intrinsic to the joint itself, while others are produced by muscle action which in turn is influenced by the emotional state. The effective management of pain in the lumbopelvic-hip region which is associated with dysfunction requires attention to all four components – form closure, force closure, motor control, and emotions – with the goal being to guide patients towards a healthier way to live and move. This text will focus on the assessment and treatment of the first three components of this model and its application to the lumbar spine, pelvic girdle, and hip.

Chapter 6

Biomechanics of the lumbopelvic–hip region

The primary function of the lower quadrant is to move and simultaneously to provide a stable base from which the upper extremity can function (transfer load). Together, the trunk and the lower extremities have the potential for multidirectional movement with a minimum of energy expenditure (Abitbol 1995, 1997, McNeill 1995, 1997). Neuromusculoskeletal harmony is essential for optimal lumbopelvic-hip function. In 1911, Meisenbach stated that:

> When the trunk is moved to one side quickly there are direct opposing forces of the lumbar and spinal muscles against the pelvic and leg muscles. Normally these work in harmony and are resisted by the strong pelvic ligaments and fascia to a certain extent. If the harmony of these muscles is disturbed from some cause or another, or if the ligamentous support is weakened, other points of fixation must necessarily yield.

It is traditional to study both anatomy and biomechanics in a regional manner. For example, the lumbar spine is often considered separately from the pelvic girdle which in turn is investigated separately from the hip. This approach yields information as to how the parts function but not as to how the parts work together. While it is necessary to consider the function of the individual parts, rehabilitation is unsuccessful without consideration of how these parts achieve the harmonious action noted by Meisenbach almost a century ago. After studying individually the biomechanics of the lumbar spine, pelvic girdle, and hip, the collective biomechanics will be presented. Hopefully, a more integrated perspective of the biomechanics of the lumbopelvic-hip region can be achieved. First, a description of the terminology used is required.

TERMINOLOGY

The terms kinematics (the study of movement) and kinetics (the study of forces) come from the science of kinesiology, the study of biomechanics. The prefixes *osteo* and *arthro* are Greek derivatives meaning bone and joint respectively.

Osteokinematics refers to the study of motion of bones regardless of the motion of the joints. These motions are named according to the axis about which they occur. Flexion/extension occurs when one or more bones rotate about a coronal axis. This terminology is consistent throughout the spinal column and peripheral joints. When the trunk bends forward/backward in a sagittal plane about a coronal axis, this is called forward/backward bending. Within the pelvic girdle, the accepted terms for flexion and extension of the sacrum are nutation and counternutation respectively. Forward rotation of the innominate about a coronal axis is termed anterior rotation, backward rotation is termed posterior rotation. Nutation/counternutation and anterior/posterior rotation of the innominate should be reserved to describe motion between the sacrum and the innominate. When the two innominates and the sacrum rotate as a unit (pelvic girdle) about a coronal axis through the hip joint, this is called an anterior or posterior pelvic tilt.

Abduction/adduction occurs when one or more appendicular (peripheral) bones rotate about a sagittal axis. Within the spinal column, sideflexion occurs when an axial bone (skull, vertebral column) rotates about a sagittal axis. Motion of the trunk in the coronal plane about a sagittal axis is called lateral bending. When the two innominates and the sacrum rotate as a unit (pelvic girdle) about a sagittal axis, this is called a lateral pelvic tilt.

Medial/lateral or internal/external rotation occurs when one or more appendicular (peripheral) bones rotate about a vertical or longitudinal axis. Axial rotation occurs when an axial bone (skull, vertebral column) rotates about a vertical or longitudinal axis. A twist of the body about a vertical axis is also called axial rotation.

The bones can also translate along the same axes resulting in posteroanterior, anteroposterior, mediolateral, lateromedial, and vertical (distraction–compression) translation.

Arthrokinematics refers to the study of motion of joints regardless of the motion of the bones. "Intra-articular kinematics or arthrokinematics has to do

with the movement of one articular surface upon another … Articular surfaces can spin and/or slide upon each other" (MacConaill & Basmajian 1977). These motions are referred to as pure spins and pure and impure swings. A pure spin occurs when the only motion of a point on the articular surface is a rotation around the mechanical axis of the bone. A pure swing occurs when the only motion of a point on the articular surface is a slide along the shortest possible line (the chord) between two points. An impure swing occurs when a point on the articular surface slides along any other curved line (an arc) between two points such that an element of spin also occurs.

Arthorkinetics refers to the study of forces met by the joint during static and dynamic function.

KINEMATICS WITHIN THE LUMBAR SPINE

Newton's second law states that the motion of an object is directly proportional to the applied force and occurs in the direction of the straight line in which the force acts. Translation occurs when a single net force causes all points of the object to move in the same direction over the same distance (Bogduk 1997). Rotation occurs when two unaligned and opposite forces cause the object to move around a stationary center or axis (Bogduk 1997). In mechanical terms, the lumbar vertebrae have the potential for 12 degrees of freedom (Levin 1997) (Fig. 6.1), as motion can occur in a positive and negative direction along and about three perpendicular axes. However, this model does not account for the anatomical factors which modify and restrict the actual motion which can occur. Clinically, the lumbar spine appears to exhibit four degrees of freedom of motion: flexion, extension, rotation/sideflexion right, and rotation/sideflexion left (Pearcy & Tibrewal 1984, Vicenzino & Twomey 1993, Bogduk 1997). Throughout the spine, flexion/extension is an integral part of forward/backward bending of the head or trunk while rotation/sideflexion occurs during any other motion.

FLEXION/EXTENSION

In the lumbar spine, the coronal axis is dynamic rather than static and moves forward with flexion such that flexion couples with a small degree (1–3 mm) of anterior translation (Figs 6.2 and 6.3)

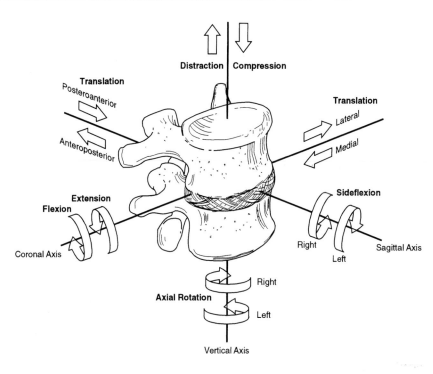

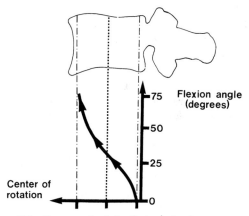

Figure 6.1   In mechanical terms, there is the potential for 12 degrees of motion of the lumbar vertebrae (Bogduk 1997, Levin 1997).

Figure 6.3   The coronal axis for flexion/extension moves anteriorly with increasing degrees of flexion.

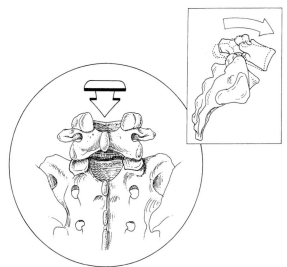

Figure 6.2   Flexion/anterior translation at L5–S1.

(White & Panjabi 1978, Gracovetsky et al 1981, Gracovetsky & Farfan 1986, Bogduk 1997). Conversely, extension couples with posterior translation during backward bending of the trunk.

At the zygapophyseal joints, the arthrokinematics of flexion and extension are impure swings. During flexion, the inferior articular processes of the superior vertebra glide superiorly and anteriorly along the superior articular processes of the inferior vertebra/sacrum (Bogduk 1997). During extension, the inferior articular processes of the superior vertebra glide inferiorly and posteriorly along the superior articular processes of the inferior vertebra/sacrum. The total amplitude of this glide is about 5–7 mm.

ROTATION/SIDEFLEXION

Motion coupling of the vertebral column during rotation or lateral bending of the trunk was first recorded by Lovett in 1903. He noted that a flexible rod bent in one plane could not bend in another without twisting. The direction of this motion coupling has been a controversial issue.

In 1984, Pearcy & Tibrewal reported on a three-dimensional radiographic study of lumbar motion during rotation and lateral bending of 10 men under 30 years of age. Their findings of coupled motion (Fig. 6.4) were consistent with those of Gracovetsky & Farfan (1986) except at the lumbosacral junction where lateral bending coupled with ipsilateral axial rotation. L4–L5 was noted to be transitional and followed the movement pattern of either L3–L4 or L5–S1. This study did not investigate the coupling of motion when lateral bending was introduced from a position of flexion or extension.

According to Bogduk (1997), 3° of *pure* axial rotation of a lumbar motion segment is possible. At this point, all of the fibers of the annulus fibrosus that are aligned in the direction of the rotation are under stress, the sagittal component of the contralateral zygapophyseal joint is compressed, and the ipsilateral zygapophyseal joint capsule is tensed. The axis of motion is vertical through the posterior part of the vertebral body. After 3° of rotation, the axis shifts to the impacted zygapophyseal joint and the upper vertebra pivots about this new axis. The vertebral body swings posterolaterally, imposing a lateral translation force on the intervertebral disk. The impacted inferior articular process swings backwards and medially, further stretching the capsule and ligaments. Further rotation can result in failure of any of the stressed or compressed components. According to Bogduk (1997), 35% of the resistance to torsion is provided by the intervertebral disk and 65% by the posterior elements of the neural arch.

Bogduk (1997) supports Pearcy & Tibrewal's (1984) model of motion coupling and concurs that for the upper three segments axial rotation is accompanied by contralateral sideflexion. This motion is unidirectional about an oblique axis and also involves slight flexion or extension of the segment (Fig. 6.5). He agrees that at L5–S1 the pattern tends to be ipsilateral (Fig. 6.6) and that L4–L5 is variable. In addition, he notes that individual variation exists and resists any rules for segmental motion patterning.

Vicenzino & Twomey (1993) investigated the conjunct rotation which occurred during lateral

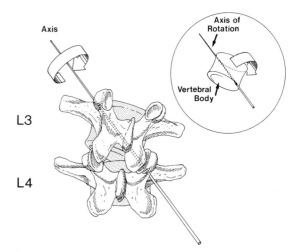

Figure 6.5   Left rotation of the L3–L4 joint complex couples with contralateral sideflexion.

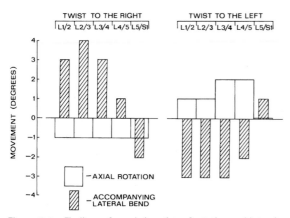

Figure 6.4   Findings of coupled motion of rotation and lateral bending in the lumbar spine. At the lumbosacral junction, lateral bending occurs in the same direction as the induced rotation. (Redrawn from Pearcy & Tibrewal 1984.)

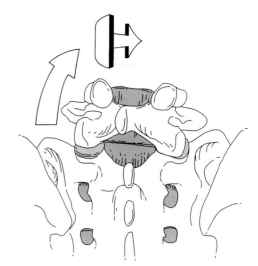

Figure 6.6   During right rotation, the L5 vertebra rotates/sideflexes to the right.

bending of the lumbar spine and noted that in 64% of their specimens no conjunct rotation occurred at L5–S1. In the remainder, the direction of rotation was always the same as sideflexion. This coupling of motion was consistent when the segment was sideflexed from a flexed, neutral, or extended position. Above L5–S1 an interesting pattern emerged. In extension, L1–L2 and L3–L4 rotated opposite to the direction of sideflexion. In flexion, L1–L2 and L3–L4 rotated in the same direction as the sideflexion. Conversely, in extension, L2–L3 and L4–L5 rotated in the same direction as the sideflexion and in flexion L2–L3 and L4–L5 rotated in the opposite direction! The conclusion from this study was that the coupling of motion in the lumbar spine was indeed complex.

The biomechanics of the lumbar spine have been shown (Farfan 1973, Kirkaldy-Willis et al 1978, White & Panjabi 1978, Kirkaldy-Willis 1983, Gilmore 1986, Grieve 1986, Stokes 1986, Twomey & Taylor 1986) to change with both age and degeneration. The instantaneous center of rotation for flexion/extension and/or rotation/sideflexion can be significantly displaced with degeneration, resulting in excessive posteroanterior and/or lateral translation during physiological motion of the trunk (White & Panjabi 1978, Stokes 1986). Consequently, "on the intersegmental level … normal loads may in fact be acting about a displaced IAR [instantaneous axis of rotation], thus locally producing abnormal motion" (Gilmore 1986).

In summary, even if the biomechanics of the lumbosacral junction were confirmed and conclusive, the potential for altered biomechanics to exist is high, rendering "perceptive clinical observation of a patient [as] the most direct way to assess spine motion clinically, despite its lack of objectivity" (Stokes 1986).

KINEMATICS WITHIN THE PELVIC GIRDLE

Mobility of the sacroiliac joint (SIJ) has been recognized since the seventeenth century. Since the middle of the nineteenth century, both postmortem and in vivo studies have been done in an attempt to clarify the movements of the SIJs and the pubic symphysis and the axes about which these movements occur (Meyer 1878, Goldthwait & Osgood 1905, Albee 1909, Sashin 1930, Weisl 1954, 1955, Colachis et al 1963, Egund et al 1978, Wilder et al 1980, Lavignolle et al 1983, Walheim & Selvik 1984, Miller et al 1987, Sturesson et al 1989, 2000, Vleeming et al

1990a, b, Kissling & Jacob 1997, Sturesson 1997, Hungerford et al 2001, Hungerford 2002).

The investigative methods include: manual manipulation of the SIJ both at surgery and in a cadaver (Jarcho 1929, Chamberlain 1930, Lavignolle et al 1983); X-ray analysis in various postures of the trunk and lower extremity (Albee 1909, Brooke 1924); roentgen stereophotogrammetric and stereoradiographic imaging after the insertion of tantalum balls into the innominate and sacrum (Egund et al 1978, Walheim & Selvik 1984, Sturesson et al 1989, 2000, Sturesson 1997); and after the attachment of surface markers to the femur, sacrum, and innominate (Hungerford et al 2001, Hungerford 2002), inclinometer measurements in various postures of the trunk and lower extremity, after the insertion of Kirschner wires into the innominate and sacrum (Pitkin & Pheasant 1936, Colachis et al 1963, Jacob & Kissling 1995, Kissling & Jacob 1997), and computerized analysis using a Metrecom skeletal analysis system (Smidt 1995). Clinical theories (DonTigny 1985, 1990, 1997, Hesch et al 1992, Lee 1992, 1999, Hesch 1997) have also contributed significantly towards the research in this region. The results of these studies have led to proposals concerning both function and dysfunction of the pelvic girdle. The following section will detail the current status of the biomechanics of the pelvic girdle.

Motion of the pelvic girdle as a unit can occur in all three body planes: anterior and posterior pelvic tilt in the sagittal plane, lateral tilt in the coronal plane, and axial rotation in the transverse plane. A combination of all of these motions occurs during the normal gait cycle (Greenman 1990, 1997). In addition, motion occurs *within* the pelvis. While mobility of the SIJ is small, movement has been shown to occur (Walheim & Selvik 1984, Miller et al 1987, Sturesson et al 1989, 2000, Sturesson 1997, Hungerford et al 2001, Hungerford 2002) throughout life (Vleeming et al 1992b, 1997). In the past, the quantity of motion available at the SIJ has been debated. In 1983, Lavignolle et al reported 10–12° of posterior rotation of the innominate (coupled with 6 mm of anterior translation), and 2° of anterior rotation (coupled with 8 mm of anterior translation), in an in vivo study of two women and three men under 25 years of age. This study was conducted in the non-weight-bearing position and Vleeming et al (1990a) note that this is probably a significant factor in the quantity of motion reported. Sturesson et al (1989, 2000) used roentgen stereophotogrammetric analysis (RSA) to investigate SIJ mobility in 21 women from 19 to 45 years of age and four men from 18 to 45 years of age. They found only 2.5° of innominate rotation (coupled with 0.5–1.6 mm of translation). This in vivo study was conducted in the weight-bearing position. Sturesson et al (2000) felt that the other authors (Weisl 1954, 1955, Colachis et al 1963, Lavignolle et al 1983) had overestimated the mobility of the SIJ.

Jacob & Kissling's (1995) findings of SIJ mobility using the RSA technique supported those of Sturesson et al (1989, 2000). The average values for rotation and translation were low, being 1.8° of rotation (coupled with 0.7 mm of translation) for the men and 1.9° of rotation (coupled with 0.9 mm translation) for the women. No statistical differences were noted for either age or gender. They postulated that more than 6° of rotation and 2 mm of translation should be considered pathologic (Jacob & Kissling 1995).

In 1995, Buyruk et al (1995a, b) established that the Doppler imaging system could be used to measure stiffness of the SIJ. This research has recently been repeated and confirmed by Leonie Damen et al (2002a). Doppler imaging of vibrations across the SIJ has shown (Buyruk et al 1995a, b, 1997, 1999, Damen et al 2002a) that stiffness of the SIJ is variable between subjects and therefore the range of motion is potentially variable. This research has also revealed that stiffness of the SIJ is symmetric when the left and right sides are compared in subjects without pelvic pain and asymmetric in subjects with pelvic pain. These studies will be discussed in greater depth later. In conclusion, we know that the SIJs are capable of a small amount of both angular (1–4°) and translatoric motion (1–3 mm), that the amplitude of this motion is variable between subjects; however, within one subject it should be symmetric between sides.

NUTATION/COUNTERNUTATION OF THE SACRUM

Nutation and counternutation are osteokinematic terms that describe how the sacrum moves relative to the innominates regardless of how the pelvic girdle is moving relative to the lumbar spine and femora. Nutation of the sacrum occurs when the sacral promontory moves forward into the pelvis about a coronal axis through the interosseous ligament (Fig. 6.7). Conversely, counternutation of the sacrum occurs when the sacral promontory moves backward about this coronal axis (Fig. 6.8). The sacrum is counternutated in supine lying (Sturesson et al 2000) and nutates in sitting or standing (Sturesson

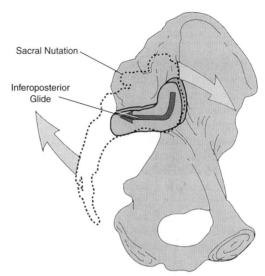

Figure 6.7 When the sacrum nutates, its articular surface glides inferoposteriorly relative to the innominate.

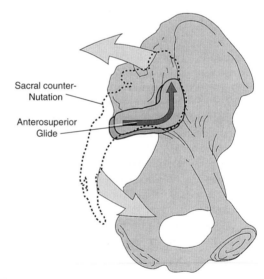

Figure 6.8 When the sacrum counternutates, its articular surface glides anterosuperiorly relative to the innominate.

et al 2000). In other words, whenever an individual is vertical, the sacrum is nutated relative to the innominates. The amount of sacral nutation depends on *how* the individual is sitting or standing. In an optimal posture, the sacrum should be suspended between the two innominates in slight nutation but not completely nutated (Levin 1997). During the initial stages of forward or backward bending, the sacrum completely nutates between the innominates and should remain there throughout the full range of motion. On returning to standing, the sacrum remains nutated between the innominates until the erect posture is reached. At this point, the sacrum counternutates slightly (remaining relatively nutated) to become suspended once again between the two innominates. When an individual stands in a collapsed posture (excessive kypholordosis or sway back), the sacrum can be completely nutated between the innominates. No further nutation will occur during forward or backward bending since the total available range of motion has been exhausted. When an individual sits in a collapsed posture (slouched), the sacrum can be completely counternu-tated (forced by weight-bearing through the coccyx).

Arthrokinematically, when the sacrum nutates relative to the innominate, a linear motion or transla-tion between the two joint surfaces can occur. To date, there have been no studies to validate the following arthrokinematics proposed to occur when the sacrum nutates relative to the innominate. During nutation, the proposal is that the the sacrum glides inferiorly down the short arm (S1) and posteriorly along the long arm (S2, S3) of the articular surface (Fig. 6.7). The amplitude of this translation is extremely small yet can be palpated. This motion is resisted by the wedge shape of the sacrum, the ridges and depres-sions of the articular surface, the friction coefficient of the joint surface and the integrity of the inter-osseous and sacrotuberous ligaments (Vleeming et al 1990a, b) (Fig. 6.9). This is the close-packed or self-braced position of the SIJ – the most stable position for transferring intermittent, high loads. The inter-osseous and sacrotuberous ligaments are supported during nutation by the muscles which not only insert into them but compress the pelvic girdle transversely.

During counternutation, it is proposed that the sacrum glides anteriorly along the long arm and superiorly up the short arm (Fig. 6.8). This motion is resisted by the long dorsal sacroiliac ligament (Fig. 4.15) (Vleeming et al 1996). This ligament is sup-ported by the contraction of the multifidus which acts to nutate the sacrum. The multifidus and levator ani appear to act as a force couple to control sacral nutation/counternutation (Snijders et al 1997).

FLEXION/EXTENSION OF THE COCCYX

Bo et al (2001) used MRI to investigate the function of the pelvic floor muscles and in this study noted that a contraction of the pelvic floor caused the coccyx to move in a ventral and cranial direction (flexion). During a Valsalva, or straining, they noted that the coccyx moved caudal and dorsal (extension).

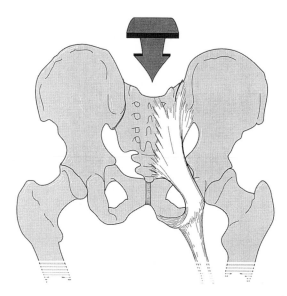

Figure 6.9   Sacral nutation is the forward motion of the sacral promontory into the pelvis. This motion is resisted by the interosseous and sacrotuberous ligaments. (Redrawn from Vleeming et al 1997.)

POSTERIOR ROTATION OF THE INNOMINATE

Posterior rotation of the innominate is an osteokine-matic term used to describe motion of the innomin-ate relative to the sacrum and occurs about a coronal axis through the interosseous ligament of the SIJ. Using reflective surface markers on 15 bony land-marks of the femur, innominate, and sacrum and a sophisticated imaging system (six-camera Expert vision motion analysis hi res 5.0 system), Hungerford (2002) noted that when an individual transferred weight through one leg and flexed the contralateral femur (Fig. 6.10), the supporting innominate (weight-bearing side) either posteriorly rotated or remained posteriorly rotated relative to the sacrum (sacrum is therefore relatively nutated). The SIJ is thus close-packed in preparation for load transfer. The non-weight-bearing innominate (side of hip flexion) also posteriorly rotated relative to the sacrum (Figs 6.10 and 6.11) during this motion. Sturesson et al (2000) initially reported this osteokinematic pattern of intrapelvic motion during one-leg standing and this research confirms their findings. Hungerford also described a conjunct osteokinematic motion which occurred in association with posterior rotation of the innominate. On both the non-weight-bearing and weight-bearing sides, posterior rotation of the innominate was associated with sideflexion

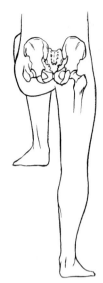

Figure 6.10 The one-leg standing test (Gillet): the individual transfers weight through one leg and flexes the contralateral hip joint to approximately 90°.

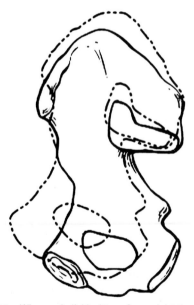

Figure 6.11 When an individual transfers weight through one leg and flexes the contralateral hip, the innominate on the non-weight-bearing side rotates posteriorly (dotted lines) relative to the sacrum (osteokinematics). The innominate glides anterosuperior and lateral (possibly reflects decompression of the joint) relative to the sacrum (arthrokinematics) (Hungerford 2002). Note the dotted line of the articular surface. The amplitude of the osteokinematic and arthrokinematic motion has been exaggerated in this illustration for visual purposes. In reality, the amplitude of osteokinematic motion is less than 5° coupled with 2–3 mm of translation.

(Fig. 6.12a, b) and rotation (Fig. 6.12c, d) of the innominate. Sideflexion and rotation of the innominate were coupled in a countralateral sense, although some variability was noted.

Hungerford also investigated the translatoric motion (arthrokinematics) between the innominate and sacrum during posterior rotation of the innominate on both the non-weight-bearing and weight-bearing sides. She was able to confirm part of what was originally proposed in the second edition of this text (Lee 1999); that is, during posterior rotation of the *non-weight-bearing innominate* (side of hip flexion), the innominate glides anterosuperiorly relative to the sacrum (Fig. 6.11). On the weight-bearing side, the relative translatoric glide was *posterior* and superior relative to the sacrum (Fig. 6.13). Concurrently, a medial translation was noted, which may reflect increased articular compression during loading. In other words, when the pelvic girdle is self-braced and compressed by the passive and active elements, the direction of the translation is not as predicted (Lee 1999). Posterior and superior translation of the articular surface of the innominate relative to the sacrum would effectively "lock in" the SIJ similar to the engagement of gears in a bicycle. Motion would be prevented and stability ensured for load transfer when the articular surfaces engage in this manner.

ANTERIOR ROTATION OF THE INNOMINATE

Anterior rotation of the innominate is an osteokinematic term used to describe motion of the innominate relative to the sacrum and occurs about a coronal axis through the interosseous ligament of the SIJ (Fig 6.14). Hungerford did not investigate anterior rotation of the innominate in healthy subjects; consequently the following is still a proposal. In health, anterior rotation of the innominate occurs during extension of the freely swinging leg. When the innominate anteriorly rotates, it glides inferiorly down the short arm and posteriorly along the long arm of the SIJ (Fig. 6.14).

In conclusion, we now know that in non-weight-bearing an arthrokinematic glide between the innominate and the sacrum occurs during posterior rotation of the innominate and is physiological (i.e., follows the articular surfaces). In weight-bearing, the close-packing of the SIJ precludes this physiological glide. The rest is still hypothesis. Sacral nutation produces the same relative arthrokinematic glide as posterior rotation of the innominate

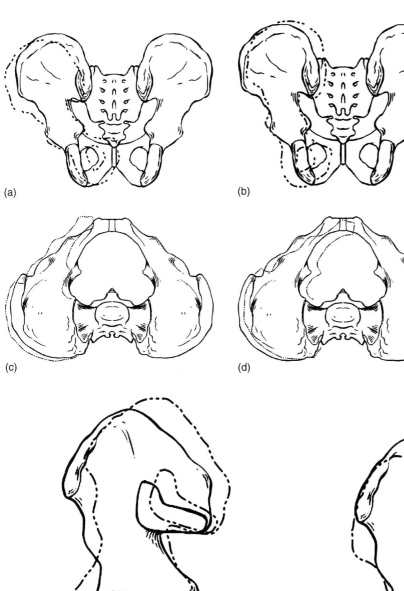

(a)

(b)

(c)

(d)

Figure 6.12 Hungerford (2002) describes a conjunct osteokinematic motion which occurs in association with posterior rotation of the innominate on both the non-weight-bearing and weight-bearing sides. The posterior rotation motion was associated with side-flexion (a: left sideflexion, b: right sideflexion) and rotation (c: left rotation, d: right rotation). The combined pattern was often contralateral (the rotation occurred contralateral to the direction of sideflexion) although this finding was variable. The amplitude of the osteokinematic motion has been exaggerated in these illustrations for visual purposes.

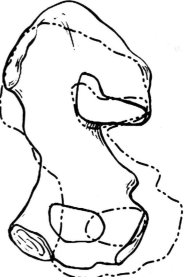

Figure 6.13 When an individual transfers weight through one leg and flexes the contralateral hip, the innominate on the weight-bearing side either remains posteriorly rotated or posteriorly rotates (dotted line) relative to the sacrum (osteokinematics). The innominate glides *posterior* and superior relative to the sacrum (note dotted line of the articular surface) (Hungerford 2002). The amplitude of the osteokinematic and arthrokinematic motion has been exaggerated in this illustration for visual purposes.

Figure 6.14 Anterior rotation of the innominate occurs during extension of the freely swinging leg. When the innominate anteriorly rotates (dotted line), it glides inferiorly down the short arm and posteriorly along the long arm of the sacroiliac joint (note dotted line of the articular surface). The amplitude of the osteokinematic and arthrokinematic motion has been exaggerated in this illustration for visual purposes.

(inferoposterior motion of the sacrum is the same as anterosuperior motion of the innominate); sacral counternutation produces the same arthrokinematic glide as anterior rotation of the innominate (anterosuperior motion of the sacrum is the same as inferoposterior motion of the innominate). Further findings from Hungerford's research on how these biomechanics are impacted in patients with pelvic pain and failed load transfer will be discussed later.

KINEMATICS OF THE HIP

The femur articulates with the innominate via a ball-and-socket joint, the hip, which is capable of circumductive motion. The hip is classified as an unmodified ovoid joint and in mechanical terms is capable of 12 degrees of freedom of motion along and about three perpendicular axes (Fig. 6.15). This classification does not account for the anatomical factors which influence the coupling of motion which actually occurs at the joint.

Osteokinematically, flexion/extension occurs when the femur rotates about a coronal axis through the center of the femoral head and neck. Although variable, approximately 100° of femoral flexion is possible, following which motion of the SIJ and intervertebral joint occurs to allow the anterior thigh to approximate the chest (Williams 1995). Approximately 20° of femoral extension is possible (Kapandji 1970). When rotation of the femoral head occurs purely about this axis (i.e., without conjoined abduction/adduction or medial/lateral rotation), the motion is arthrokinematically described as a pure spin.

Abduction/adduction is an osteokinematic term used when the femur rotates about a sagittal axis through the center of the femoral head. Approximately 45° of femoral abduction and 30° of femoral adduction are possible, following which the pelvic girdle laterally tilts beneath the vertebral column (Kapandji 1970). When the femur rotates purely about this sagittal axis, the head of the femur arthrokinematically transcribes a superoinferior chord within

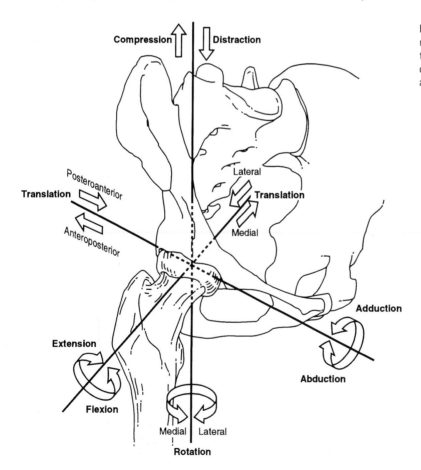

Figure 6.15 The osteokinematic motion of the femur. In mechanical terms, the femur is capable of 12 degrees of freedom of motion along and about three perpendicular axes.

the acetabulum (i.e., the shortest distance between two points); therefore this motion is described as a pure swing.

Medial/lateral rotation is an osteokinematic term used when the femur rotates about a longitudinal axis. The location of this axis depends on whether the foot is fixed on the ground. When the pelvic girdle rotates about a firmly planted foot, the longitudinal axis of rotation runs from the center of the femoral head through to the lateral femoral condyle. When the foot is off the ground, the femur can rotate about a variety of longitudinal axes, all of which pass through the femoral head and the foot (Williams 1995). Approximately 30–40° of medial rotation and 60° of lateral rotation are possible (Kapandji 1970). Pure femoral rotation about this axis causes the femoral head arthrokinematically to transcribe an anteroposterior chord within the acetabulum and this motion is described as a pure swing.

Functionally, movement of the femur relative to the innominate does not produce pure arthrokinematic motion. Rather, combinations of movement are the norm. The habitual pattern of motion for the non-weight-bearing lower extremity is a combination of flexion, abduction, and lateral rotation and extension, adduction, and medial rotation. Arthrokinematically, both motions are impure swings. The close-pack position (most stable) of the hip is extension, abduction, and internal rotation.

INTEGRATED BIOMECHANICS OF THE LUMBOPELVIC–HIP REGION

Functional movements of the lumbopelvic-hip region are part of the clinical examination, consequently the integrated biomechanics need to be understood.

FORWARD BENDING

Forward bending of the trunk results in a posterior displacement of the pelvic girdle as a unit. This motion shifts the center of gravity behind the pedal base (Figs 6.16 and 6.17). The pelvic girdle anteriorly tilts on the femoral heads about a transverse axis through the hip joints (hip joint flexes). The lumbar spine flexes in a superoinferior direction until L5 flexes on the sacrum.

Within the pelvic girdle itself, there is no relative anterior or posterior rotation between the innominates during forward bending. Both innominates

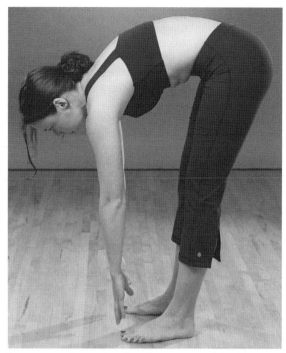

Figure 6.16 Forward bending of the trunk. Optimally, the apex of the forward bending curve should be in the mid-buttock. This model demonstrates a lack of anterior tilt of the pelvic girdle on the femoral heads due to insufficient lengthening of the hamstrings. (Reproduced with permission from © Diane G. Lee Physiotherapist Corp.)

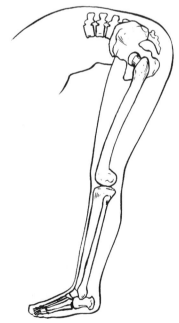

Figure 6.17 The osteokinematic motion of the lumbopelvic-hip region during forward bending of the trunk.

should travel an equal distance as the pelvic girdle anteriorly tilts on the femoral heads. During the initial stages of forward bending, the sacrum completely nutates between the innominates and should remain there throughout the full range of motion. On returning to standing, the sacrum remains nutated between the innominates until the erect posture is reached. At this point, the sacrum counternutates slightly (remaining relatively nutated) to become suspended once again between the two innominates.

The muscles which eccentrically control forward bending of the trunk and the pelvic girdle include the erector spinae, multifidus, quadratus lumborum, and the hip joint extensors (gluteus maximus and the hamstrings). Contributions from the hip joint rotators, abductors, and adductors as well as from the deep back muscles function to stabilize and coordinate the motion between the lumbar spine, pelvic girdle, and hip. Prior to this motion, stabilization of the lumbar segments and the pelvic girdle is required from the local stabilizing system, in particular, the transversus abdominis, multifidus, and pelvic floor.

BACKWARD BENDING

Backward bending of the trunk (Figs 6.18 and 6.19) results in an anterior displacement of the pelvic girdle and a shift of the center of gravity anterior to the pedal base. The pelvic girdle posteriorly tilts on the femoral heads about a transverse axis through the hip joints (hip joint extends). The thoracolumbar spine extends in a superoinferior direction until L5 extends on the sacrum.

Within the pelvic girdle itself, there is no relative anterior or posterior rotation between the innominates during backward bending. Both innominates should travel an equal distance as the pelvic girdle posteriorly tilts on the femoral heads. The sacrum should remain in its nutated position relative to the innominates.

The muscles which eccentrically control backward bending of the trunk include the abdominals, the quadriceps, the tensor fascia latae, and the psoas major. Contributions from the hip joint rotators, abductors, and adductors as well as the deep back muscles function to stabilize and coordinate the motion between the lumbar spine, pelvic girdle, and hip. Prior to this motion, stabilization of the lumbar segments and the pelvic girdle is required from the local stabilizing system, in particular the transversus abdominis, multifidus, and the pelvic floor.

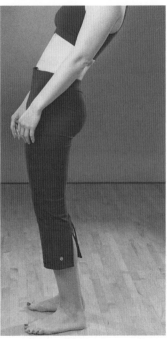

Figure 6.18 Backward bending of the trunk. Optimally, the apex of the backward bending curve should be at the level of the iliofemoral ligament of the hip joint. (Reproduced with permission from © Diane G. Lee Physiotherapist Corp.)

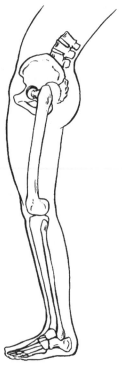

Figure 6.19 The osteokinematic motion of the lumbopelvic-hip region during backward bending of the trunk.

LATERAL BENDING

Left lateral bending of the trunk is initiated by displacing the upper legs to the right, thus maintaining the line of gravity central within the pedal base (Fig. 6.20). The apex of this lateral bending curve should be at the level of the greater trochanter. The pelvic girdle as a unit laterally tilts to the left such that the left femur abducts and the right femur adducts. Within the pelvis a slight right intrapelvic torsion can occur. The right innominate posteriorly rotates relative to the left innominate and the sacrum rotates to the right. The lumbar spine laterally bends

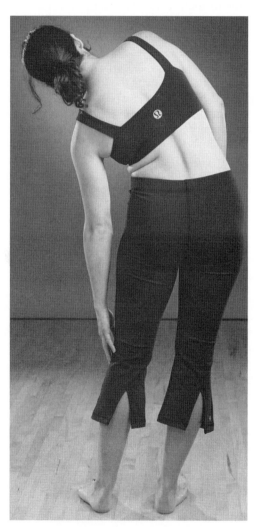

Figure 6.20 Lateral bending of the trunk. Optimally, the apex of the lateral bending curve should be at the level of the greater trochanter. (Reproduced with permission from © Diane G. Lee Physiotherapist Corp.)

to the left. The segmental conjunct rotation is variable. Clinically, L5 appears to rotate/sideflex congruently with the sacrum.

The muscles which eccentrically control lateral bending of the trunk include the contralateral abdominals, erector spinae, multifidus, quadratus lumborum, iliacus, psoas, tensor fascia latae, gluteus medius, gluteus minimus, and the ipsilateral adductors of the hip. Contributions from the hip joint rotators as well as the deep back muscles function to stabilize and coordinate the motion between the lumbar spine, pelvic girdle, and hip. Prior to this motion, stabilization of the lumbar segments and the pelvic girdle is required from the local system.

AXIAL ROTATION

Axial rotation of the pelvic girdle, together with axial rotation of the vertebral column, knees, and feet, allows the eyes to scan 360° from a stationary point. During left axial rotation, the femora twist to the left about a midline vertical axis, resulting in an anteromedial displacement of the proximal right femur and a posteromedial displacement of the proximal left femur. Simultaneously, the pelvic girdle as a unit rotates to the left on the displaced femoral heads, resulting in extension and lateral rotation of the right femur and flexion and medial rotation of the left femur. The twist continues in an inferosuperior direction, producing intrapelvic torsion. The right innominate anteriorly rotates relative to the left innominate and the sacrum rotates to the left. The lumbar spine rotates to the left; the segmental conjunct rotation is variable. Clinically, L5 appears to rotate/sideflex congruently with the sacrum.

WALKING

Walking is an excellent example of the integrated model in motion. When function is optimal and one's mood is light and confident, walking is effortless and the individual glides through space with minimal displacement of the center of gravity. This requires optimal form closure, force closure, and motor control of multiple regions. The individual's emotional state can be reflected in an individual's gait pattern.

This section will review the osteokinematics of the lumbopelvic–hip region during one cycle of gait. The integrated biomechanics presented here comes from clinical extrapolation (Greenman 1997, Gracovetsky 1997, Lee 1999) since detailed osteokinematic research is lacking, especially for motion between the sacrum and the innominate (intrapelvic motion). During gait, there is motion within the lumbar spine and pelvic girdle as well as motion of the pelvic girdle as a unit relative to the lumbar spine and femur. The amplitude and patterning of each motion are individual; however, optimal gait requires the following components (Table 6.1).

Femoral motion

During the swing phase of the right lower extremity (toe-off to heel strike), the right femur moves from an extended to a flexed position. The habitual femoral movement pattern is not an arthrokinematic pure spin at the hip joint but rather an arcuate (impure) swing and therefore conjoined osteokinematic motions also occur. At toe-off, the femur is extended and medially rotated relative to the innominate (abduction/adduction is variable) and some of the ligaments of the hip joint are taut. As the femur flexes, it rotates laterally relative to the innominate due to the left transverse rotation of the pelvic girdle as a unit (see below); consequently,

the path of femoral motion is in the pure sagittal plane.

During the stance phase of the right lower extremity (heel strike to toe-off), the femur moves from a flexed to an extended position. Again, this motion is not a pure spin at the hip joint but rather an arcuate or impure swing. The conjoined motion includes medial rotation, although as mentioned above, the medial femoral rotation is due to right transverse rotation of the pelvic girdle and therefore the path of femoral motion is in the pure sagittal plane. Adduction/abduction during this motion is variable. The ligaments are progressively wound around the femoral neck as the body weight passes anterior to the hip joint. Through the mid-stance position, the winding of the ligaments of the hip joint, together with the myokinetic forces, increases compression of the femoral head into the acetabular fossa. This increase in force closure augments the form closure of the hip joint as the load transfer requirements increase. Adequate stride length requires optimal mobility of the hip joint which requires a centered femoral head (neither displaced anteriorly nor posteriorly) during all motion. Effective load transfer requires harmonious action of the local and global systems of the entire lumbopelvic-hip region (force closure and motor control).

Table 6.1 One gait cycle for the right lower extremity

	Right toe-off (Fig. 6.21)		Right heel strike (Fig. 6.22)		Right mid-stance (Fig. 6.24)
Femora	Right extended and internal rotation at hip joint	Left slightly flexed and external rotation at hip joint	Right flexed and external rotation at hip joint	Left extended and internal rotation at hip joint	Right and left are approaching vertical beneath the pelvic girdle
Pelvic girdle as a unit	Rotated in transverse plane to the right		Rotated in transverse plane to the left		Neither rotated left or right
Intrapelvic motion					
Right innominate	Anterior rotated relative to sacrum and left innominate		Posterior rotated relative to sacrum and left innominate		Anterior rotating relative to sacrum
Left innominate	Posterior rotated relative to the right innominate		Anterior rotated relative to the right innominate		Posterior rotating relative to the sacrum and right innominate
Sacrum	Left rotated between the innominates		Right rotated between the innominates		Left rotating between the innominates

Pelvic girdle motion

At right toe-off, the pelvic girdle as a unit is rotated in the transverse plane to the right. Through the right swing phase, the pelvic girdle as a unit rotates transversely to the left. At right heel strike, the pelvic girdle as a unit is rotated in the transverse plane to the left. Through the right stance phase, the pelvic girdle as a unit rotates transversely to the right.

Within the pelvis, an alternating intrapelvic torsion occurs. At right toe-off (Fig. 6.21), the right innominate is anteriorly rotated relative to the sacrum and the left innominate. The sacrum is left-rotated between the innominates. Through the right swing phase, the right innominate posteriorly rotates relative to the sacrum and also relative to the left innominate. The sacrum rotates to the right between the innominates.

At right heel strike (Fig. 6.22), the right innominate is posteriorly rotated relative to the sacrum. The sacrum is right-rotated between the innominates. The sacrum is nutated on the right relative to the right innominate (right innominate is posteriorly rotated) and also nutated on the left relative to the left innominate (due to the right sacral rotation). Therefore both SIJs are self-braced (the left one is already under load and the right one is preparing for load). Posterior rotation of the right innominate (or sacral nutation) increases the tension of the sacrotuberous and interosseous ligament and prepares the joint for heel strike (Fig. 6.23). The increase in tension contributes to the force closure mechanism, augments the form closure mechanism, and therefore

increases compression through the SIJ and thus its stability. Inman et al (1981) have shown that the hamstrings become active just before heel strike. Contraction of the biceps femoris muscle increases

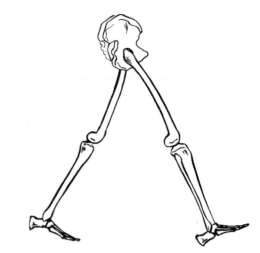

Figure 6.22 Walking: osteokinematics of the femora and pelvic girdle at heel strike phase of the right lower extremity.

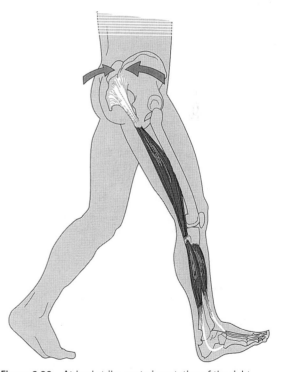

Figure 6.23 At heel strike, posterior rotation of the right innominate increases the tension of the right sacrotuberous ligament. Contraction of the biceps femoris further increases tension in this ligament, preparing the sacroiliac joint for impact. (Redrawn from Vleeming et al 1997.)

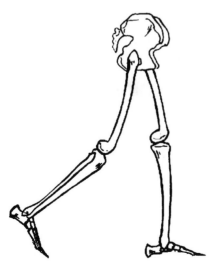

Figure 6.21 Walking: osteokinematics of the femora and pelvic girdle at toe-off phase of the right lower extremity.

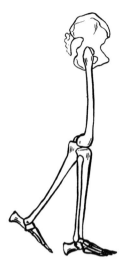

Figure 6.24 Walking: osteokinematics of the femora and pelvic girdle at mid-stance phase of the right lower extremity.

the tension in the sacrotuberous ligament, further contributing to the force closure mechanism.

From heel strike to mid-stance (Fig. 6.24), the right innominate anteriorly rotates relative to the sacrum. Simultaneously, the sacrum left-rotates between the two innominates. It is possible for the sacrum to left-rotate as the right innominate anteriorly rotates, thus maintaining sacral nutation on the right side. As the body moves from double support to single-leg support, force closure of the pelvis is extremely important and the system relies on effective motor control (both within the local and global systems) for stability.

From mid-stance to toe-off, the right innominate continues to rotate anteriorly relative to the sacrum. This motion unlocks the right SIJ and allows the sacrum to continue to left-rotate between the innominates. Through the mid-stance phase, the hamstring muscles relax and the gluteus maximus muscle becomes more active (Inman et al 1981). This occurs in conjunction with a counterrotation of the trunk and firing of the contralateral latissimus dorsi muscle (Gracovetsky 1997, Vleeming et al 1997). Together, these two muscles tense the thoracodorsal fascia and facilitate the force closure mechanism through the SIJ (Fig. 5.14).

In optimal gait, the unlocking of the SIJs allows for slight mobility which dissipates some of the rotation force away from the lumbosacral junction and facilitates shock absorption within the pelvis. The locking of the SIJs facilitates stability during times of high load. Optimally, the center of gravity should

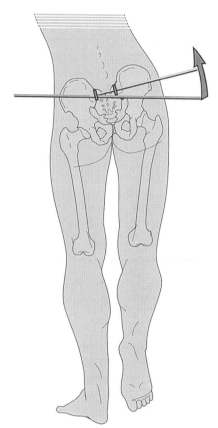

Figure 6.25 Compensated Trendelenburg.

travel along a smooth sinusoidal curve both vertically and laterally and the displacement in both planes should be no more than 5 cm (Inman et al 1981). This displacement is exaggerated when the pelvic girdle is unable to transfer load (insufficient in either form closure or force closure) (Lee 1997a). The patient attempts to compensate by reducing the forces through the pelvic girdle. In a fully compensated gait, the patient transfers weight laterally over the involved limb (compensated Trendelenburg), thus reducing the vertical shear forces through the SIJ (Fig. 6.25). In a non-compensated gait pattern, the patient tends to demonstrate a true Trendelenburg (Fig. 6.26). The pelvic girdle adducts excessively (on the weight-bearing leg). The femur abducts relative to the foot, thus bringing the center of gravity closer to the SIJ, which reduces the vertical shear force.

Lumbar motion

During gait, the lower lumbar vertebrae rotate in the same direction as the posteriorly rotating innominate. The axis about which lumbar rotation occurs is

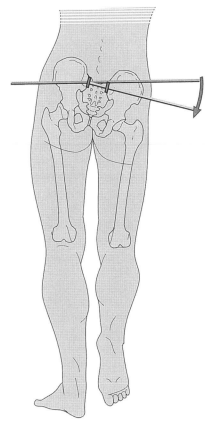

Figure 6.26 True Trendelenburg.

oblique (see Fig. 6.5) such that sideflexion occurs in conjunction with the rotation (Gracovetsky & Farfan 1986, Bogduk 1997). The direction of sideflexion can be variable: commonly L5–S1 rotates and sideflexes in an ipsilateral direction (Fig. 6.6) and L4–L5 in a contralateral direction (Pearcy & Tibrewal 1984).

LIFTING

Lifting is another example of the integrated model in motion during potentially high loading. McGill (2002) has quantified the moments and loads for both the active and passive elements of the spine during a squat lift of 27 kg (59.5 lb). The forces necessary to support the load can induce a compressive load on the spine of over 7000 N (1568 lb)! Therefore, optimal technique which balances tension and reduces compression is essential for injury prevention. This will require optimal form closure, force closure, and motor control if loads are to be transferred and moved safely. Repetitive incorrect

lifting technique is often responsible for the onset of low back and/or pelvic pain (McGill 2002).

Moving an object from the floor to a higher surface initially requires forward bending. Optimally, full spine flexion should be avoided to minimize passive tissue tension. Forward bending of the trunk should occur by flexing the hip joints and the spine should be maintained in neutral. This requires the coordinated action of both the local and global systems. The pars thoracis extensors are powerful extenders and when combined with activation of the oblique abdominals (powerful flexors) help to maintain the proper thoracopelvic position. In addition, they have a strong posterior shear moment on the lumbar spine and this counteracts the anterior shear force produced by gravity and the lifted load (McGill 2002). Underneath this, the local system functions to control intersegmental motion, particularly shear within the neutral zone.

The tension of the thoracodorsal fascia (generated by activation of the muscles which insert into it as well as the hydraulic amplification mechanism of those beneath it) contributes to force closure of the low back and SIJs and the maintenance of stability during loading. The moment the trunk inclines forward, the sacrum completely nutates between the innominates (Sturesson et al 2000) (SIJs self-locked), and the interosseous and sacrotuberous ligaments are taut. These ligaments are supported by the activation of the local and global muscles which insert into them.

McGill (2002) considers "motor control errors" to be the most common cause of injury during lifting.

Cholewicki noted that the risk of such an event was greatest when high forces were developed by the large muscles and low forces by the small intersegmental muscles (a possibility with our power lifters) or when all muscle forces were low such as during a low-level exertion. Thus injury from quite low intensity bending is possible. Adams and Dolan (1995) noted that passive tissues begin to experience damage with bending moments of 60 Nm. This can occur simply from a temporary loss of muscular support when bending over. This mechanism of motor control error resulting in temporary inappropriate neural activation explains how injury might occur during extremely low load situations, for example picking up a pencil from the floor following a long day at work performing a very demanding job.   (McGill 2002)

Returning to erect standing is initiated by backward rotation of the pelvis. This motion is produced by the concentric contraction of the gluteus maximus.

Load transference through the trunk is maintained by a coordinated action of the local and global systems. The sacrum should remain nutated between the innominates and supported. Pelvic stability for load transference is maintained by the force closure mechanism provided by the tension in the thoracodorsal fascia caused by contraction of the latissimus dorsi, the transversus abdominis, internal oblique, multifidus, and gluteus maximus. The gluteus maximus muscle has a considerable mechanical advantage in humans as compared to other primates, given the increased anteroposterior depth of the human pelvis. In addition, more than half of the muscle inserts into the iliotibial band distally which increases its leverage on the hip joint, especially when the band is taut. The size and anatomy of this muscle render it an excellent "lifter."

In summary, optimal and therefore safe loading and unloading of the lumbopelvic-hip region during activities of daily living can only occur when the force closure/motor control mechanisms support the bones and joints (form closure) they stabilize and move. The coordinated muscle response depends on complex peripheral and central feedback and feedforward mechanisms which integrate the osseous, articular, and muscular function.

PREGNANCY

The impact of pregnancy on the biomechanics of the pelvic girdle warrants consideration. The joints of the pelvic girdle become lax secondary to relaxation of the ligaments of the SIJs and the pubic symphysis during pregnancy (Brooke 1930, Young 1940, Hagen 1974, Kristiansson 1997, Buyruk et al 1999, Damen et al 2001). This process begins during the 4th month and continues until the 7th month of pregnancy, following which only a slight increase in mobility occurs. Great variation in the degree of both transverse and superoinferior widening of the pubic symphysis has been noted radiologically (Brooke 1930, Hagen 1974), with the average increase being 5 mm. Whereas widening of the pubic symphysis is universally found in postpartum women (Wurdinger et al 2002), a correlation between this widening and pelvic pain either during pregnancy or in the postpartum phase has not been found (Ostgaard 1997, Wurdinger et al 2002). Similarly, Damen et al (2002b) have shown that there is no statistical correlation between increased laxity of the SIJs and pelvic pain in pregnancy. There is a correlation; however, between asymmetric laxity of the SIJ and pelvic pain in pregnancy (Damen et al 2001).

According to Hagen (1974), relaxation of the pelvic girdle in pregnancy is due to the presence of a specific high-molecular-weight hormone, relaxin, which together with oestrogen causes "depolymerization of hyaluronic acid … Compressive, shearing and tensile forces constitute a chronic trauma increasing the concentration of hyaluronidase … This interferes with the humoral conditions needed for pelvic stability and very likely also plays a certain role as a pathogenetic factor in pelvic relaxation." This has been confirmed by Kristiansson (1997). Consequently, the self-bracing mechanism of the pelvic girdle is less effective, thus increasing the strain on the ligaments of both the SIJs and the pubic symphysis. The morphological changes within the pelvic girdle associated with pregnancy are universal and often occur without symptoms (Damen et al 2001, 2002b).

Occasionally, women present between the 26th and 28th weeks with increasing tenderness over the SIJ and/or pubic symphysis secondary to loss of force closure. Damen et al (2002b) have shown that if a woman presents at this time with moderate to severe (7/10 on a visual analog scale) pelvic pain and has asymmetric laxity of the SIJs, then this can be predictive of ongoing pelvic pain into the postpartum period (8 weeks postpartum).

Chapter 7

Pain, dysfunction, and healing

CHAPTER CONTENTS

MANUAL THERAPY AND PAIN

In the late 1970s and early 1980s, the emphasis of manual therapy was on the detection and treatment of painful joints. Using specific manual techniques, Jull was able to identify painful cervical zygapophyseal joints 100% of the time in a blinded study in which the painful joints were confirmed with anesthetic joint blocks (Jull et al 1988). Jull was able to verify that the manual therapy techniques she used during this study were valid and specific. To date, a similar study has not been conducted for painful sacroiliac joints (SIJs); in fact, up until the mid-1990s, there was still debate regarding the ability of the SIJ to cause low back or pelvic pain. This issue was laid to rest in 1994 when Fortin et al (1994a, b) investigated the location of pain which resulted when healthy SIJs were injected with an irritant solution. From these two studies, the SIJ is now known to cause pain directly over the posterior aspect of the joint and tends to refer pain down the posterolateral buttock and thigh (Fig. 7.1). Rarely does the pain refer below the knee. Schwarzer et al (1995) and Maigne et al (1996) demonstrated, via formal studies using intraarticular SIJ anesthetic blocks, that 15–21% of people with low back pain had a contribution from the SIJ.

Maigne et al (1996) also investigated the validity of certain manual techniques thought to provoke pain from the SIJ. Of 67 participants, 54 had at least 75% of their pain relieved when the SIJ was injected under fluoroscopy. All participants had suffered from their pain for more than 50 days. These subjects then had several SIJ pain provocation tests applied

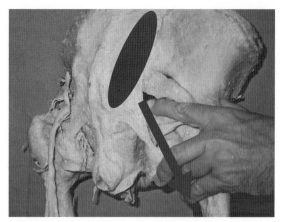

Figure 7.1 The pattern of pain produced when the sacroiliac joint is irritated (Fortin et al 1994a, b). (Reproduced with permission from © Diane G. Lee Physiotherapist Corp.)

to their pelvic girdle (compression, sacral pressure, Gaenslen, Patrick, pain on resisting external rotation of the hip, pressure directly over the pubic symphysis, distraction); the response was noted and correlated with the findings from the joint block. The authors note:

> There was no statistically significant association between response to blocks and any single clinical parameter. No pain provocation test was a useful predictor of sacroiliac joint pain.   (Maigne et al 1996)

Dreyfuss et al (1996) were also unsuccessful in identifying either a consistent medical history or relevant SIJ test (as determined by a multidisciplinary expert panel) for detecting individuals who had 90% of their pain relieved with anesthetic joint blocks. The tests in this study included:

1. pain drawing depicting pain over the SIJ
2. pain drawing depicting pain into the buttock
3. pain drawing depicting pain into the groin
4. pointing to within 5 cm (2 measured inches) of the posterior superior iliac spine to indicate the site of maximal pain
5. sitting with partial elevation from the chair of the buttock on the affected side
6. Gillet test
7. thigh thrust
8. Patrick's test
9. Gaenslen's test
10. midline sacral thrust
11. sacral sulcus tenderness
12. joint play

They emphatically state that "The results of the present study vindicate [these] reservations and offer little support to proponents of the use of physical examination for diagnosis." This belief was supported internationally by respected authors in this subject (Laslett & Williams 1994, Bogduk 1997, Buyruk et al 1997, Laslett 1997, Mooney 1997). Bogduk's (1997) interpretation of this work is that "although SIJ pain is common in patients with chronic low back pain, it can only be diagnosed using diagnostic local anesthetic blocks."

MANUAL THERAPY AND DYSFUNCTION

Fortunately, the last 5 years have seen the development of some reliable, valid, sensitive, and specific physical examination tests for identifying those individuals with impaired *function* of the lumbar spine and pelvis (Ch. 8). When these tests are used as inclusion criteria for investigating pelvic pain patients; reliability, sensitivity, and specificity can be found. Vleeming et al (2002) have confirmed that the long dorsal ligament is a significant pain generator in patients with peripartum pelvic pain (sensitivity 76%). When a combination of pain severity, pain provocation tests, and functional tests was applied to tighten the inclusion criteria (severe pelvic pain coupled with a positive posterior pelvic pain provocation test (Ostgaard et al 1994, Ostgaard 1997) and a positive active straight leg raise test (Mens et al 1999, 2001, 2002; see Ch. 8) the sensitivity was 98%.

In 1999, it was proposed (Lee 1999) that:

> Perhaps we have not yet "discovered" the right manual tests for the SIJ. How can we be so accurate with respect to the cervical spine and so inaccurate in the pelvic girdle? Dreyfuss et al (1996) put forth this challenge: "If proponents of other tests believe that their tests are superior, they have the responsibility and the means to validate those tests by challenging them with diagnostic, intra-articular SIJ blocks as described in this study."

Slowly but surely we are doing just that (Ch. 8). Manual therapists have long advocated "joint play" tests (passive accessory mobility tests) for analyzing joint mobility/stability. Recently, Doppler studies (Buyruk et al 1999, Damen et al 2001, 2002a–d, Richardson et al 2002) have established stiffness values for the SIJ under different conditions (Ch. 8). It is only a matter of time until we can test our manual tests of "joint play" (the "manual Doppler" test) against this technology. However, these tests evaluate function, not pain, and this is where the integrated model of function differs from those which seek to identify pain generators. Pain is not predicatible because it is an emotional experience and depends on both mechanical and biopsychosocial factors. Those which initiate the pain response (mechanical and/or chemical deformation of nociceptors in pain-sensitive tissues) can be quite different from those which maintain the perception (Butler 2000, Butler & Moseley 2003, Hodges & Moseley 2003).

PAIN, DYSFUNCTION, AND HEALING

Pain disability is a form of pain behavior (Vlaeyen et al 1997, Waddell 1998, Butler 2000) constantly influenced by social and psychological conditions. According to Vlaeyen et al (1997) pain disability shifts from a structural/mechanical control to a cognitive/environmental control over a period of 4–8 weeks. It is interesting to note that all of the subjects in the Maigne et al (1996) and Dreyfuss et al (1996) studies had low back pain for longer than 8 weeks. With respect to low back pain, Moseley has been able to show that a combination of physiotherapy (as outlined in this text) and education regarding the neurophysiology of pain is effective in producing both symptomatic and functional change in the moderately disabled chronic group (Moseley 2002). He also notes that health professionals often believe that patients will not understand the neurophysiology of chronic pain and therefore hold back this valuable information (Moseley 2003). A new book, *Explain Pain*, co-authored by Lorimer Moseley and David Butler (www.noigroup.com), intends to bridge this gap.

The prefix "dys" is Greek for abnormal, the word "function" is Latin for performance. Abnormal performance has little to do with pain perception, although it is known that pain and fear of pain have a negative impact on motor control (Hides et al 1994, Hodges & Richardson 1996, Danneels et al 2000, Hodges & Moseley 2003). Several studies (Mattila et al 1986, Bullock-Saxton et al 1994, Uhlig et al 1995, Hides et al 1996, Hodges & Richardson 1996, Dangaria & Naesh 1998) have shown that changes in muscle fiber type, muscle bulk, and recruitment patterns occur with pain and pathology. It is clear that relieving pain does not necessarily restore optimum function (Bullock-Saxton et al 1994, Hides et al 1996, Hodges & Moseley 2003). Many people have abnormal joint function (stiffness – arthrodesis, looseness – instability) and no pain from these

joints. Others have apparently full function in terms of mobility and stability and yet intraarticular joint blocks relieve their pain (Buyruk et al 1997). Stiff joints put extra stress on those above and below them, and over time symptoms may appear. Maigne et al (1996) do concede that "It remains possible that a major part of the so-called SIJ pathology is a pathology of the soft tissues surrounding the joint." Or maybe, the joints above and/or below the ones which are *dysfunctional* are responsible for the pain.

When treating *dysfunction*, it is important to restore optimal form closure (mobility and stability), force closure, and motor control so that the injured soft tissue which may be responsible for some of the nociception can heal, while remaining cognizant of other factors (emotions and psychological state) which can impact the pain experience and rate of recovery.

THE SOFT–TISSUE HEALING PROCESS

When an injury has occurred either directly (macro-trauma over a short period of time) or indirectly (microtrauma over a long period of time) to the soft tissues of the body, the principles of treatment follow those of the body's natural healing process. Since it is doubtful that anything can be done to accelerate the normal response for wound repair, the intent of therapy is to prevent and/or reverse the factors which tend to retard recovery and facilitate the factors which restore the neurophysiology that accompanies the injury. The aim is to restore the function and treat the soft tissue according to the stage of its recovery.

Approximately three billion years ago when living organisms were unicellular, death of the cell meant death of the organism. With the evolution of multicellular organisms, so followed the process of repair after injury. Ultimately this repair process was perfected so that complete regeneration of an amputated limb was possible. Some lower vertebrates such as lizards and newts have retained this capability. The evolution of more complex life forms (e.g., the mammal) has occurred at the expense of total regenerative ability. For example, in humans, cardiac muscle does not regenerate after infarction, neural tissue does not regenerate after cellular death, skin does not regenerate after full-thickness injury, and an amputated finger does not grow back. With few exceptions, mammalian tissue responds to injury by repair rather than regeneration.

In most tissues, repair occurs by fibrous tissue proliferation regardless of which tissue has been damaged. Although the healing process is not a state, it can be divided into three phases: the substrate phase, the fibroblastic phase, and maturation.

SUBSTRATE PHASE

The substrate phase (also called the lag, latent, or productive phase) extends from the time of injury to the 4th to 6th day. It is characterized by the inflammatory response which prepares the wound for subsequent healing by removing the debris, necrotic tissue, and bacteria. At the same time, fibroblasts migrate to the wound site. Exactly how these cells are attracted to the wound is unknown; however, several investigators (Bassett 1968, Kappel et al 1973, Peacock 1984) feel that an electric potential exists at the injury site which influences their migration. During this phase, the wound is held together by the gluing action of fibrin which has a very low breaking strength.

FIBROBLASTIC PHASE

The fibroblastic phase begins between the 4th and 6th day after injury and can last up to 4–10 weeks (Peacock 1984). At this time, the proliferating fibroblasts begin to synthesize collagen, mucopolysaccharides, and glycoproteins. Regardless of the location of the wound, the fibroblasts carry on the process of wound repair by replacing the damaged structures with fibrous tissue. Tropocollagen is secreted from the fibroblasts and quickly aggregates into collagen fibers. The orientation of the fibers at this stage has been shown (Bassett 1968, Peacock 1984) to be influenced by the mechanical forces existing at the wound site. The tensile strength of the wound during the fibroblastic phase is proportional to the quantity of collagen present rather than the cross-linking between the collagen fibers.

MATURATION PHASE

These is no sharp demarcation between the end of the fibroblastic phase and the beginning of the maturation phase. Peacock (1984) states that the quantity of collagen within the wound ceases to increase between the 3rd and 4th week after injury. Although the collagen content within the wound remains constant or even decreases after the stage of fibroplasia, the wound continues to gain in tensile strength. This strength gain is due to two factors: the intramolecular/intermolecular cross-linking of the collagen fibers, and remodeling of the wound by the dissolution and reformation of the collagen fibers to give a stronger weave. The quantity of collagen is constant; it is the organization that is undergoing change. This process of remodeling may require 6–12 months for completion.

CLINICAL APPLICATION TO TREATMENT

Following an acute soft-tissue injury, functional disability can be caused by the synthesis and deposition of scar tissue and the way in which the physical properties of collagen differ from the unwounded tissue it replaces. In addition, the impact of pain on motor control must be considered. The aim of treatment, therefore, must be to control and guide the repair process such that optimal structure and function are restored.

During the stage of fibroplasia, the tensile strength of the wound is proportional to the rate of collagen accumulation. Webster et al (1980) have shown that ultrasound can increase the quantity of collagen synthesized, thereby increasing the tensile strength of the scar. Research (Mester 1971, Abergel 1984) on the effects of lasers indicates that facilitation of the optimal rate of healing is possible with this modality. However, whether it is possible to shorten the total length of time required for maturation of the scar is controversial. What can be done; however, is to prevent the undesirable factors which tend to retard the healing process. The fibrosis can also be controlled and directed during the stages of synthesis, deposition, and remodeling, such that a more functional scar subserves the tissue it replaces as best it can.

Tendon

To illustrate, compare the structural characteristics of the tendon of the piriformis muscle with those of the peroneus longus muscle. The tendon of piriformis is relatively short and is not enclosed in a synovial sheath (Fig. 7.2). The collagen fibers within the tendon are oriented in a longitudinal regular manner (Fig. 7.3), consistent with the lines of stress produced when the muscle contracts. Since the type I collagen which is present in tendon is inelastic, this

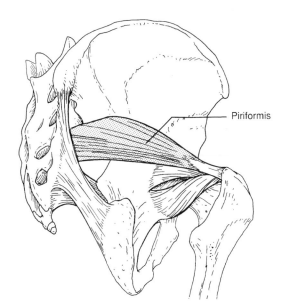

Figure 7.2   The piriformis muscle and its tendon.

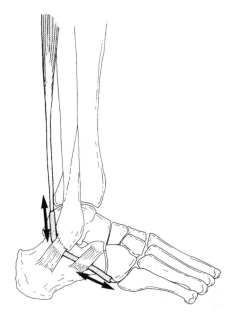

Figure 7.4   The peroneus longus muscle, its tendon and synovial sheath.

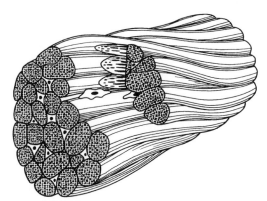

Figure 7.3   Both tendons and ligaments are composed of a regular longitudinal arrangement of collagen fibers. (Redrawn from Williams 1995.)

arrangement allows the force generated by contraction of the muscle to be efficiently transmitted to the bony insertion on the greater trochanter. Minimal gliding of the tendon on the adjacent structures is required for normal function.

Conversely, the tendon of the peroneus longus muscle is long and is enclosed within a synovial sheath passing beneath several fibrous tunnels on the lateral aspect of the ankle as well as within the sole of the foot (Fig. 7.4). The collagen fibers within the tendon are also oriented in a longitudinal manner consistent with the lines of stress produced when the muscle contracts. Again, this arrangement

facilitates the transmission of force from the muscle belly to the bone efficiently. However, when the muscle contracts, the tendon is required to glide extensively between the adjacent structures and the restoration of this function is critical to the success of treatment.

The repair process following injury to either of these tendons is the same. The inflammatory response of the substrate phase is followed by the proliferation of fibroblasts and the production of collagen, mucopolysaccharides, and glycoproteins. The orientation of the new collagen fibers at this stage of repair is influenced by mechanical deformation of the wound. Exactly how tension affects the orientation process is controversial; however, research (Bassett 1968, Kappel et al 1973) suggests that the electrical field surrounding the injury site may influence both healing and regeneration of tissue.

In 1880, Pierre and Jacques Curie discovered that when a quartz crystal was stressed, a potential difference was produced across its faces. This was called the piezoelectric effect. It is felt (Bassett 1968, Kappel et al 1973, Peacock 1984) that since collagen is crystalline in nature, a potential difference, or field of electricity, is produced when the fibers are deformed. Perhaps this deformation produces the piezoelectric current which subsequently directs the newly formed collagen fibrils. Bassett (1968) has described the cellular effects of electrical current and believes these to be the trigger of wound repair. Clinically, this appears to be the most effective stage in which to implement electrical, ultrasonic, light, and/or manual therapy if optimal function is to be achieved.

The tendons of the piriformis and peroneus longus muscles contain type I collagen fibers which lie in a longitudinal direction in series with the muscle fibers. Therefore, during the fibroblastic stage of healing, treatment should be directed towards orienting the collagen fibers of both tendons longitudinally. Passive physiological mobilizations and exercise programs which *gently* stress the tendon should be started at this stage. Vigorous exercises or aggressive passive mobilizations will prevent the revascularization of the tendon and retard the healing process, so "gentle" is the key word at this time. As well, since there is minimal intramolecular or intermolecular cross-linking of collagen fibers at this stage, strong stretching or forcing of the wound is contraindicated. More pain will definitely lead to less gain. Both ultrasound and laser can facilitate the synthesis of collagen and are useful adjunctive modalities.

The maturation phase is the stage when things can definitely go wrong. The structure may be restored and extremely resistant to tensile forces but the function may be completely devastated. Consider the torn peroneus longus tendon in the foot. Collagen cannot differentiate between the tendon, the synovium, and the fibrous tunnel. The new collagen fibers uniting the tendon will indiscriminately cross-link with those restoring the structure of the sheath or the fibrous tunnel beneath which it passes. Stability is thus restored at the expense of mobility. Since this tendon must glide extensively for normal function, a 50% reduction in gliding ability will have profound effects on the function of the foot. By contrast, the tendon of the piriformis muscle requires little mobility between itself and the adjacent structures, and loss of this mobility will have less effect on the overall function.

There are two kinds of adhesions which can occur subsequent to the healing process – restrictive and non-restrictive. Restrictive adhesions are regularly organized with a compact arrangement of collagen fibers oriented in a longitudinal manner. Non-restrictive adhesions are randomly organized with small-fiber bundles. Although the evidence is not conclusive, it is felt (Peacock 1984) that longitudinal slippage or friction-induced instability of collagen fibers and fibrils is the most probable method by which additional length in the scar is gained.

This information can be applied to healing tissue in the following manner. If the injured tendon is stressed repetitively during the therapeutic exercise program, an excellent environment will be created for lateral intertissue cross-linking. This facilitates tensile strength but a restrictive adhesion will also be encouraged. If, however, transverse mobilizations (or frictions) of the tendon are also incorporated into the therapy session, elongation of the entire adhesion will be promoted as the collagen fibers are "teased" apart and longitudinal slippage of the fibers occurs. The adhesion is therefore non-restrictive and both tensile strength and mobility are encouraged.

To summarize, tendon tensile strength can be effectively restored by exercise programs which apply stress to the tendon. These programs can be graduated from gentle passive stretching to vigorous eccentric loading depending upon the stage of healing. If tendon mobility is also required, attention must be directed to the lateral attachments which bind the tendon down, otherwise the stage is set for chronic repeated microtears of scar tissue such as those seen in chronic tennis elbow or chronic peroneal tendinitis following old inversion injuries of the ankle.

Ligament

Ligaments structurally resemble tendons and therefore the tensile requirements are the same. They must, however, be free to move on the bones they cross. If a restrictive adhesion is allowed to develop, chronic repeated microtears will occur. If the adhesion can be elongated via transverse frictions, the mobility and the elasticity of the ligament will be restored. Manipulation of adhesions is a destructive treatment technique since the adhesion rarely releases where it is intended. More commonly, a fresh tear between the adhesion and normal tissue occurs which sets up another inflammatory response. If the fibroblastic phase and the maturation phase of collagen synthesis, deposition, and remodeling are now treated appropriately, a new elongated adhesion will be formed which allows the necessary mobility.

Fibrous joint capsule

The structural characteristics and functional requirements of a fibrous joint capsule are quite different from those of either a tendon or ligament. The outer layer of the joint capsule is composed of an irregular random arrangement of collagen fibers (Fig. 7.5) unlike the tendon or ligament which displays a regular longitudinal arrangement. This is a good example of function governing structure. The primary function of a ligament is to resist tensile forces between two bones, and the anatomy suits its needs ideally. The fibrous capsule; however, must be extensible to allow mobility of the joint, and since collagen is inextensible, a longitudinal arrangement would inhibit mobility.

The random, irregular orientation of the collagen fibers permits mobility. When the capsule is stretched, the fibers orient themselves along the lines of tension produced by the stretch. Ultimately, the collagen fibers set the limit to the amount of extensibility

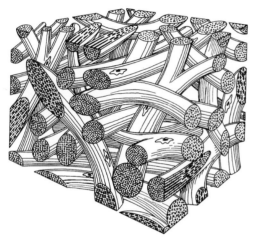

Figure 7.5 The outer layer of the joint capsule is composed of an irregular random arrangement of collagen fibers. (Redrawn from Williams 1995.)

permitted (Fig. 7.6). This anatomical arrangement promotes mobility while the physical characteristics of the collagen fiber itself afford end-range stability.

The repair process following capsular injury is identical to the one previously described. The initial inflammatory response is clinically apparent as traumatic arthritis. Fibroplasia and collagen synthesis follows 4–6 days after injury. The orientation of the new fibers will not automatically assume a random arrangement if tensile forces are applied to the wound. If the patient is started on an exercise program designed to restore full range of motion, and that exercise program puts tension through the wound, longitudinal orientation of new collagen fibers will be promoted, leading to increased lateral cross-linking and restricted mobility. This is not an adhesion, but rather the restoration of structure with tissue that does not subserve the joint capsule's function. The treatment given to any tissue is governed by the functional requirements of the damaged tissue. In this instance, both extensibility and tensile strength require restoration.

The challenge is to preserve the extensibility of the joint capsule by creating a random arrangement of small-fiber collagen bundles while simultaneously increasing the tensile strength. An extensible scar is more likely to develop if stresses are induced in a multitude of directions across the wound. Three-dimensional exercise programs, together with physiological active and passive mobilization techniques, will theoretically facilitate the random arrangement of the new collagen fibers.

The principles and progressions for exercise instruction will be covered in detail in Chapter 10.

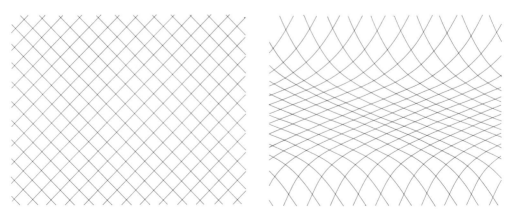

Figure 7.6 The orientation of the collagen fibers within the joint capsule influences the degree of extensibility permitted. The random irregular orientation initially permits mobility (left). When placed under tension the reorientation of the fibers (right) ultimately restricts the motion.

Summary

Left alone, wounded tissue will repair. However, wound repair is not necessarily accompanied by the restoration of function. Recent research has increased our understanding of the impact of low back and pelvic pain on both articular function (form closure) and neuromyofascial function (force closure and motor control). Changes in the proprioceptive and motor control systems alter movement patterns and strategies of load transfer. The result is less efficient movement, suboptimal function, a higher risk for recurrence of pain and injury, and altered joint forces (due to altered axes of joint rotation) that may lead to earlier degenerative changes and pain. The effective management of low back and/or pelvic pain requires assessment of the impact of the injury and consequences of the subsequent pain state on the form closure, force closure, motor control, and emotional state of the patient.

Chapter **8**

Diagnosing the lumbopelvic–hip dysfunction

Diane Lee   Linda-Joy Lee

When the integrated model is used to treat patients with dysfunction, the primary focus is the restoration of function: the location and behavior of pain become less relevant to the assessment and subsequent treatment. However, to ignore completely the patient's complaints is to fail to address the psychosocial factors of the patient's experience. Dreyfuss et al (1996) note: "Patients with sacroiliac joint (SIJ) pain exhibit no characteristic feature such as aggravation or relief of their pain by sitting, walking, standing, flexion, or extension." This research is not consistent with clinical experience; however, it is not surprising if pain was used to indicate dysfunction. Clinically, activities which aggravate or relieve symptoms tend to follow common patterns when patients with similar pelvic *impairments*, and not pain patterns, are considered. Thus, it is important to investigate the symptom behavior as this will address the patient's psychosocial needs as well as provide a preliminary indication of the underlying impairment once clinical expertise is attained. Therapists who take the time to develop a disciplined examination technique will be rewarded later with the ability to recognize similar patterns of impairment quickly. The purpose of this section is to describe and illustrate the basic subjective and objective examination for the lumbar spine, pelvic girdle, and hip. Chapter 9 will elaborate further on the significance of the findings from these tests.

SUBJECTIVE EXAMINATION (Table 8.1)

MODE OF ONSET

- How did the problem begin – suddenly or insidiously? With respect to wound repair

Table 8.1   Subjective examination

Name		Age		Doctor	
Mode of onset					
Past history			Past treatment		
Pain/dysesthesia location					
Aggravating activities					
Relieving activities					
Sleep surface/position			Status in a.m.		
Occupation/leisure activities/sport					
General health			Medication		
Results of adjunctive tests					

(Ch. 7), is the patient presenting during the substrate, fibroblastic, or maturation phase of healing?

- Was there an element of trauma? If so, was there a major traumatic event over a short period of time, such as a fall, or was there a series of minor traumatic events over a prolonged period of time, such as the habitual use of improper lifting technique?
- Is this the first episode requiring treatment or has there been a similar past history of events? If this is a repeat episode, how long did it take to recover from the previous one and was therapy necessary at that time? If so, what therapy was beneficial, if any?
- Is the problem a consequence of a pregnancy and/or delivery? If so, when did the symptoms begin, what was the nature of the delivery, and how much trauma occurred to the pelvic floor?

PAIN/DYSESTHESIA

- Exactly where is the pain/dysesthesia? Is it localized or diffuse and can its quality be described?

- How far down the limb or limbs do the symptoms radiate?
- Which activities (including how much) will aggravate the symptoms?
- What effect does prolonged sitting, standing, walking, stair-climbing and descent, rolling over in bed, getting in/out of a chair/car, cough, and/or sneeze have on the pain/dysesthesia? Does the aggravating activity induce more vertical or horizontal loading (or both)?
- What activities (including how much) provide relief?

SLEEP

- Are the symptoms interfering with sleep? Does rest provide relief?
- What kind of bed is being slept in and what position is most frequently adopted?

OCCUPATION/LEISURE ACTIVITIES/SPORT

- What level of physical activity does the patient consider normal and essential for return to full function?

- What are the patient's goals from therapy? The specifics of both the patient's occupation and sport are required if rehabilitation is to be successful and complete.

GENERAL INFORMATION

- What is the status of the patient's general health?
- Is the patient currently taking any medication for this or any other condition?
- What are the results of any adjunctive diagnostic tests (i.e., X-ray, computed tomography (CT) scan, magnetic resonance imaging, laboratory tests, etc.)?
- Is there any urinary incontinence? If so, is it stress, urge, or mixed?

OBJECTIVE EXAMINATION

Bogduk (1997) states that biomechanical diagnoses require biomechanical criteria. He notes that "Pain on movement is not that criteria." Tests which aim to analyze the mobility and stability of a joint are required to fulfill these criteria. Several biomechanical tests of the SIJ have been criticized with regard to their reliability, validity, and specificity (Potter & Rothstein 1985, Carmichael 1987, Herzog et al 1989, Dreyfuss et al 1994, 1996, Laslett & Williams 1994, Paydar et al 1994, Maigne et al 1996, Bogduk 1997, Buyruk et al 1997, Laslett 1997). From this research, it has been suggested that manual testing of the SIJ is unreliable and therefore should be abandoned. This conclusion has not been reached with other joints of the body. Stability tests for the knee joint (Lachman's and the anterior drawer tests) are commonly accepted amongst both physiotherapists and orthopedic surgeons (Reid 1992) even though their reliability, validity, and specificity have been questioned (Cooperman et al 1990). The results from the latter intertester reliability study clearly showed poor agreement in all areas. In spite of this research, the Lachman's test remains widely used for evaluation of stability at the knee joint.

Wurff et al (2000) conducted a systematic literature review of the reliability studies for both pain provocation and mobility tests for the SIJ. They conclude that individually there is no reliability for any test! They suggest that a multitest score would likely be more reliable and a valid method for detecting SIJ pain and dysfunction. Intertester reliability has long been an issue and there is some suggestion (Strender et al

1997, Herrington 2000, Damen et al 2002a) that tester experience and standardization of testing are strong variables which influence the reliability of any test.

The tests for spinal and SIJ function (i.e., mobility/stability, not pain) continue to evolve and as we understand more about the factors which influence the test findings, hopefully they will be able to withstand the scrutiny of scientific research and take their place in a clinical evaluation which follows an integrated model of function. The tests presented in this chapter follow this model and are presented with good intention, recognizing their failure to respond in isolation to reliability and validity studies. They remain the best we have and when a clinical reasoning process is applied to their findings, a logical diagnosis can be made with respect to load transfer through the low back, pelvis, and hip.

The objective examination is divided into tests for function, form closure (lumbar spine, pelvic girdle, and hip), force closure, and motor control, specific neurological conduction and mobility tests, vascular tests, and adjunctive imaging tests (Table 8.2). This chapter will outline the details of how to perform these tests. The clinical interpretation of the test findings will be discussed in Chapter 9.

FUNCTION: GAIT

Careful observation of the patient's gait can be informative since walking requires optimal lumbo-pelvic-hip function (see Ch. 6). Initially, deviation of the top of the head in the vertical and/or coronal planes is noted. When gait is optimal, there is minimal deviation of the head in either plane. Failed load transfer through the pelvis and/or hip joint manifests as a deviation in the coronal plane of either the entire body (Trendelenburg gait: Fig. 6.25) or of the pelvis relative to the lumbar spine and hip (subtle hip drop/Trendelenburg sign) (Fig. 6.26). Alterations in stride length and timing can be indicative of mobility or stability dysfunction within the lumbo-pelvic-hip complex.

FUNCTION: POSTURE

Postural asymmetry is not necessarily indicative of pelvic girdle dysfunction; however, pelvic girdle dysfunction is often reflected via postural asymmetry. The *impact* of a specific impairment (intrinsic or extrinsic to the pelvic girdle) is often reflected in the patient's posture. Optimal posture requires the following. In the sagittal plane, a vertical line should

Table 8.2 Objective examination

Function
Gait
Posture
Regional movement tests
    Forward bending in standing
    Backward bending in standing
    Lateral bending in standing
    Axial rotation in standing
    One-leg standing

Form closure – lumbar spine
Lumbar spine: positional tests
    Flexion
    Extension
Lumbar spine: passive tests of osteokinematic function (PIVM)
    Flexion/extension
    Sideflexion/rotation
Lumbar spine: passive tests of arthrokinematic function (PAVM)
    Superoanterior glide – zygapophyseal joint
    Inferoposterior glide – zygapophyseal joint
Lumbar spine: passive tests of arthrokinetic function
    Compression
    Rotation
    Anterior translation
    Posterior translation
    Lateral translation

Form closure – pelvic girdle
Pelvic girdle: positional tests
    Innominate
    Sacrum
Pelvic girdle: passive tests of osteokinematic function (PIVM)
    Anterior/posterior rotation – innominate
    Nutation/counternutation – sacrum
Pelvic girdle: passive tests of arthrokinematic function (PAVM)
    Inferoposterior glide – sacroiliac joint
    Superoanterior glide – sacroiliac joint
Pelvic girdle: passive tests of arthrokinetic function
    Horizontal translation – sacroiliac joint and pubic symphysis
    Vertical translation – sacroiliac joint and pubic symphysis
    Vertical translation – pubic symphysis
Pelvic girdle: pain provocation tests
    Long dorsal ligament
    Sacrotuberous ligament
    Anterior distraction – posterior compression
    Posterior distraction – anterior compression

Form closure – hip
Hip: positional tests
Hip: passive tests of osteokinematic function (PIVM)
    Flexion
    Extension

(Contd over column)

    Abduction/adduction
    Lateral/medial rotation
    Combined movement test (in flexion)
    Combined movement test (in extension)
Hip: passive tests of arthrokinematic and arthrokinetic function (PAVM)
    Lateral/medial translation
    Distraction/compression
    Anteroposterior/posteroanterior translation
Hip: pain provocation and global stability
    Torque test
    Inferior band of the iliofemoral ligament
    Iliotrochanteric band of the iliofemoral ligament
    Pubofemoral ligament
    Ischiofemoral ligament

Force closure and motor control
Anterior abdominal fascia – test for diastasis of the linea alba
Deep fibers of multifidus
Active straight leg raise test
    Simulation of the local system
    Simulation of the global system
Active bent leg raise test
Local system – co-contraction analysis
Local system and the neutral zone
Real-time ultrasound analysis
Global system slings – strength analysis
    The posterior oblique sling
    The anterior oblique sling
    The lateral sling
Global system slings – length analysis
    The posterior oblique sling and the latissimus dorsi
    The anterior oblique sling and the oblique abdominals
    The longitudinal sling and the erector spinae
    The longitudinal sling and the hamstrings
    Psoas major, rectus femoris, tensor fascia latae, adductors
    Piriformis/deep external rotators of the hip
Pain provocation tests – contractile lesions

Neurological conduction and mobility tests
Motor conduction tests
Sensory conduction tests
Reflex tests
Dural/neural mobility tests
    Femoral nerve
    Sciatic nerve

Vascular tests

Adjunctive tests

pass through the external auditory meatus, the bodies of the cervical vertebrae, the glenohumeral joint, slightly anterior to the bodies of the thoracic vertebrae transecting the vertebrae at the thoracolumbar junction, the bodies of the lumbar vertebrae, the sacral promontory, slightly posterior to the hip joint and slightly anterior to the talocrural joint and naviculo-calcaneo-cuboid joint (Fig. 8.1). The primary spinal curve should be maintained, i.e., lumbar lordosis, thoracic kyphosis. The innominates should not be rotated excessively relative to one another and the sacrum should not be rotated between them. The anterior superior iliac spine (ASIS) of the innominate should lie in the same coronal plane as the pubic symphysis such that the innominate is vertical over the femoral shaft.

In the coronal plane, the clavicles should be symmetrical and slightly elevated, the manubrium and sternum vertical (with the manubriosternal junction in the same plane as the pubic symphysis and ASISs of the innominate), and the scapulae should rest in slight upward rotation (abduction) with the inferior angle on the chest wall.

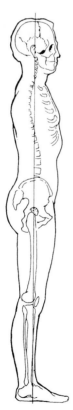

Figure 8.1 Optimal posture in standing. (Reproduced with permission from Lee & Walsh 1996.)

FUNCTION: REGIONAL MOVEMENT TESTS

These tests examine the integrated biomechanics (Ch. 6) of the low back, pelvis, and hip. Effective load transfer requires optimal function of the passive (form closure), active (force closure), and neural systems (motor control).

Forward bending in standing

Initially, the patient is instructed to forward bend and the ease with which the patient does so is noted (Fig. 6.16). Repeat the test three to four times. Note the apex of the sagittal curve for the whole body and then specifically note:

1. the relative intersegmental mobility of the lumbar spine (segmental kyphosis/lordosis or rotation). The spinal segments should flex symmetrically without shifting or hinging.

2. the paravertebral fullness. It should be equal on the left and right sides of the spinal column.

3. the relative mobility of the pelvic girdle on the femoral heads (the hip joint can be palpated anteriorly for this). The pelvic girdle should anteriorly tilt symmetrically over the femoral heads.

4. any intrapelvic rotation. Palpate both innominates at the inferior aspect of the posterior superior iliac spine (PSIS) and at the iliac crest (Fig. 8.2). No intrapelvic rotation or torsion should occur.

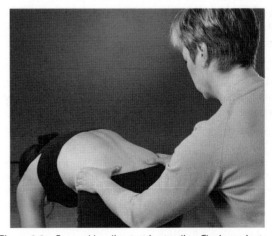

Figure 8.2 Forward bending test in standing. The innominates are palpated at the posterior superior iliac spine and the iliac crest. There should be no relative rotation between the two innominates, i.e., the pelvic girdle should anteriorly tilt as a unit on the femoral heads bilaterally. (Reproduced with permission from © Diane G. Lee Physiotherapist Corp.)

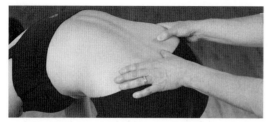

Figure 8.3 Forward bending test in standing. The innominate is palpated with one hand and the sacrum with the other (either at the median sacral crest at S2 or the inferior lateral angle). In the first few degrees of forward bending the sacrum nutates relative to the innominate (may or may not be felt) and should remain nutated throughout the full forward bend. (Reproduced with permission from © Diane G. Lee Physiotherapist Corp.)

5. the maintenance of sacral nutation throughout the full forward bend. Palpate the innominate with one hand (as in #4 above) and the median sacral crest at S2, or the inferior lateral angle (ILA) of the sacrum, with the other (Fig. 8.3). As the trunk bends forward there is an increase in the activation of multifidus. If the sacral base is palpated directly parallel to the PSIS (lateral to the median sacral crest), the bulging of the sacral multifidus pushes your thumb posteriorly (Fig. 5.12) and it is easy to interpret this as counternutation of the sacrum when in fact deep to the multifidus the sacrum is actually nutating. Therefore, the median sacral crest at S2, or the ILA, is a more reliable point to palpate the sacrum since there are no muscle fibers here to confuse the tester. The sacrum may be felt to nutate during the first few degrees of the forward bend (depending on the starting position of the sacrum) and should remain nutated throughout the forward bend.

Note the consistency/inconsistency of any positive findings during the repeated testing and the ease with which the patient is able to forward bend repeatedly.

Backward bending in standing

Initially, the patient is instructed to backward bend and the ease with which the patient does so is noted (Fig. 6.18). Repeat the test three to four times. Note the apex of the sagittal curve for the whole body and then specifically note:

1. the relative intersegmental mobility of the lumbar spine (segmental kyphosis/lordosis or rotation). The spinal segments should extend symmetrically without shifting or hinging.

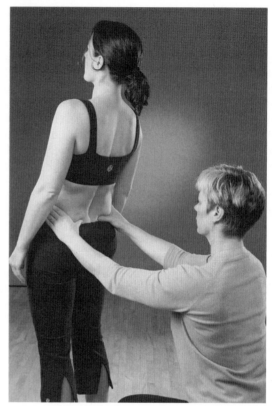

Figure 8.4 Backward bending test in standing. The innominates are palpated at the posterior superior iliac spine and the iliac crest. There should be no relative rotation between the two innominates, i.e., the pelvic girdle should posteriorly tilt as a unit on the femoral heads bilaterally. (Reproduced with permission from © Diane G. Lee Physiotherapist Corp.)

2. the relative mobility of the pelvic girdle on the femoral heads (the hip joint can be palpated anteriorly for this). The pelvic girdle should posteriorly tilt symmetrically on the femoral heads.

3. any intrapelvic rotation. Palpate both innominates at the inferior aspect of the PSIS and at the iliac crest (Fig. 8.4). No intrapelvic rotation or torsion should occur.

Note the consistency/inconsistency of any positive findings during the repeated testing and the ease with which the patient is able to backward bend repeatedly.

Lateral bending in standing

Initially, the patient is instructed to laterally bend (Fig. 6.20) and the ease with which the patient does so is noted. Repeat the test three to four times. Note the apex of the coronal curve for the whole body and then specifically note:

1. the relative intersegmental mobility of the lumbar spine (segmental sideflexion/rotation). The spinal segments should sideflex symmetrically.
2. the relative mobility of the pelvic girdle on the femoral heads (the hip joint can be palpated). The pelvic girdle should laterally translate and laterally tilt relative to the femora.
3. any intrapelvic rotation. Palpate both innominates at the inferior aspect of the PSIS and at the iliac crest. In a mobile individual some intrapelvic motion occurs during lateral bending in standing such that in left lateral bending the right innominate posteriorly rotates relative to the left and the sacrum rotates slightly to the right. Relatively, both sides of the sacrum remain nutated compared to the left and right innominate and therefore stability is ensured for load transfer.

Repeat the test and note the consistency/inconsistency of any positive findings and the ease with which the patient is able to lateral bend repeatedly.

Axial rotation in standing

Initially, the patient is instructed to rotate and the ease with which the patient does so is noted. Repeat the test several times and note:

1. the relative intersegmental mobility of the lumbar spine (segmental sideflexion/rotation). The spine should rotate without "kinking."
2. the relative mobility of the pelvic girdle on the femoral heads (the hip joint can be palpated anteriorly for this). The pelvic girdle should rotate such that there is relative internal rotation of the ipsilateral hip joint and external rotation of the contralateral hip joint.
3. any intrapelvic rotation. Palpate both innominates at the inferior aspect of the PSIS and at the iliac crest. In a mobile individual some intrapelvic motion occurs such that in left axial rotation the right innominate anteriorly rotates relative to the left and the sacrum rotates slightly to the left. Relatively, both sides of the sacrum are nutated compared to the left and right innominates and therefore stability is ensured for load transfer.

Repeat the test and note the consistency/inconsistency of any positive findings and the ease with which the patient is able repeatedly to rotate axially.

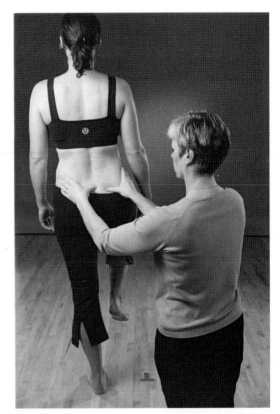

Figure 8.5 One-leg standing test: hip flexion phase. The innominate should posteriorly rotate relative to the sacrum. Arthrokinematically this requires an anterosuperior glide of the innominate relative to the sacrum (Hungerford 2002). (See also Figs 6.10 and 6.11.) (Reproduced with permission from © Diane G. Lee Physiotherapist Corp.)

One-leg standing

This test is also known as the Gillet test, stork test, or kinetic test and examines the ability of the low back, pelvis, and hip to transfer load unilaterally (support phase) as well as for the pelvis to allow intrapelvic rotation (Ch. 6) (Hungerford 2002). Initially, the patient is instructed to stand on one leg and to flex the contralateral hip and knee towards the waist (Fig. 6.10). The ability to perform this task is observed. The pelvis should not anteriorly/posteriorly/laterally tilt nor rotate in the transverse plane as the weight is shifted to the supporting limb. The test is repeated on the opposite side. Subsequently, the intrapelvic motion which occurs during this task can be examined as follows:

1. Hip flexion phase (ipsilateral kinetic test) (Fig. 8.5): With one hand, palpate the innominate at the inferior aspect of the PSIS and at the iliac

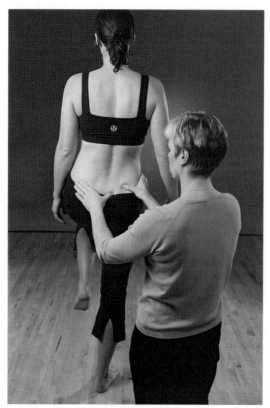

Figure 8.6 One-leg standing test: support phase. The innominate should remain posteriorly rotated relative to the sacrum. (Reproduced with permission from © Diane G. Lee Physiotherapist Corp.)

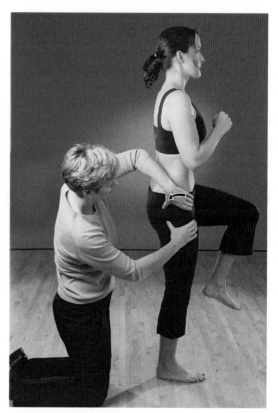

Figure 8.7 One-leg standing test: support phase. The innominate should extend relative to the femur (arrow) or remain vertical. This is a stable position for load transfer through the hip joint. (Reproduced with permission from © Diane G. Lee Physiotherapist Corp.)

crest on the non-weight-bearing side. With the other hand, palpate either the median sacral crest at S2 or the ILA of the sacrum on the same side as the innominate being palpated. Instruct the patient to flex the ipsilateral hip (same side you are palpating) and note the posterior rotation of the innominate relative to the sacrum. Compare the amplitude and quality (resistance) of this movement to the contralateral side. This is not a test for mobility of the SIJ but rather a test of osteokinematic motion of the low lumbar vertebrae, the innominate, and the sacrum. Many factors can impede osteokinematic motion: the SIJ is one.

2. Support phase:

a. On the weight-bearing side, with one hand, palpate the innominate at the inferior aspect of the PSIS and at the iliac crest. With the other hand, palpate either the median sacral crest at S2, or the ILA of the sacrum, on the same side as the innominate being palpated (Fig. 8.6). Instruct the patient to flex the contralateral hip (side you are

not palpating) and note the motion of the innominate relative to the sacrum (contralateral kinetic test). Especially note the movement that occurs as the weight is transferred on to the supporting leg (initial loading) and the contralateral leg is coming off the ground. The innominate should either posteriorly rotate or remain still *relative to the sacrum* (in a posteriorly rotated position; what is observed will depend on the starting position of the innominate).

b. On the weight-bearing side, palpate the innominate with one hand and the femur with the other (Fig. 8.7). Instruct the patient to flex the contralateral hip (side you are not palpating) and note the motion of the innominate relative to the femur. The innominate should either move towards the vertical position (extend) or remain vertical *relative to the femur*.

A positive test occurs when the innominate anteriorly rotates or internally rotates relative to the sacrum

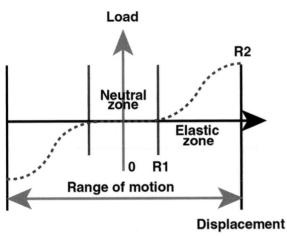

Figure 8.8 The zones of articular motion: the neutral zone (0–R1) and the elastic zone (R1–R2) (Panjabi 1992b).

(failed load transfer through the pelvic girdle) (Hungerford et al 2001, Hungerford 2002) or flexes relative to the femur (failed load transfer through the hip joint). This is a less stable position for load transfer through both the pelvis and the hip.

FORM CLOSURE: LUMBAR SPINE

The following tests examine the mobility and passive stability of the joints of the lumbar spine. Form closure analysis requires an evaluation of two zones of motion: the neutral zone and the elastic zone (Fig. 8.8) (Panjabi 1992b). The neutral zone is a small range of movement near the joint's neutral position where minimal resistance is given by the osteoligamentous structures (joint play from 0 to R1 or first resistance). The elastic zone is the part of the motion from the end of the neutral zone up to the joint's physiological limit (end-feel from R1 to R2).

Panjabi (1992b) noted that joints have non-linear load-displacement curves. The non-linearity results in a high degree of laxity in the neutral zone and a stiffening effect toward the end of the range of motion. He found that the size of the neutral zone may increase with injury, articular degeneration, and/or weakness of the stabilizing musculature and that this is a more sensitive indicator than angular range of motion for detecting instability. He used a ball and bowl illustration to represent this change in the neutral zone (Fig. 8.9). Lee & Vleeming (1998, 2004) suggest that the neutral zone is not only affected quantitatively (bigger or smaller), but also qualitatively (more or less resistance) when compression is increased or decreased across the joint

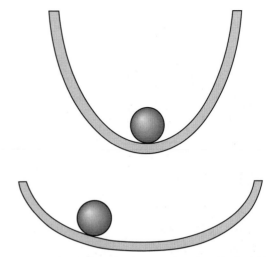

Figure 8.9 The ball and bowl concept introduced by Panjabi (1992b) to represent differences in neutral zone motion. The distance the ball can roll represents the amplitude of the neutral zone of motion under varying conditions.

(Fig. 8.10a–f). Each of the situations illustrated in Figure 8.10 will be discussed in Chapter 9.

Lumbar spine: positional tests

To determine the position of L5 relative to the sacrum, the posteroanterior relationship between the transverse processes of the L5 vertebra and the sacral base is noted in neutral, full flexion, and full extension. The influence of muscular hypertonicity and/or atrophy should be considered when interpreting the positional findings.

Flexion With the patient sitting, feet supported, and the lumbar spine fully flexed, the lateral aspect of the L5 segment and the sacral base are palpated bilaterally (Fig. 8.11). The posteroanterior relationship of the articular pillar of L5 relative to the sacral base is noted. A posterior right articular pillar of L5 relative to the sacral base is indicative of a right rotated position of L5–S1 in hyperflexion.

Extension With the patient prone and the lumbar spine fully extended, the L5 and then the sacral base are palpated laterally (Fig. 8.12). The posteroanterior relationship of the articular pillar of L5 relative to the sacral base is noted. A posterior right articular pillar of L5 relative to the sacral base is indicative of a right rotated position of L5–S1 in hyperextension.

Lumbar spine: passive tests of osteokinematic function (passive intervertebral motion: PIVM)

Flexion/extension With the patient sidelying, hips and knees flexed and supported on the therapist's

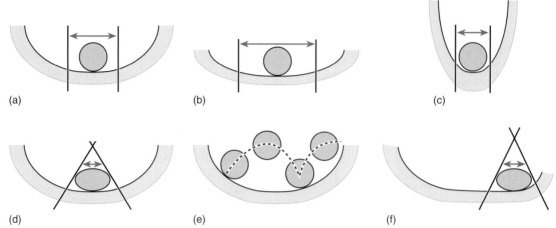

(a) (b) (c)

(d) (e) (f)

Figure 8.10 The neutral zone can be affected by altering compression across the joint. (a) A graphic illustration of the neutral zone of motion in a hypothetically normal joint. (b) A joint which is insufficiently compressed due to the loss of either form or force closure will have a relative increase in the neutral zone of motion. (c) A joint which is excessively compressed due to fibrosis will have a relative decrease in the neutral zone of motion. (d) A joint which is excessively compressed due to overactivation of the global system will also have a relative decrease in the neutral zone of motion. (e) When there is an intermittent motor control deficit, *passive* motion within the neutral zone can be normal since the dysfunction is dynamic. The bouncing ball reflects the intermittent loss of compression during functional activities (dynamic instability). (f) A joint which is fixated (subluxed) is excessively compressed and no neutral zone of motion can be palpated (complete joint block).

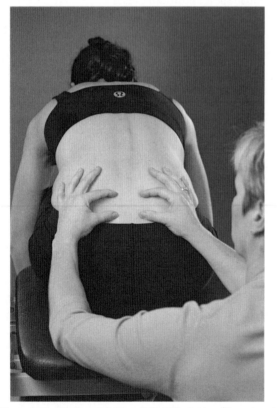

Figure 8.11 Positional testing of L5–S1 in flexion. (Reproduced with permission from © Diane G. Lee Physiotherapist Corp.)

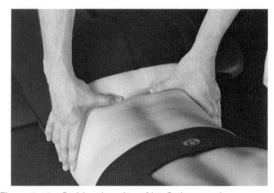

Figure 8.12 Positional testing of L5–S1 in extension. (Reproduced with permission from © Diane G. Lee Physiotherapist Corp.)

abdomen, palpate the interspinous space of the lumbar segment being tested (Fig. 8.13). With your caudal arm and hand, support the patient's legs. Passively flex/extend the lumbar segment and note the quantity and quality of intersegmental motion. Repeat the test for the other lumbar segments.

Sideflexion/rotation: L3–L4 With the patient side-lying, top hip and knee slightly flexed, bottom hip and knee extended, weave your cranial arm between the patient's arm and thorax and palpate lateral to the interspinous space of L3–L4 with the index and middle fingers. Your cranial hand should

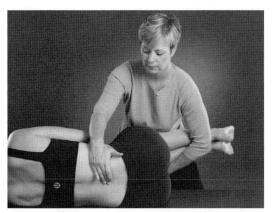

Figure 8.13 Passive test for osteokinematic flexion/extension of the lumbar spine. (Reproduced with permission from © Diane G. Lee Physiotherapist Corp.)

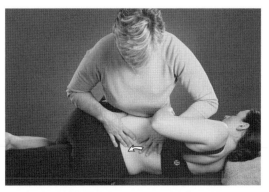

Figure 8.15 Passive test for the arthrokinematic superoanterior glide of the left zygapophyseal joint at L4–L5. The lumbar spine is purely sideflexed (arrow indicates the direction of the induced sideflexion) to produce the superoanterior glide. (Reproduced with permission from © Diane G. Lee Physiotherapist Corp.)

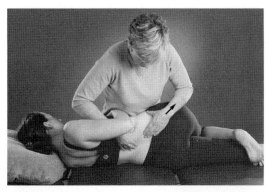

Figure 8.14 Passive test for osteokinematic left sideflexion combined with right rotation at L3–L4. The arrow indicates the direction of force applied by the therapist's caudal hand. (Reproduced with permission from © Diane G. Lee Physiotherapist Corp.)

be directly dorsal to the L3–L4 zygapophyseal joint (Fig. 8.14). Palpate the pelvic girdle in an obliquely distolateral direction with the caudal arm. With the index and middle fingers of this hand, palpate L4. Passively sideflex and contralaterally rotate L3–L4 using an oblique force through both arms. Note the quantity and quality of segmental motion. Repeat the test for the other lumbar segments and then test sideflexion/rotation in the opposite direction by laying the patient on the opposite side.

Lumbar spine: passive tests of arthrokinematic function (passive accessory vertebral motion: PAVM)

Superoanterior glide: left zygapophyseal joint L4–L5
A superoanterior glide of the left zygapophyseal

joint occurs during flexion and right sideflexion L4–L5. With the patient in right sidelying, left hip and knee slightly flexed, right hip and knee extended, weave your cranial arm between the patient's left arm and thorax. This will give you good control of the thoracolumbar region during this test. With the cranial hand, palpate lateral to the interspinous space of L4–L5. With the caudal hand, palpate L5 (Fig. 8.15). Passively sideflex the segment to the right (i.e., produce a superoanterior glide of the left zygapophyseal joint). Analyze the two zones of motion (neutral zone from 0 to R1, and elastic zone from R1 to R2) for amplitude, resistance to motion, and end-feel.

Inferoposterior glide: right zygapophyseal joint L4–L5
An inferoposterior glide of the right zygapophyseal joint occurs during extension and right sideflexion L4–L5. With the patient in left sidelying, right hip and knee slightly flexed, left hip and knee extended, weave your cranial arm between the patient's right arm and thorax. This will give you good control of the thoracolumbar region during this test. With the index finger of the cranial hand, palpate lateral to the interspinous space of L4–L5 (Fig. 8.16). Passively sideflex the segment to the right (i.e., produce an inferoposterior glide of the right zygapophyseal joint). Analyze the two zones of motion (neutral zone, from 0 to R1, and elastic zone, from R1 to R2) for amplitude, resistance to motion, and end-feel.

Lumbar spine: passive tests of arthrokinetic function

Compression   With the patient lying supine and the hips and knees flexed, the lower extremities are

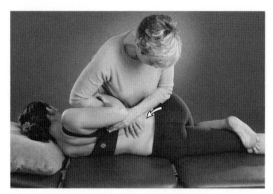

Figure 8.16 Passive test for the arthrokinematic inferoposterior glide of the right zygapophyseal joint at L4–L5. The pelvic girdle is purely sideflexed beneath the lumbar spine to produce the inferoposterior glide. The arrow indicates the direction of the induced sideflexion. (Reproduced with permission from © Diane G. Lee Physiotherapist Corp.)

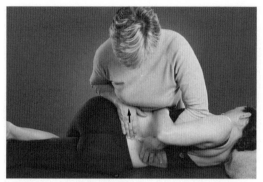

Figure 8.18 Arthrokinetic test of left segmental rotation at L4–L5. Note that the rotation induced at the lumbar segment is about a pure vertical axis and is therefore unphysiological. The arrow indicates the direction of force applied by the therapist's caudal hand. (Reproduced with permission from © Diane G. Lee Physiotherapist Corp.)

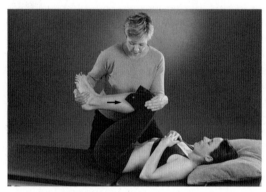

Figure 8.17 Arthrokinetic test of compression of the lumbar spine. The arrow indicates the force produced by the therapist's hands. (Reproduced with permission from © Diane G. Lee Physiotherapist Corp.)

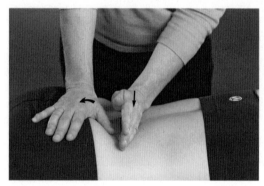

Figure 8.19 Arthrokinetic test of anterior translation at L4–L5. The arrows indicates the direction of force applied by the therapist's hands. (Reproduced with permission from © Diane G. Lee Physiotherapist Corp.)

cradled. Compression is applied to the lumbar segments by applying a cranial force parallel to the table through the flexed lower extremities (Fig. 8.17). Note the provocation of pain and/or spasm during compression loading.

Rotation: left rotation L4–L5 With the patient in right sidelying, left hip and knee slightly flexed, right hip and knee extended, palpate the left side of the spinous process of L4 with the cranial hand. With the long and ring fingers of the caudal hand, palpate the right side of the spinous process of L5 (Fig. 8.18). Left rotation, or left segmental torsion, is tested by fixing L4 and right-rotating L5 about a pure vertical axis beneath the L4 vertebra (the L4–L5 segment relatively left-rotates). Note the amplitude of the neutral zone, the resistance to motion within the neutral and the elastic zones, the quality of the

end-feel of the elastic zone, and the provocation of pain or spasm.

Anterior translation: L4–L5 With the patient lying prone, palpate the spinous process of L4 with the pisiform of one hand. With the other hand, stabilize the sacrum and L5 with a caudal force (to prevent extension of the spine) (Fig. 8.19). Apply an anterior translation force to the L4 vertebra. Note the amplitude of the neutral zone, the resistance to motion within the neutral and the elastic zones, the quality of the end-feel of the elastic zone, and the provocation of pain or spasm. This test may also be done in the sidelying position by fixing the spinous process of the superior vertebra and taking the inferior vertebra posteriorly by applying compression along the flexed femurs.

Posterior translation: L4–L5 With the patient sitting in a neutral lumbar spine position, arms crossed,

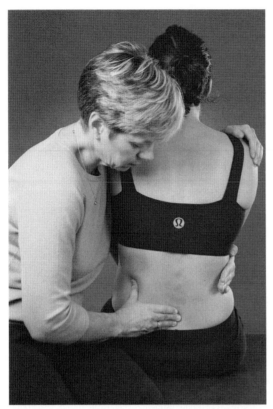

Figure 8.20   Arthrokinetic test of posterior translation at L4–L5. L4–L5 is in neutral and the lumbar spine is flexed above. Right hand: the index finger palpates the interspinous space and the middle and ring fingers fix L5. Left hand: applies a posterior translation force through the lumbar spine. (Reproduced with permission from © Diane G. Lee Physiotherapist Corp.)

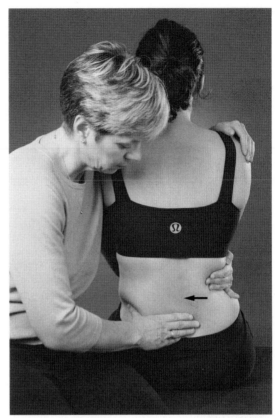

Figure 8.21   Arthrokinetic test of lateral translation at L3–L4. Right hand: the thumb and index finger fix L4. Left hand: applies a lateral translation force (arrow indicates the direction of the applied force). (Reproduced with permission from © Diane G. Lee Physiotherapist Corp.)

palpate the interspinous space of L4–L5. To localize the force, flex the lumbar spine down to L3–L4, ensuring that L4–L5 remains in a neutral position. Fix L5 with the caudal hand and apply a pure posterior translation force through the trunk with the other arm/hand (Fig. 8.20). The amplitude of the neutral zone, the resistance to motion within the neutral and the elastic zones, the quality of the end-feel of the elastic zone, and the provocation of pain or spasm are noted.

Lateral translation: L3–L4   With the patient sitting in a neutral lumbar spine position, arms crossed, palpate and stabilize L4 with an open web space grip. Fix L4 with this hand and apply a pure lateral translation force through the trunk with the other arm/hand (Fig. 8.21). The amplitude of the neutral zone, the resistance to motion within the neutral and the elastic zones, the quality of the end-feel of the elastic zone, and the provocation of pain or spasm are noted.

FORM CLOSURE: PELVIC GIRDLE

The following tests examine the mobility and passive stability of the joints of the pelvic girdle. Form closure analysis requires an evaluation of two zones of motion, the neutral zone and the elastic zone (Fig. 8.8) (Panjabi 1992b), but first, positional analysis is required. When interpreting the mobility findings, the position of the bone at the beginning of the test should be correlated with the subsequent mobility, since alterations in joint mobility may merely be a reflection of an altered starting position. If the innominate is posteriorly rotated relative to the sacrum, then the amplitude of the neutral zone will be reduced compared to the other side. Buyruk et al (1997) and Damen et al (2002b) have shown that asymmetrical stiffness (or laxity) of the SIJs correlates with and is prognostic for pelvic impairment and pain. Since it is not possible to know exactly

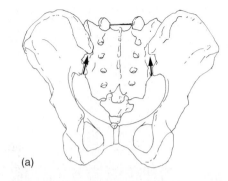

(a)

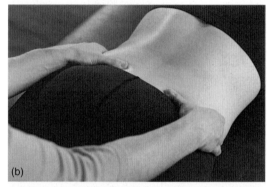

(b)

Figure 8.23 (a, b) Points of posterior palpation and hand position for positional testing of the innominate. The arrows indicate the resting point of the heels of the hands. (Reproduced with permission from © Diane G. Lee Physiotherapist Corp.)

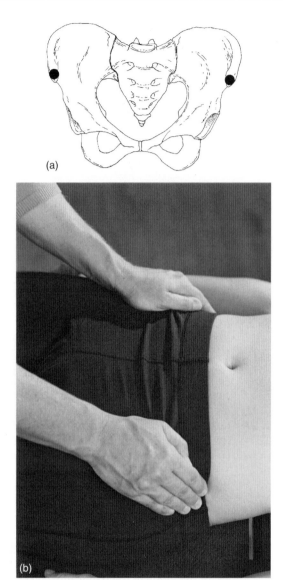

(a)

(b)

Figure 8.22 (a, b) Points of anterior palpation and hand position for positional testing of the innominate. Cup the innominate by resting the heels of your hands over the anterior superior iliac spines (dots). (Reproduced with permission from © Diane G. Lee Physiotherapist Corp.)

how *much* movement an individual should have, form closure analysis relies on comparing one side to the other. If consideration isn't given to the starting position of the joint, then the findings from the mobility tests are easily misinterpreted.

Pelvic girdle: positional tests

Innominate When analyzing the position of the innominate bones, it is more reliable to use the entire hand to gain information rather than visualizing one point of the bone (i.e., ASIS or PSIS). With the patient lying supine, legs extended, palpate the ASIS of both innominates with the heels of your hands. Let the rest of your hand "mold" to the innominate (Fig. 8.22a, b) and with your eyes initially closed, gain an impression as to whether the pelvis feels twisted (intrapelvic torsion) or sheared in a craniocaudal or anteroposterior plane. Then, open your eyes and palpate the inferior aspect of the ASIS bilaterally and/or the superior aspect of the pubic tubercles to confirm or negate your initial impression. Make sure that you keep your head and neck very still while making this judgment. Sideflexion of your own craniovertebral joints will change your perception and could alter your visual findings.

With the patient lying prone, palpate the inferior aspect of the PSIS of both innominates with your thumbs. Let the rest of your hand "mold" to the innominate and repeat your analysis from this position (Fig. 8.23a, b). To confirm a superior shear of the innominate, palpate the inferior aspect of the

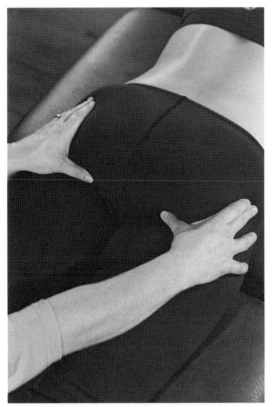

Figure 8.24 Positional testing of the ischial tuberosities. Ensure that the most inferior aspect of the ischial tuberosity is palpated. (Reproduced with permission from © Diane G. Lee Physiotherapist Corp.)

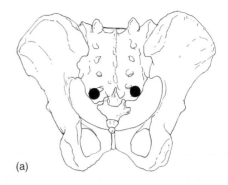

(a)

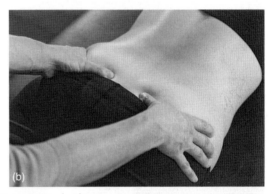

(b)

Figure 8.25 (a, b) Points of palpation and hand position for positional testing of the sacrum. (Reproduced with permission from © Diane G. Lee Physiotherapist Corp.)

ischial tuberosity bilaterally. Initially use the heels of both hands and then palpate the ischial tuberosity with the thumbs (Fig. 8.24). Ensure that you are on the most *inferior* aspect of the tuberosity since a rotated innominate can change the apparent craniocaudal relationship between the left and right sides if you are palpating the dorsal aspect of the ischial tuberosity.

Sacrum The most reliable place for positional testing of the sacrum is the dorsal aspect of the ILA (Fig. 8.25a, b) since at the sacral base the size and tone of multifidus can influence the findings. To determine the position of the sacrum, a comparison is made of the posteroanterior relationship of the ILA bilaterally. To find the ILA, begin by palpating the median sacral crest. Follow the crest inferiorly until you reach the sacral hiatus (unfused spinous processes of S4 and S5). From this point, palpate laterally until you feel the lateral edge of the sacrum: this is the ILA. A posterior left ILA is indicative of a left rotated sacrum.

Pelvic girdle: passive tests of osteokinematic function (PIVM)

Anterior/posterior rotation: innominate With the patient in sidelying, hips and knees slightly flexed, palpate the ASIS of the innominate with the cranial hand. Let the fingers of this hand mold around as much of the innominate as possible. With the heel of the other hand, palpate the ischial tuberosity. Let the fingers of this hand mold around as much of the innominate as possible (Fig. 8.26). Passively anteriorly and posteriorly rotate the innominate relative to the sacrum (remember the amplitude of SIJ movement is very small) and note the quantity and quality of the motion.

Nutation/counternutation: sacrum With the patient lying prone, palpate the apex of the sacrum with one hand and the midline of the sacral base with the other (Fig. 8.27). Passively nutate and counternutate the sacrum relative to the innominates and note the quantity and quality of the motion.

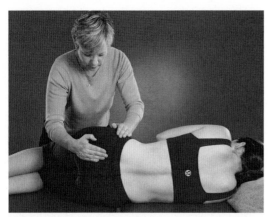

Figure 8.26   Passive test for osteokinematic anterior/posterior rotation of the innominate. (Reproduced with permission from © Diane G. Lee Physiotherapist Corp.)

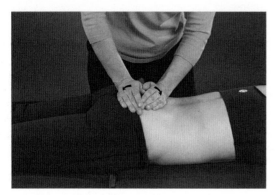

Figure 8.27   Passive test for osteokinematic nutation and counternutation of the sacrum. The arrows indicate the direction of force applied by the therapist's hands to produce nutation (arrow on therapist's left hand) and counternutation (arrow on the therapist's right hand). (Reproduced with permission from © Diane G. Lee Physiotherapist Corp.)

Pelvic girdle: passive tests of arthrokinematic function (PAVM)

Inferoposterior glide: SIJ   An inferoposterior glide of the innominate relative to the sacrum occurs at the SIJ during non-weight-bearing anterior rotation of the innominate (see Fig. 6.14). The patient is in crook lying with the knees comfortably supported over a bolster and arms by the sides. It is important to ensure that the patient is as relaxed as possible since even minimal activation of the local system (as well as activation of the longitudinal and oblique slings) can change the stiffness value of the SIJ. This has been confirmed via Doppler imaging under varying conditions of muscle contraction (Van Wingerden et al 2001, submitted, Richardson

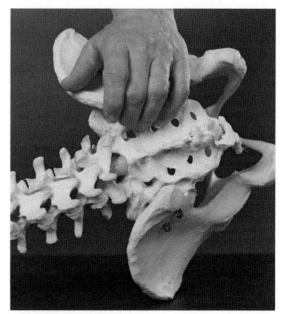

Figure 8.28   Position of the posterior hand for palpation of mobility and stability of the SIJ. (Reproduced with permission from © Diane G. Lee Physiotherapist Corp.)

et al 2002). The goal is to have the lumbopelvic region in a neutral position. Check to ensure that the pubic symphysis is level with the ASISs (no posterior pelvic tilt) and gently move the ribcage laterally from side to side to ensure the oblique abdominals and erector spinae muscles are not overactive. Once you are sure that the patient is relaxed, palpate the medial aspect of the posterior iliac crest (just above and medial to the PSIS) (Fig. 8.28) by sliding your cranial hand beneath the pelvis. Do not press too deeply into the multifidus muscle to avoid nutating the sacrum. With the heel of the other hand, palpate the ipsilateral ASIS and with the rest of this hand, the iliac crest. The first step is to determine the plane of the joint since there is a high degree of individual variance (Ch. 4). Apply a gentle oscillatory force in an anteroposterior direction varying the inclination from slightly medial to slightly lateral. One of those planes will meet with the least amount of resistance: this is the joint plane. Once the plane of the joint is found, apply a small anterior rotation force (Fig. 8.29) to the innominate to produce an inferoposterior glide of the innominate relative to the sacrum at the SIJ. Analyze the two zones of motion (neutral zone from 0 to R1, and elastic zone from R1 to R2) for amplitude, resistance to motion, and end-feel. Compare the findings to the opposite side: symmetry is the norm, while

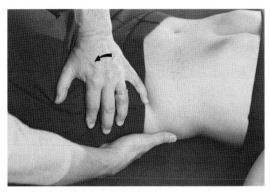

Figure 8.29 An inferoposterior glide of the innominate relative to the sacrum occurs when the innominate is anteriorly rotated. The arrow indicates the direction of force applied by the therapist's hand. (Reproduced with permission from © Diane G. Lee Physiotherapist Corp.)

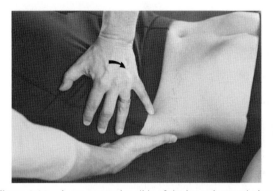

Figure 8.30 A superoanterior glide of the innominate relative to the sacrum occurs when the innominate is posteriorly rotated. The arrow indicates the direction of force applied by the therapist's hand. (Reproduced with permission from © Diane G. Lee Physiotherapist Corp.)

asymmetry of stiffness, or laxity, is indicative of dysfunction (Buyruk et al 1997, Damen et al 2002b).

Superoanterior glide: SIJ   A superoanterior glide of the innominate relative to the sacrum occurs at the SIJ during non-weight-bearing posterior rotation of the innominate (see Fig. 6.11) (Hungerford 2002). The patient's position and therapist's palpation points are identical to that described for testing the inferoposterior glide at the SIJ. The first step is to determine the plane of the joint since there is a high degree of individual variance (Ch. 4). Apply a gentle oscillatory force in an anteroposterior direction, varying the inclination from slightly medial to slightly lateral. One of those planes will meet with the least amount of resistance; this is the joint plane. Once the plane of the joint is found, apply a small posterior rotation force (Fig. 8.30) to the innominate

to produce a superoanterior glide of the innominate relative to the sacrum at the SIJ. Analyze the two zones of motion (neutral zone – from 0 to R1, and elastic zone – from R1 to R2) for amplitude, resistance to motion and end-feel. Compare the findings to the opposite side; symmetry is the norm, asymmetry of stiffness, or laxity, is indicative of dysfunction (Buyruk et al 1997, Damen et al 2002b).

Pelvic girdle: passive tests of arthrokinetic function

These tests are also used to detect a change in the neutral zone of motion of the SIJ or the pubic symphysis. They specifically evaluate the ability of the SIJ and pubic symphysis to resist vertical and horizontal plane translation (Lee 1992, 1997b, Lee & Walsh 1996). Individually, neither vertical nor horizontal translation occur physiologically, therefore these are unphysiological translatoric tests of stability. Clinically, they appear to be more sensitive to changes in the neutral zone than angular motion (anterior/posterior rotation).

Horizontal translation: SIJ and pubic symphysis   The patient's position and therapist's palpation points are identical to that described for testing the inferoposterior glide at the SIJ. The first step is to determine the plane of the SIJ since there is a high degree of individual variance (Ch. 4). Apply a gentle oscillatory force in an anteroposterior direction, varying the inclination from slightly medial to slightly lateral. One of those planes will meet with the least amount of resistance: this is the SIJ plane. Once the plane of the joint is found, apply a small posterior translation force (Fig. 8.31a, b) to the innominate. Analyze the two zones of motion (neutral zone from 0 to R1, and elastic zone from R1 to R2) for amplitude, resistance to motion, and end-feel. Compare the findings to the opposite side: symmetry is the norm, while asymmetry of stiffness, or laxity, is indicative of dysfunction (Buyruk et al 1997, Damen et al 2002b).

Vertical translation: SIJ and pubic symphysis   The patient's position and therapist's posterior palpation points are identical to that described for testing horizontal translation at the SIJ. The therapist's caudal hand palpates the distal end of the femur or knee (Fig. 8.32a, b). The first step is to determine the plane of the joint since there is a high degree of individual variance (Ch. 4). Apply a gentle oscillatory force through the femur in a craniocaudal direction, varying the inclination from directly cranial to cranial and slightly lateral. One of those planes will

Stability Tests – Pure Plane

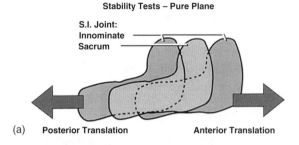

S.I. Joint:
Innominate
Sacrum

(a)   Posterior Translation   Anterior Translation

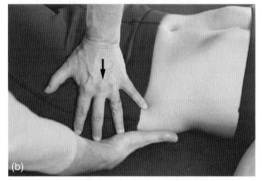

(b)

Figure 8.31   (a, b) This test examines the ability of the sacroiliac (S.I.) joint to resist a horizontal posterior translation force. The arrow indicates the direction of force applied by the therapist's hand. (Reproduced with permission from © Diane G. Lee Physiotherapist Corp.)

Stability Tests – Pure Plane

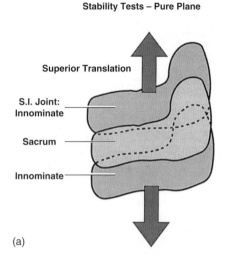

Superior Translation

S.I. Joint:
Innominate

Sacrum

Innominate

(a)

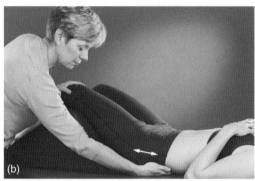

(b)

Figure 8.32   (a, b) This test examines the ability of the sacroiliac (S.I.) joint to resist a vertical translation force. The arrows indicate the resultant force on the innominate produced through "pushing and pulling" the femur. (Reproduced with permission from © Diane G. Lee Physiotherapist Corp.)

meet with the least amount of resistance: this is the SIJ plane. Once the plane of the joint is found, apply a small cranial and then caudal translation force to the innominate through the femur. Analyze the two zones of motion (neutral zone from 0 to R1, and elastic zone from R1 to R2) for amplitude, resistance to motion, and end-feel. Compare the findings to the opposite side: symmetry is the norm, while asymmetry of stiffness, or laxity, is indicative of dysfunction (Buyruk et al 1997, Damen et al 2002b).

Stability is *not* about *how much* movement there is or is not but rather about the symmetry of stiffness. Buyruk et al (1995b) as well as Damen et al (2001) found that unstable SIJs had lower stiffness values and that symptomatic individuals demonstrated asymmetry in the values between their left and right sides. While the Doppler studies suggest that the stiffness value for the SIJ should be symmetric, they do not determine if the amount of stiffness in the vertical plane should equal that in the horizontal plane. Clinically, it appears that an individual can have more or less stiffness in one plane than the other and yet still be symmetric when the planes are compared. For example, the stiffness found on

testing vertical translation is comparable left and right and the stiffness found on testing horizontal translation is comparable left and right; however, the stiffness found on vertical translation is more or less than that found on horizontal translation. It appears that an individual can have differing amounts of form closure for different directions of force. Therefore, when applying these tests, the therapist should compare the stiffness value left and right for a particular direction of translation and not compare the stiffness value for vertical translation with horizontal translation on the same side; they may not necessarily be the same, yet may be quite normal and functional for that individual.

The neutral zone is analyzed by comparing the sense of ease with which the innominate glides in a parallel manner relative to the sacrum until the

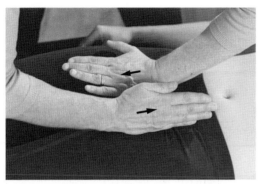

Figure 8.33   This test examines the ability of the pubic symphysis to resist a direct vertical translation force. The arrows indicate the direction of force applied by the therapist's hands. (Reproduced with permission from © Diane G. Lee Physiotherapist Corp.)

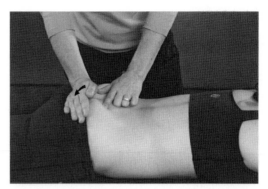

Figure 8.34   Pain provocation test for the long dorsal ligament, counternutation of the sacrum. In this photo, the model's arms are overhead to facilitate viewing of the technique. Clinically, the arms should be by the sides to reduce any tension in the posterior oblique slings. The arrow indicates the direction of force applied by the therapist's hand. (Reproduced with permission from © Diane G. Lee Physiotherapist Corp.)

point of first resistance. The elastic zone is analyzed from R1 to R2 and the quality of the resistance is assessed as well as the provocation of any pain or muscle spasm. The findings are then compared to the patient's opposite side, comparing the antero-posterior glide left and right and the craniocaudal glide left and right. We cannot make any judgments regarding *amplitude of motion* (stiff, loose, normal) with this test since it has been shown that the range of motion at this joint is highly variable and making a statement regarding the amplitude implies knowledge of what is "normal." It is not possible to know what the patient's normal should be. We can only compare the left to the right side of the pelvis and look for symmetry.

Vertical translation: pubic symphysis   The pubic symphysis can be specifically tested for vertical stability. With the heel of one hand, palpate the superior aspect of the superior ramus of one pubic bone. With the heel of the other hand, palpate the inferior aspect of the superior ramus of the opposite pubic bone (Fig. 8.33). Fix one pubic bone and apply a slow, steady vertical translation force to the other. Analyze the two zones of motion (neutral zone from 0 to R1, and elastic zone from R1 to R2) for amplitude, resistance to motion, and end-feel as well as the reproduction of any symptoms.

Pelvic girdle: pain provocation tests

Pain provocation tests have shown good intertester reliability (Laslett & Williams 1994, Laslett 1997), although their validity and specificity have been questioned (Dreyfuss et al 1994, 1996, Wurff et al

2000). When combined with tests of function, certain provocation tests are useful when developing inclusion criteria for research (Vleeming et al 2002). They can also help to explain to patients why certain activities/exercises may be provocative to their condition. On occasion, it is necessary to treat the painful structure before function can be restored, particularly if the exercises being taught are aggravating a painful, inflamed structure.

Long dorsal ligament   This structure is commonly tender to palpation in patients with pelvic pain (Vleeming et al 2002). The patient is lying prone with the head neutral and arms by the sides. With one hand, palpate the iliac crest at approximately the level of L3. Follow the iliac crest posteriorly until you drop off the PSIS. At this point, you should be dorsal to the long dorsal ligament, which can be felt as a vertically oriented band (Fig. 4.14). Note any tenderness to palpation. Continue to palpate the ligament with one hand and apply a counternutation force to the sacrum (Fig. 8.34). You should feel an increase in tension in the long dorsal ligament. If this is associated with increased pain, then this structure is a likely pain generator.

Sacrotuberous ligament   Although the sacrotuberous ligament can be injured during a fall on the buttock, this structure is less often a source of pelvic pain. The patient is lying prone with the head neutral and arms by the sides. Palpate the ischial tuberosity with one thumb. From this point, palpate medially and cranially until you reach the inferior arcuate band (medial band) of the sacrotuberous ligament (Figs 4.16 and 8.35a, b). It should feel like

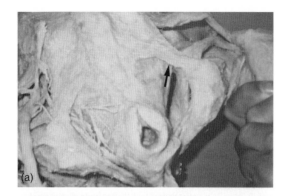

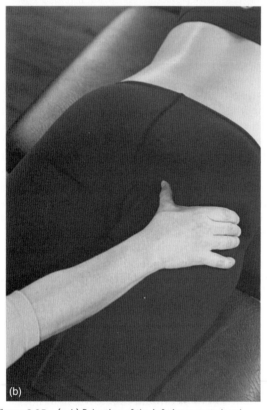

Figure 8.35 (a, b) Palpation of the inferior arcuate band (medial band) of the sacrotuberous ligament. (Reproduced with permission from © Diane G. Lee Physiotherapist Corp.)

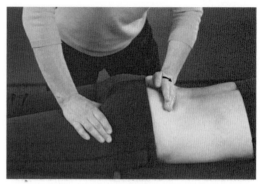

Figure 8.36 Pain provocation test for the sacrotuberous ligament, nutation of the sacrum. In this photo, the model's arms are overhead to facilitate viewing of the technique. Clinically, the arms should be by the sides to reduce any tension in the posterior oblique slings. The arrow indicates the direction of force applied by the therapist's hand. (Reproduced with permission from © Diane G. Lee Physiotherapist Corp.)

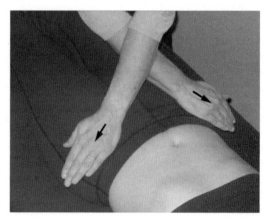

Figure 8.37 This pain provocation test stresses the anterior structures of the pelvic girdle and compresses those posterior. The arrows indicate the direction of force applied by the therapist's hands. (Reproduced with permission from © Diane G. Lee Physiotherapist Corp.)

a taut guitar string when you pronate and supinate your forearm. Continue to palpate the ligament and apply a nutation force to the sacrum (Fig. 8.36). You should feel an increase in tension in the sacrotuberous ligament. If this is associated with increased pain, then this structure is a likely pain generator.

Anterior distraction: posterior compression This test is not intended to stress a particular structure but rather tests for pain provocation when the pelvic girdle is compressed posteriorly and distracted anteriorly. If the SIJ is inflamed and an intraarticular synovitis is present, this test markedly increases the patient's pain. With the patient lying supine, the medial aspect of the ASIS is palpated bilaterally with the heels of the crossed hands (Fig. 8.37). A slow, steady, posterolateral force is applied through the ASISs, thus distracting the anterior aspect of the SIJ and pubic symphysis and compressing the posterior structures. The force is maintained for 5 s and the provocation and location of pain are noted.

Posterior distraction: anterior compression This test is not intended to stress a particular structure but

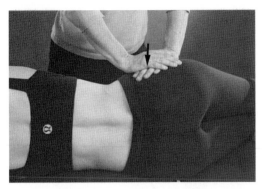

Figure 8.38 This pain provocation test stresses the posterior structures of the pelvic girdle and compresses those anterior. Ensure that the applied force is anteromedial thus gapping the sacroiliac joint posteriorly and compressing it anteriorly. The arrow indicates the direction of force applied by the therapist's hands. (Reproduced with permission from © Diane G. Lee Physiotherapist Corp.)

rather tests for pain provocation when the pelvic girdle is compressed anteriorly and distracted posteriorly. If an intraarticular synovitis of the SIJ is present, this test also increases the patient's pain. With the patient sidelying, hips and knees comfortably flexed, the anterolateral aspect of the uppermost iliac crest is palpated (Fig. 8.38). A slow, steady, medial force is applied through the pelvic girdle, thus distracting the posterior structures of the SIJ and compressing the anterior. The force is maintained for 5 s and the provocation and location of pain are noted.

FORM CLOSURE: HIP

The following tests examine the mobility and passive stability of the hip joint. As with the lumbar spine and pelvic girdle, form closure analysis requires an evaluation of two zones of motion: the neutral zone and the elastic zone (Fig. 8.8); however, before any interpretation of mobility can be made, the position of the femoral head with respect to the acetabulum must be determined. The hip joint is under the influence of several large muscles and imbalance can cause a displacement of the femoral head and thus give the appearance of restricted articular range of motion.

Hip: positional tests

With the patient standing, palpate the contour of the posterolateral buttock behind the greater trochanter and the anterior hip joint at the level of the inguinal ligament (Fig. 8.39). If there is a large "divot" in the

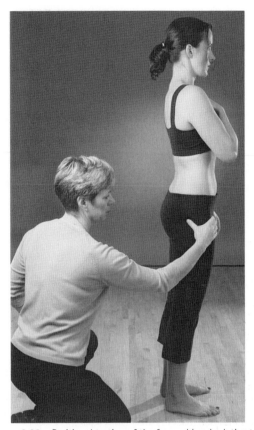

Figure 8.39 Positional testing of the femoral head relative to the innominate in weight-bearing. When the femoral head is positioned anteriorly in the actebulum there is a "divot" in the posterolateral buttock (Fig. 8.40) and the head of the femur is easily palpated anteriorly. (Reproduced with permission from © Diane G. Lee Physiotherapist Corp.)

posterolateral buttock (Fig. 8.40) and the anterior hip structures feel like they are under considerable tension, it is likely that this individual is gripping with the deep external rotators of the hip. Overactivation of these muscles forces the femoral head anteriorly and has marked consequences for mobility at the hip, low back, and pelvis (Fig. 8.41). We call these people "butt grippers." Try this simple experiment. Stand with your feet under your hips and with one hand, palpate just posterior to the greater trochanter. With the other hand, palpate the anterior aspect of the hip at the level of the inguinal ligament. Keep your feet firmly planted on the floor and actively externally rotate your femoral head in the acetabulum bilaterally. You will feel the development of the "divot" posteriorly as well as the anterior displacement of the femoral head. You have become a butt gripper too! Maintain this contraction

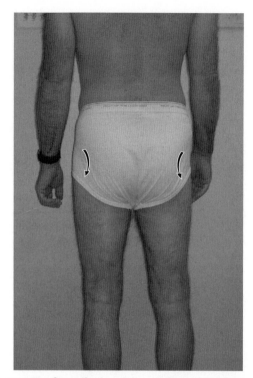

Figure 8.40 Overactivation of the external rotators of the hip causes "butt gripping." Note the large "divots" (arrows) in the posterolateral buttock. (Reproduced with permission from © Diane G. Lee Physiotherapist Corp.)

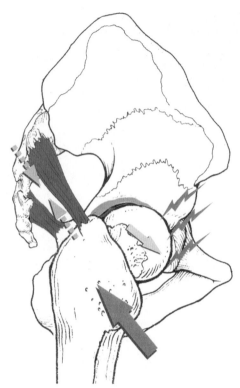

Figure 8.41 Overactivation of the deep external rotators of the hip pulls the greater trochanter posteriorly (large arrow) and forces the femoral head anteriorly. (Reproduced with permission from Lee 2001a.)

and try to forward bend. It's no wonder that the pelvic girdle and low back become sore when this method of stabilization is used.

With the patient supine, note the resting position of the legs. Overactivation of the external rotators of the hip will cause the legs to lie in external rotation at rest. Palpate the anterior femoral head in this position. If the femoral head is displaced anteriorly, its prominence will be very superficial and the structures between your hand and the femoral head can be quite tender. It is not uncommon for individuals to have a bilateral pattern of overactivation of the external rotators, therefore comparing to the opposite side is not always an option.

Since there is a wide individual variation of coxa vara, coxa valga, and angle of inclination of the femoral neck, specific measurements of where the greater trochanter is in relation to the ASIS is not always a reliable indicator of displacement of the femoral head. Clinically, consideration must be given to both the mobility findings and the positional findings to understand the significance of this positional test.

Hip: passive tests of osteokinematic function (PIVM)

Flexion With the patient lying supine, the flexed knee of the lower extremity to be tested is palpated with the caudal hand. The femoral head is palpated anteriorly with the other hand (Fig. 8.42). The femur is passively flexed at the hip joint until posterior rotation of the ipsilateral innominate begins. At that point, the limit of available range for femoral flexion has occurred. Both the quantity of motion and the end-feel are noted. The test is repeated on, and compared to, the other side.

Extension With the patient supine lying at the end of the table, one femur is flexed, held by the patient, and supported against the therapist's lateral thorax. Ensure that no intrapelvic torsion has occurred. The anterior aspect of the iliac crest and the ASIS of the limb being tested are palpated with the cranial hand. With the caudal hand, the therapist guides the femur into extension until anterior rotation of the ipsilateral innominate begins (Fig. 8.43). At that point, the limit of available range for femoral

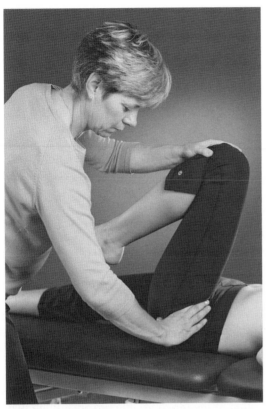

Figure 8.42   Passive test for osteokinematic flexion of the hip. (Reproduced with permission from © Diane G. Lee Physiotherapist Corp.)

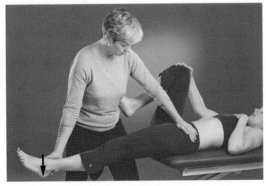

Figure 8.43   Passive test for osteokinematic extension of the hip. (Reproduced with permission from © Diane G. Lee Physiotherapist Corp.)

extension has occurred. Both the quantity of motion and the end-feel are noted. The test is repeated on, and compared to, the opposite side.

Abduction/adduction   With the patient supine, lying at the end of the table, one femur is flexed, held by the patient, and supported against the therapist's

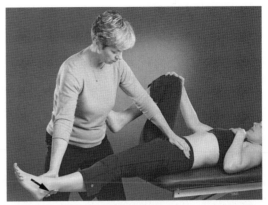

Figure 8.44   Passive test for osteokinematic abduction of the hip. Lateral tilting of the pelvic girdle beneath the lumbar spine indicates all available range of motion at the hip joint has occurred. (Reproduced with permission from © Diane G. Lee Physiotherapist Corp.)

lateral thorax. The anterior aspect of the iliac crest and the ASIS of the limb being tested are palpated with the cranial hand. With the caudal hand, the therapist guides the femur into abduction/adduction (Fig. 8.44) until lateral bending of the pelvic girdle beneath the vertebral column begins. At that point, the limit of femoral abduction/adduction has been reached. Both the quantity of motion and the end-feel are noted. The test is repeated on, and compared to, the opposite side.

Lateral/medial rotation   With the patient lying supine, the lower extremity to be tested is palpated above the ankle with the caudal hand. The test can be performed in varying degrees of hip flexion/extension to assist in the differentiation between an articular and myofascial restriction. The anterior aspect of the iliac crest and the ASIS are palpated with the cranial hand. The femur is passively laterally/medially rotated (Fig. 8.45) until rotation of the innominate begins. At that point, the limit of available range for femoral rotation has occurred. Both the quantity of motion and the end-feel are noted. The test is repeated on, and compared to, the opposite side.

Combined movement test (in flexion)   With the patient lying supine, the flexed knee of the lower extremity to be tested is palpated with the caudal hand. The anterior aspect of the iliac crest and the ASIS are palpated with the cranial hand. The femur is passively flexed, adducted, and medially rotated (Fig. 8.46). If the femoral head is displaced anteriorly secondary to overactive external rotators, impingement will occur, and the patient will likely complain of anterior groin pain.

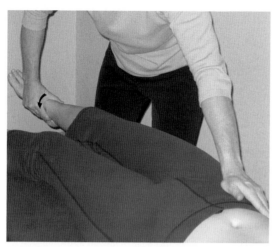

Figure 8.45 Passive test for osteokinematic medial rotation of the hip. The arrow indicates the direction of force applied by the therapist's hand. (Reproduced with permission from © Diane G. Lee Physiotherapist Corp.)

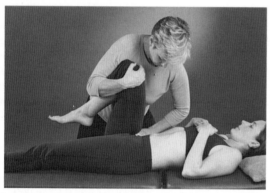

Figure 8.46 Combined movement test for anterior impingement of the hip. (Reproduced with permission from © Diane G. Lee Physiotherapist Corp.)

Combined movement test (in extension) With the patient lying prone, the extended knee of the lower extremity to be tested is palpated with the caudal hand. The posterior aspect of the greater trochanter is palpated with the cranial hand. The femur is passively extended, medially rotated, and then adducted or abducted. If the femoral head is displaced anteriorly and the joint is stiff, a restriction of extension will occur. If the femoral head is displaced anteriorly and the anterior aspect of the capsule/labrum is lax, excessive extension will occur.

Hip: passive tests of arthrokinematic and arthrokinetic function (PAVM)

Linear translation is relatively limited at the hip joint due to its high degree of form closure. Consequently,

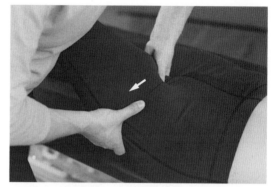

Figure 8.47 Arthrokinematic tests at the hip: an inferolateral force glides the superior and inferior aspects of the femoral head laterally and distracts the fovea. The arrow indicates the direction of force applied by the therapist's hands. (Reproduced with permission from © Diane G. Lee Physiotherapist Corp.)

movement analysis of linear translation (arthrokinematics: PAVMs) will be less informative than analysis of the osteokinematic motion (PIVMs). With respect to stability, it is the elastic zone analysis which reveals the most information (quality of the end-feel).

Lateral distraction/compression With the patient lying supine and the femur flexed to 30° (resting position of the hip joint), the proximal thigh is palpated. The joint is translated laterally by applying an inferolateral force parallel to the neck of the femur (Fig. 8.47). The superior and inferior aspects of the head of the femur translate laterally in relation to the acetabulum while the fovea is distracted. Compression is applied by approximating the femur superomedially into the medial aspect of the acetabular fossa. Analyze the two zones of motion (neutral zone from 0 to R1, and elastic zone from R1 to R2) for amplitude, resistance to motion, and end-feel.

Superoinferior glide With the patient lying supine and the femur flexed to 30°, the proximal thigh is palpated. The superior aspect of the joint is distracted (the inferior aspect is compressed) by applying an inferior force along the longitudinal axis of the femur (Fig. 8.48). The superior aspect of the joint is compressed (the inferior aspect is distracted) by approximating the femur superiorly into the superior aspect of the acetabular fossa. Analyze the two zones of motion (neutral zone from 0 to R1, and elastic zone from R1 to R2) for amplitude, resistance to motion, and end-feel.

Anteroposterior glide With the patient lying supine and the femur flexed to 30°, the proximal thigh is palpated. An anteroposterior glide is induced by applying a posterolateral force in the

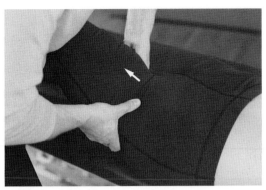

Figure 8.48 Arthrokinematic tests at the hip: an inferior force distracts the superior aspect of the femoral head. The arrow indicates the direction of force applied by the therapist's hands. (Reproduced with permission from © Diane G. Lee Physiotherapist Corp.)

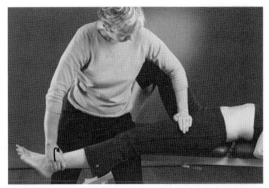

Figure 8.50 Pain provocation test for all the ligaments of the hip joint: torque test. The femur is held extended and medially rotated (arrow) as a posterolateral force is applied to the proximal femur. (Reproduced with permission from © Diane G. Lee Physiotherapist Corp.)

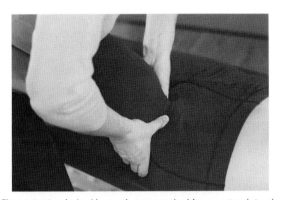

Figure 8.49 Arthrokinematic tests at the hip: a posterolateral force distracts the anterior aspect of the femoral head. (Reproduced with permission from © Diane G. Lee Physiotherapist Corp.)

plane perpendicular to the line of the femoral neck (Fig. 8.49). Analyze the two zones of motion (neutral zone from 0 to R1, and elastic zone from R1 to R2) for amplitude, resistance to motion, and end-feel.

Hip: pain provocation and global stability

Torque test This is a global test of passive stability and a pain provocation test for the ligaments of the hip joint. The intent is to stress all of the capsular ligaments simultaneously. If the test is painless, then the subsequent tests which help to differentiate the individual ligaments are not required. With the patient supine, lying close to the edge of the table, the ipsilateral femur is extended until anterior rotation of the innominate begins. The femur is then medially rotated to the limit of the physiological range of motion. The proximal thigh is palpated and

a slow, steady, posterolateral force is applied along the line of the neck of the femur to stress the capsular ligaments further (Fig. 8.50). The amplitude of the neutral zone (should be zero), the resistance to motion within the elastic zone (should be very firm), the quality of the end-feel of the elastic zone, and the provocation of pain or spasm are noted.

Inferior band of the iliofemoral ligament This ligament is taut when the femur is fully extended. If passive femoral extension elicits the greatest amount of pain, this ligament may be a nociceptive source.

Iliotrochanteric band of the iliofemoral ligament With the patient supine, lying close to the edge of the table, the ipsilateral femur is slightly extended, *adducted*, and fully laterally rotated. The distal femur is fixed against the therapist's thigh and the proximal femur is palpated. A slow, steady distraction force is applied along the line of the neck of the femur and the provocation of local pain is noted.

Pubofemoral ligament With the patient lying supine, the ipsilateral femur is slightly extended, *abducted*, and fully laterally rotated. The distal femur is fixed against the therapist's thigh and the proximal femur is palpated. A slow, steady distraction force is applied along the line of the neck of the femur and the provocation of local pain is noted.

Ischiofemoral ligament This ligament primarily limits internal rotation as well as adduction of the flexed hip (Hewitt et al 2002). With the patient lying supine, the ipsilateral femur is flexed, adducted, and fully *medially* rotated. A slow, steady distraction force is applied along the line of the neck of the femur and the provocation of local pain is noted. This position can also create anterior impingement so noting the location of the pain is critical for differentiation.

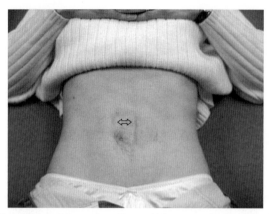

Figure 8.51 A large three-fingerwidth postpartum diastasis of the linea alba. (Reproduced with permission from © Diane G. Lee Physiotherapist Corp.)

FORCE CLOSURE AND MOTOR CONTROL

The following tests examine the integrity of the myofascial systems which provide dynamic stability for the lumbopelvic-hip region. Force closure and motor control analysis evaluate the patient's ability specifically to recruit both the local and global systems appropriately (the right amount at the right time: see Chs 5 and 6). In addition, tests are required to assess the impact of the force closure mechanism on form closure in both the lumbar spine and pelvic girdle.

The impact of an effective contraction of the local system on force closure of the lumbar spine and pelvic girdle depends on an intact anterior and posterior fascial connection. Anteriorly, this requires integrity of the abdominal fascia and posteriorly, multifidus must be of sufficient bulk to generate tension in the thoracodorsal fascia when it contracts.

Anterior abdominal fascia – test for diastasis of the linea alba

Pregnancy is a common, but not the only, cause for diastasis of the linea alba. The fascial anatomy (see Ch. 4) renders the abdomen vulnerable just below the umbilicus, although separation of the fascia can occur along the entire length of the midline from the pubis to the xyphoid (Fig. 8.51). With the patient in crook lying, palpate the linea alba in the midline. Ask the patient to do a slow curl-up (activate the abdominals anyway the patient knows how) and palpate for separation of the midline fascia. The separation is measured in fingerwidths. According to Sapsford

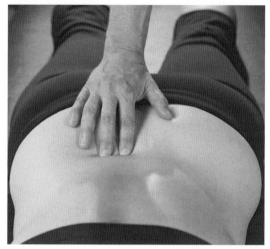

Figure 8.52 Palpation of the deep fibers of the multifidus. In this figure the therapist's index finger is palpating the spinous process and the middle finger is sinking into a "hole" on the right side in the gutter between the spinous process and the transverse process. This hole is due to atrophy of the deep fibers of multifidus. (Reproduced with permission from © Diane G. Lee Physiotherapist Corp.)

et al (1998), it is normal to feel 1–2 cm separation in the linea alba above the umbilicus and less below.

Deep fibers of multifidus

The deep fibers of multifidus are palpated with the patient in prone lying, head in neutral. In the lumbar spine, the "gutter" between the spinous process and the transverse process is palpated (Fig. 8.52). In the pelvis, the deep fibers of the multifidus are palpated just lateral to the median sacral crest. The superficial and lateral fibers of multifidus belong to the global system (Moseley et al 2002) and in the pelvis attach to the posterior iliac crest lateral to the deep fibers (Figs 4.27 and 4.33). Press firmly but gently into the tissue and note the quality of the tissue (firmness) and the size of the muscle. Compare the firmness/size to the contralateral side and to levels above and below. In dysfunction, it is common to find atrophy of the deep (medial) fibers and hypertonicity of the superficial or lateral fibers of multifidus.

Active straight leg raise test

The supine active straight leg raise (ASLR) test (Mens et al 1997, 1999, 2001, 2002) has been validated as a clinical test for measuring effective load transfer between the trunk and lower limbs. When

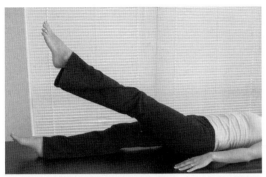

Figure 8.53 An optimal active straight leg raise. The only joint moving is the hip joint. The thorax, lumbar spine, and pelvic girdle remain stable due to co-activation of the local and global systems; this is optimal tensegrity.

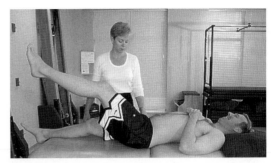

Figure 8.54 Active straight leg raise with loss of lumbopelvic stability – note the abdominal bulging, anterior pelvic tilt, and thoracic extension as well as the extreme effort required to lift the left leg. (Reproduced with permission from © Diane G. Lee Physiotherapist Corp.)

the lumbopelvic-hip region is functioning optimally, the leg should rise effortlessly from the table (effort can be graded from 0 to 5) (Mens et al 1999) and the pelvis should not move (flex, extend, laterally bend, or rotate) relative to the thorax and/or lower extremity (Fig. 8.53). This requires proper activation of the muscles (both in the local and global systems) which stabilize the thorax, low back, and pelvis. Several compensation strategies have been noted (Lee 1999, 2001a, Richardson et al 1999) when stabilization of the lumbopelvic region is lacking. The ASLR test can be used to identify these strategies. The application of compression to the pelvis has been shown (Mens et al 1999) to reduce the effort necessary to lift the leg for patients with pelvic pain and instability. It is proposed (Lee 2002) that by varying the location of this compression during the ASLR (see below), further information can be gained which will assist the clinician when prescribing exercises to improve motor control and stability (see Ch. 10: restoring force closure/motor control).

The supine patient is asked to lift the extended leg off the table and to note any effort difference between the left and right leg (does one leg seem heavier or harder to lift?). The strategy used to stabilize the thorax, the low back, and the pelvis during this task is observed. The leg should flex at the hip joint and the pelvis should not rotate or laterally, anteriorly or posteriorly tilt relative to the lumbar spine (Fig. 8.54 and see Fig. 8.56). The ribcage should not draw in excessively (overactivation of the external oblique muscles) (Fig. 8.55a–c), nor should the lower ribs flare out excessively (overactivation of the internal oblique muscles). Overactivation of the external and internal oblique will result in a braced, rigid ribcage that limits lateral costal expansion on inspiration. The thoracic spine should not extend (overactivation of the erector spinae) (Fig. 8.56), nor should the abdomen bulge (breath-holding: Valsalva) (Fig. 8.57). In addition, the thorax should not shift laterally relative to the pelvic girdle. The provocation of any pelvic pain is also noted at this time.

Simulation of the local system The pelvis is then compressed passively and the ASLR is repeated; any change in effort and/or pain is noted. The location of the compression can be varied to simulate the force which would be produced by optimal function of the local system. Although still a hypothesis, clinically it appears that compression of the anterior pelvis at the level of the ASISs (Fig. 8.58) simulates the force produced by contraction of lower fibers of transversus abdominis and compression of the posterior pelvis at the level of the PSISs (Fig. 8.59) simulates that of the sacral multifidus. Compression of the anterior pelvis at the level of the pubic symphysis (Fig. 8.60) simulates the action of the anterior pelvic floor whereas compression of the posterior pelvis at the level of the ischial tuberosities simulates the action of the posterior pelvic wall and floor. Compression can also be applied to one side anteriorly and simultaneously to the opposite side posteriorly (Fig. 8.61). You are looking for the location where more (or less) compression reduces the effort necessary to lift the leg – the place where the patient notes: "That feels marvelous!"

Simulation of the global system The thorax and pelvis are compressed obliquely to simulate the action of the oblique slings of the global system. Compression of the right anterolateral thorax towards the left side of the pelvis (Fig. 8.62) simulates the action of the left rotators of the trunk which include (but are not limited to) the right external oblique and the left internal oblique. Alternately,

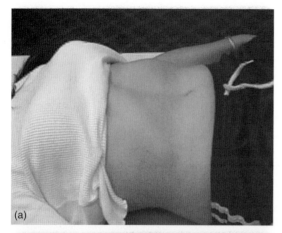

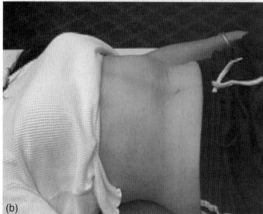

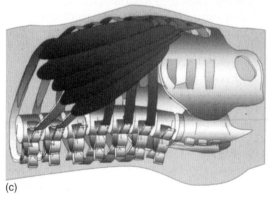

Figure 8.55 Active straight leg raise (ASLR) with excessive activation of the external oblique muscles resulting in narrowing of the infrasternal angle of the ribcage. (a) Abdomen at rest; (b) abdomen during the ASLR: note the narrowing of the infrasternal angle and the transverse abdominal crease which occurs as the thorax flexes relative to the pelvis. (Reproduced with permission from © Diane G. Lee Physiotherapist Corp.) (c) Schematic drawing reflecting the consequences of overactivating the external oblique during loading. Note the depression of the upper abdomen, bulging of the lower abdomen, flexion of the thoracolumbar spine, and posterior pelvic tilt. (Courtesy of Dr. Paul Hodges.)

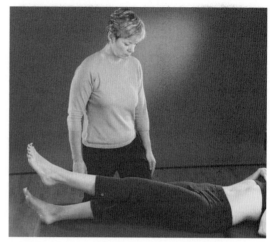

Figure 8.56 Active straight leg raise with excessive activation of the erector spinae causing the thorax to extend relative to the lumbar spine and pelvis. This model has also lost the rotation control of the pelvic girdle (pelvis is left-rotated). A combination of patterns is commonly seen. (Reproduced with permission from © Diane G. Lee Physiotherapist Corp.)

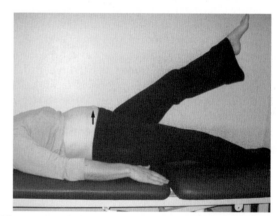

Figure 8.57 Active straight leg raise with excessive abdominal bulging (arrow) and breath-holding: a Valsalva maneuver. (Reproduced with permission from © Diane G. Lee Physiotherapist Corp.)

lengthening of a particular sling may be required. Decompression of the left anterolateral thorax away from the right side of the pelvis (Fig. 8.63) simulates a release of the right rotators of the trunk. Once again, you are looking for the location where more (or less) compression reduces the effort necessary to lift the leg.

Active bent leg raise test

Further analysis of both muscle recruitment and timing is necessary to confirm the findings of the ASLR

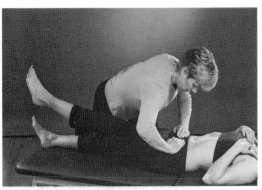

Figure 8.58 Compression of the anterior pelvis at the level of the ASISs simulates the action of the transversus abdominis. (Reproduced with permission from © Diane G. Lee Physiotherapist Corp.)

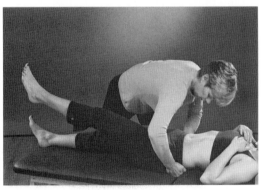

Figure 8.59 Compression of the posterior pelvis at the level of the PSISs simulates the action of the sacral multifidus. (Reproduced with permission from © Diane G. Lee Physiotherapist Corp.)

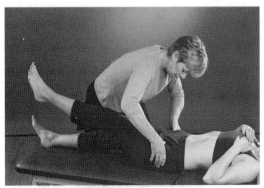

Figure 8.60 Compression of the anterior pelvis at the level of the pubic symphysis simulates the action of the anterior pelvic floor muscles. (Reproduced with permission from © Diane G. Lee Physiotherapist Corp.)

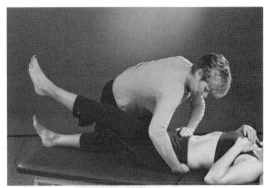

Figure 8.61 Compression of the right anterior pelvis and left posterior pelvis simulates the action of the right transversus abdominis and the left sacral multifidus. (Reproduced with permission from © Diane G. Lee Physiotherapist Corp.)

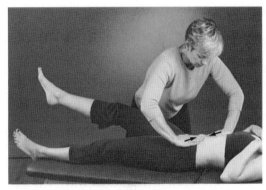

Figure 8.62 Compression applied obliquely between the thorax and pelvis simulates the action of the oblique sling system. The arrows indicate the direction of force applied by the therapist's hands. (Reproduced with permission from © Diane G. Lee Physiotherapist Corp.)

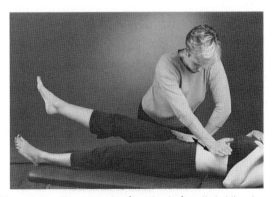

Figure 8.63 Decompression (lengthening) applied obliquely between the thorax and pelvis simulates releasing the oblique sling system. The arrows indicate the direction of force applied by the therapist's hands. (Reproduced with permission from © Diane G. Lee Physiotherapist Corp.)

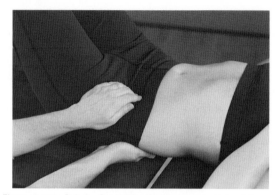

Figure 8.64 Points of palpation for transversus abdominis and multifidus for evaluating co-contraction during low loading. (Reproduced with permission from © Diane G. Lee Physiotherapist Corp.)

and to plan an effective exercise program. With the patient in crook lying, palpate the transversus abdominis deep in the abdomen approximately 2.5 cm (1 in.) medial to the ASIS. When the transversus abdominis contracts, an increase in tension (not bulging) is felt at this point. When the internal oblique contracts, a distinct bulging is felt. With the other hand, palpate multifidus at the level where atrophy was noted (Fig. 8.64). Ask the patient to lift the foot off the table, keeping the hip and knee flexed. Note the impact of this lesser load on the motor control strategy used to stabilize the lumbopelvic region. Note the ability to maintain a stable low back and pelvic girdle and, in addition, note the recruitment pattern of the lower abdominals (deep tension of transversus abdominis versus a fast bulging of internal oblique) and deep (slow tonic swelling) versus superficial (fast phasic bulging) multifidus. Both the local and global systems are required to achieve this task; however, in dysfunction the global system commonly dominates over the local.

Local system: co-contraction analysis

In health, the local system should co-contract in response to a command which begins with intention. This system is anticipatory (for the research, see Ch. 5) and should respond prior to the activation of the global system. Global muscles *do* things (move joints) whereas the local muscles prepare the region for the impending load and respond to the *thought* of doing something. Therefore imagining or thinking about (preparing), but not actually doing a movement, appears to be a more effective way of accessing the appropriate neural pathways to the local system.

With the patient in crook lying, palpate the transversus abdominis deep in the abdomen approximately 2.5 cm (1 in.) medial to the ASIS. With the other hand, palpate multifidus at the level where atrophy was noted (Fig. 8.64). To test the integrity of the neural pathway to transversus abdominis, multifidus, and the pelvic floor the following verbal cues are given and the response of the local system is noted:

1. "Slowly and gently draw your lower abdomen in."
2. "Slowly and gently squeeze the muscles around your urethra as if to stop your urine flow."
3. "Slowly and gently draw your vagina (or testicles) up into your body."
4. "Imagine there is a wire connecting your hip bones anteriorly [ASISs] from the left to right side. Think about generating a force which would draw these two bones together."
5. "Imagine there is a wire connecting your hip bones posteriorly [PSISs] from the left to right side. Think about generating a force which would draw these two bones together."
6. See Chapter 10 for further verbal cues which can help to activate the local system – there are an infinite number, you just have to find the cue that works for your patient!

If the patient is able to connect and to co-contract the muscles of the local system, you should feel a deep, light tension develop in the transversus abdominis and a slow, tonic swelling posteriorly in the deep fibers of multifidus. You should not feel a fast, phasic bulging of the internal oblique, nor a rapid superficial contraction from the superficial fibers of multifidus. The lumbopelvic region should remain still – no motion should be seen. Palpate both sides and look for equal contraction and timing for both sides of the transversus abdominis and multifidus in response to these verbal cues. This is the analysis of the "circle of integrity" (see Ch. 5, Fig. 5.13).

The functional pelvic floor (muscles and the fascia) can only be properly assessed with internal palpation techniques; however, the impact of the functional floor on bladder position and support can be assessed via real-time ultrasound (RTUS) imaging. RTUS (see below) is a useful way to visualize some of the abdominal musculature (internal oblique, transversus abdominis), multifidus, and pelvic floor during verbal cuing (using intention) as well as during functional load transfer activities (ASLR).

If the patient is able to isolate the muscles of the local system appropriately, the endurance of the local system can be assessed. The patient should be able to maintain the co-contraction for 10s repeated 10 times while breathing normally. The co-contraction should also be maintained when loads are added; this ability can be assessed by adding leg loading (i.e., heel slides, hip flexion) while palpating transversus abdominis and multifidus and ensuring that co-contraction is maintained. Further detail regarding loading progressions for assessment and treatment will be covered in Chapter 10.

Local system and the neutral zone

When the force closure mechanism is effective, co-contraction of the muscles of the local system should compress the joints of the lumbar spine (Hodges et al 2003b) and the SIJs (Richardson et al 2002), thereby increasing stiffness. To test the status of the active force closure mechanism, the patient is first instructed to recruit the local system (transversus abdominis, multifidus, and pelvic floor) (see Ch. 10: restoring force closure/motor control). This instruction may take a few sessions to master. Once the patient is able to sustain a tonic co-contraction of the local system, the effect of this contraction on the stiffness of the lumbar zygapophyseal/SIJ is assessed by repeating the form closure tests for translation while maintaining a gentle co-contraction of the local system. The joint stiffness should increase and no relative motion between the innominate and sacrum should be felt (the neutral zone of motion should be reduced to zero). This means that an adequate amount of compression has occurred and the force closure mechanism is effective. If the local system is contracting appropriately and has no effect on the stiffness of the joint, then the active force closure mechanism is ineffective for controlling shear. This is a poor prognostic sign for successful rehabilitation with exercise.

Global system slings: strength analysis

The global system of muscles is essentially an integrated sling system, comprising several muscles, which produces forces. A muscle may participate in more than one sling and the slings may overlap and interconnect depending on the task being demanded. The hypothesis is that the slings have no beginning or end but rather connect to assist in the transference of forces. It is possible that the slings are all part of one interconnected myofascial system and the particular sling (anterior oblique, posterior oblique, lateral, longitudinal), which is identified during any motion is merely due to the activation of selective parts of the whole sling.

The identification and treatment of a specific muscle dysfunction (weakness, inappropriate recruitment, tightness) is important when restoring global stabilization and mobility (between the thorax and pelvis or between the pelvis and legs) and for understanding why parts of a sling may be inextensible (tight) or too flexible (lacking in support). It is important to test for muscle strength and length; the reader is referred to Kendall et al (1993) for a detailed review of how to test specific muscles not covered in this text. Remember, just because a muscle *seems* weak to specific testing does not mean that the muscle *is* weak. It merely implies that the sling is not able to resist the force you are applying and it could be due to weakness (or lack of recruitment) of any muscle along that sling or an insufficient recruitment of the local system.

Four slings specific to the lumbopelvic region are described below. They reflect the anatomical connections observed by Vleeming et al (1995a, b) and are commonly involved in patients with lumbopelvic dysfunction. However, these are not the only slings which require consideration. Remember, the global system of muscles is essentially an integrated sling system, comprising several muscles, which produces forces. A muscle may participate in more than one sling and the slings may overlap and interconnect depending on the task being demanded.

The posterior oblique sling   This sling consists, in part, of the gluteus maximus and the contralateral latissimus dorsi and the intervening thoracodorsal fascia (Fig. 5.15). The lower part of this sling is tested by resisting extension of the leg (Fig. 8.65a). Watch, and feel, for the give in the sling; where the loss of control occurs. The upper part of this sling is tested by resisting terminal elevation of the arm (Fig. 8.65b). Watch, and feel, for the give in the sling; where the loss of control occurs. When the gluteus maximus is weak, the buttock appears flattened and the gluteal fold may be lower on the weak side. The gluteus maximus is specifically tested in the prone position. The patient is asked to squeeze the buttocks together and the ability to do so is palpated. If the patient is able to isolate an effective contraction, he or she is then asked to perform a concentric contraction by extending the femur with the knee flexed (Fig. 8.65c). Resistance is then applied to the extended femur. Careful observation of the effects of this contraction on the position of the lumbar spine

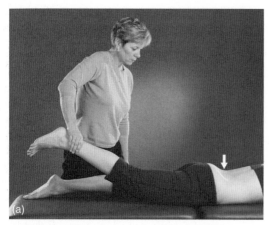

Figure 8.65a Test for the lower part of the posterior oblique sling. Note the loss of control in the lumbar spine (arrow in lumbar spine). (Reproduced with permission from © Diane G. Lee Physiotherapist Corp.)

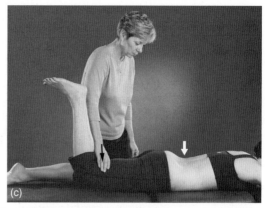

Figure 8.65c Concentric contraction of gluteus maximus in a shortened position. In this model, the gluteus maximus is holding well; however, as noted in Figure 8.65a, her region of give or loss of control is in the lumbar spine (arrow). (Reproduced with permission from © Diane G. Lee Physiotherapist Corp.)

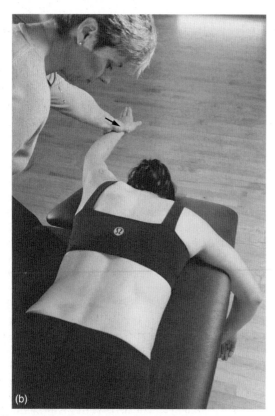

Figure 8.65b Test for the upper part of the posterior oblique sling. The arrow indicates the direction of force applied by the therapist's hand. This model is demonstrating fairly good scapular, thoracic, lumbar, and pelvic control during this test. (Reproduced with permission from © Diane G. Lee Physiotherapist Corp.)

and pelvic girdle gives the examiner further information on muscles in the rest of this sling. It is not uncommon to find positional weakness of the gluteus maximus muscle in patients with a chronically anteriorly rotated innominate. This position lengthens the gluteus maximus muscle and, when this muscle is tested in its shortened position (Fig. 8.65c), a marked weakness will be found and the femur will "give" relative to the pelvic girdle. The latissimus dorsi is isolated by resisting adduction of the extended, medially rotated arm. This muscle tends to tighten or become hypertonic and its length test will be described below.

The anterior oblique sling This sling consists, in part, of the oblique abdominals and the contralateral adductors of the thigh (Fig. 5.16). When the anterior system is weak, the ribcage appears "posteriorly rotated" in standing and extended in supine lying, especially when the trunk is loaded during the ASLR (Fig. 8.56). The anterior slings can be tested bilaterally during a sequenced curl-up (Fig. 8.66). The therapist monitors the infrasternal angle and observes the ability of the patient to flex the thorax sequentially. The patient is then asked to continue flexing the lumbar spine through to a full sit-up. When this sling is weak (or excessively resisted by hypertonicity of the posterior slings), there is an absence of sequential spinal movement (parts of the spine remain extended) and the lower extremities tend to abduct and externally rotate. Unilateral weakness presents as a thoracolumbar rotation (often associated with the lateral shift of the thorax during the curl-up).

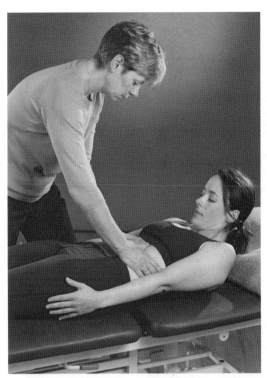

Figure 8.66   A sequenced curl-up tests the oblique abdominal portion of the anterior oblique slings bilaterally. This model was only able sequentially to flex the thorax to the thoracolumbar junction. She was not able to sit up further without extending her thoracolumbar spine. (Reproduced with permission from © Diane G. Lee Physiotherapist Corp.)

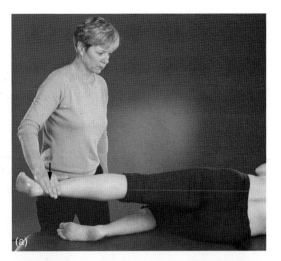

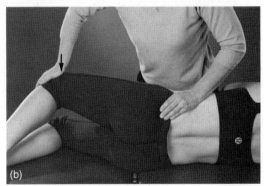

Figure 8.67   (a) Weakness during loading of the lateral sling may be indicative of insufficient recruitment of many muscles: the gluteus medius is one of them. Look and feel for the location of give (spine, pelvis, hip) during this test to gain a clearer understanding of exactly which muscle is at fault. The arrow indicates the direction of force applied by the therapist's hand. (b) The posterior fibers of gluteus medius are palpated during lateral loading of the leg in abduction and external rotation. The arrow indicates the direction of force applied by the therapist's hand. (Reproduced with permission from © Diane G. Lee Physiotherapist Corp.)

The lateral sling   The gluteus medius/minimus and the tensor fascia latae are significant muscles of this sling and work together to stabilize the pelvic girdle at the hip joint. Traditionally, gluteus medius is thought to be an abductor of the hip; however, Gottschalk et al (1989) revisted the anatomy and potential action of this muscle and propose a different functional role. They note that the gluteus medius muscle is comprised of three segments, each with its own innervation. The posterior fibers run parallel to the neck of the femur (horizontal) whereas the anterior and middle fibers are oriented more vertically. Their electromyogram (EMG) studies showed that the three parts of gluteus medius function phasically; the onset of action was sequential from posterior to anterior; the posterior fibers fire first at heel strike while the anterior fibers show the greatest amplitude of activity during stance and single-leg support. They propose that the primary function of the posterior part of the gluteus medius (and the entire gluteus minimus) is to stabilize the femoral head (by compressing it into the acetabulum) during different positions of femoral/pelvic rotation during gait. They also propose that the anterior and middle parts (have a more vertical pull) help to initiate abduction; however, the main abductor of the hip is the tensor fascia latae.

To test the left lateral sling, the patient is right sidelying. The patient is requested to abduct the left leg, maintaining neutral alignment of the lumbar spine, pelvis, and hip (Fig. 8.67a). An adduction force is applied to the limb and the response observed. Watch, and feel, for the give in the sling; where the

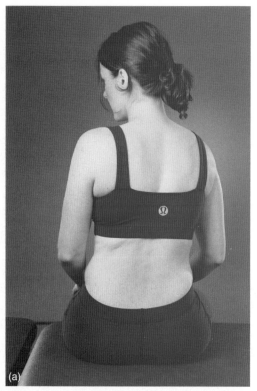
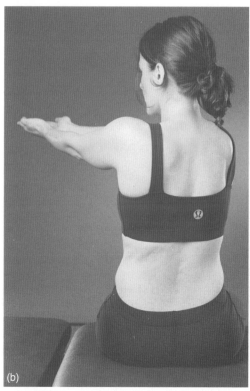

Figure 8.68a, b   Length test for latissimus dorsi and the right posterior oblique sling. (a) The amplitude of left rotation is noted with the arms at the sides. (b) Tension is increased through the right latissimus dorsi by adding flexion, external rotation, and adduction of the shoulders. When tight (or hypertonic), rotation of the trunk will be reduced with the arms maintained in this position. (Reproduced with permission from © Diane G. Lee Physiotherapist Corp.)

loss of control occurs. Look for any compensation strategies which indicate which region is giving way.

To test the posterior fibers of gluteus medius the patient is sidelying with the leg to be tested uppermost. With the knee extended, the hip is positioned in slight extension, abduction, and external rotation. The patient is requested to hold the trunk and the leg still, as support is released. The response is then observed. The patient with weak posterior fibers of gluteus medius will tend to rotate the pelvis backwards to facilitate the use of the tensor fascia latae. Alternatively, the patient may sideflex the spine in an attempt to hold the leg. In both cases, stabilization of the lumbar spine has been lost in an attempt to achieve the task demanded. If the deep fibers of the sacral multifidus are not functional, this test may be positive and yet the posterior fibers of gluteus medius are relatively strong. Alternately, the posterior fibers of gluteus medius are tested as follows. The patient is sidelying with the hips and knees slightly flexed. The patient is instructed to maintain contact between the ankles and then to lift the top knee

(externally rotate the hip). Resistance to external rotation is applied through the lateral aspect of the femur (Fig. 8.67b). When the posterior fibers of gluteus medius are weak, the leg gives way easily and the patient attempts to compensate by rotating the pelvis backwards to facilitate the use of the tensor fascia latae. Alternatively, the patient may sideflex the spine in an attempt to hold the leg. If the deep fibers of the sacral multifidus are not functional, this test may be positive and yet gluteus medius is relatively strong.

Global system slings: length analysis

Muscle shortening can adversely affect the biomechanics of the lumbopelvic-hip region. The muscles which tend to tighten in the presence of dysfunction should be assessed for their extensibility. These muscles include latissimus dorsi, erector spinae, oblique abdominals, hamstrings, psoas major, rectus femoris, tensor fascia latae, short and long adductors, and piriformis/deep external rotators of the hip.

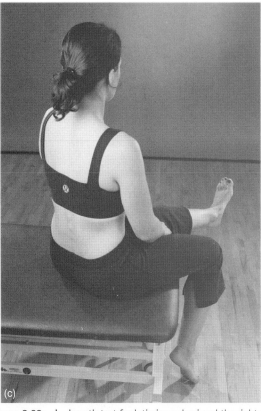 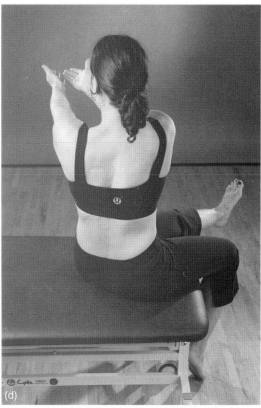

Figure 8.68c, d Length test for latissimus dorsi and the right posterior oblique sling. (c) Extending the left knee while seated increases the tension of the hamstrings. If tight or hypertonic, the pelvis will posteriorly tilt and the lumbar spine will flex to allow full knee extension. (d) The full-length test for the right posterior oblique sling. Note the loss of neutral spine (lumbar spine is flexed, thoracic spine is extended) and the excessive drawing in of the right lower ribcage. All these findings indicate insufficient length of the posterior oblique sling. The spine is responding by buckling. (Reproduced with permission from © Diane G. Lee Physiotherapist Corp.)

The posterior oblique sling and the latissimus dorsi
The patient is sitting in a neutral lumbar spine position with the arms resting by the sides. Instruct the patient to rotate the trunk to the left (Fig. 8.68a) and then to the right and note the quantity and quality of motion through the thoracic and lumbar spine. Subsequently, instruct the patient to flex the arms to 90°, and fully externally rotate and adduct the shoulders such that the hypothenar eminences are approximated. This position increases the tension through the latissimus dorsi muscle. From this position, instruct the patient to rotate the trunk to the left (Fig. 8.68b) and then to the right. The quantity and quality of the motion are noted and compared to that observed with the arms by the side. The motion is markedly reduced in this position when the latissimus dorsi muscle is tight. The length of the full posterior oblique sling can be tested by added tension to the inferior components of the sling. In the sitting position, the patient is instructed to extend the left knee (Fig. 8.68c). The ability to do so without posteriorly tilting the pelvis is observed. From this position, the arms are flexed to 90°, fully externally rotated and adducted, and the trunk is rotated to the left (Fig. 8.68d). This is a full stretch for the right posterior oblique sling.

The anterior oblique sling and the oblique abdominals
In the supine lying position, the relative position of the thorax to the pelvic girdle is noted. When the oblique abdominals are overactive, the lumbar lordosis is absent and the pelvis rests in a posteriorly tilted position. In addition, the infrasternal angle (Fig. 8.69) is narrow either bilaterally or unilaterally. Isolated overactivation of the internal oblique is less common and tends to widen the infrasternal angle.

The longitudinal sling and the erector spinae With the patient sitting, feet supported and the vertebral column in a neutral position, the patient is

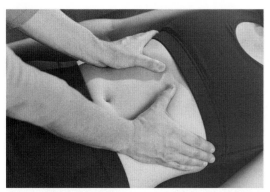

Figure 8.69 Bilateral overactivation of the oblique abdominals will narrow the infrasternal angle. Isolated activation of the internal oblique will widen the infrasternal angle. Asymmetry is common. (Reproduced with permission from © Diane G. Lee Physiotherapist Corp.)

instructed to forward bend. The quantity of the available motion, the symmetry/asymmetry of the paravertebral muscles, and the presence/absence of a multisegmental rotoscoliosis may be indicative of unilateral tightness of the erector spinae muscles.

The longitudinal sling and the hamstrings The extensibility of the longitudinal sling can be assessed in standing (Fig. 8.70a) or sitting (Fig. 8.70b). Optimally, the patient should be able to touch the toes and, with the knees extended, anteriorly tilt the pelvic girdle to at least a 90° angle relative to the femurs. Insufficient extensibility of the hamstrings is a common cause of tightness in this sling. To assess the length of the hamstrings specifically, the patient is lying supine with the lower extremity to be tested flexed at the hip joint to 90°. While maintaining the femur in this position, the knee is extended until the first resistance from the hamstrings is encountered (Fig. 8.70c). Medial and lateral rotation of the lower extremity will bias the test towards the lateral (Fig. 8.70d) or medial (Fig. 8.70e) hamstring. Both the quantity and the end-feel of motion are noted. The test is repeated on and compared to the opposite extremity. What is normal length for a functional hamstring? According to Kendall et al (1993), when hamstring length is measured with the lumbar spine in a neutral position and no motion of the pelvic girdle is allowed, the femur should flex at the hip joint to 70°. Clinically, one needs to consider the patient's functional demands. This quantity of motion would be insufficient for a dancer or for a person who works in repetitive trunk flexion or who drives a car with a low seat. If the patient presents with

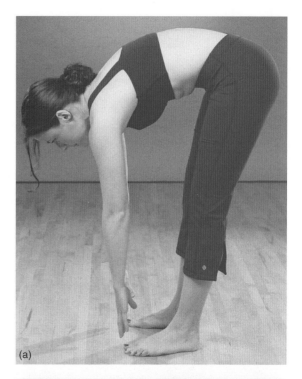

(a)

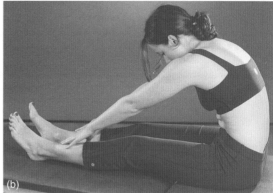

(b)

Figure 8.70a, b Test for extensibility of the longitudinal sling and the hamstrings. (a) In standing and (b) in sitting.

lumbopelvic-hip *pain* and the pain provocation tests have revealed that the pelvic ligaments are a potential source of this pain, then the hamstrings need to be extensible enough to allow full forward bending while maintaining sacral nutation between the innominates. If the biceps femoris is unable to lengthen sufficiently, it will produce a force through the sacrotuberous ligament which resists the sacral nutation. As the innominates continue to flex on the femoral heads a relative counternutation of the sacrum occurs. The SIJ is now vulnerable since it is in a less stable position.

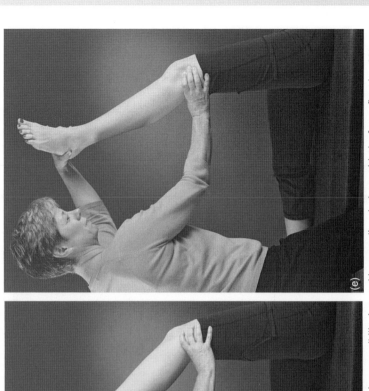

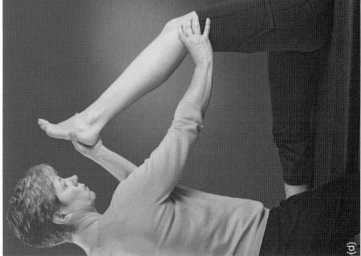

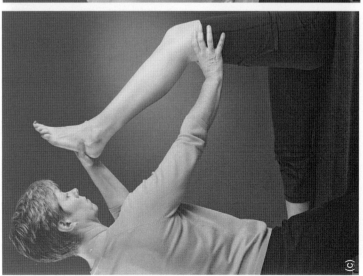

Figure 8.70c, d, e Test for extensibility of the longitudinal sling and the hamstrings. (c) The hamstring extensibility is tested by extending the knee with the femur flexed to 90°. (d) The test can be biased towards the biceps femoris by medially rotating the femur/tibia and (e) towards the medial hamstring group by laterally rotating the femur/tibia. (Reproduced with permission from © Diane G. Lee Physiotherapist Corp.)

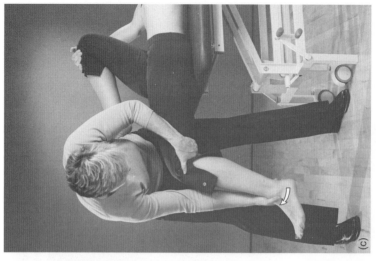

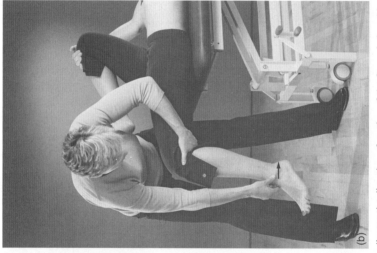

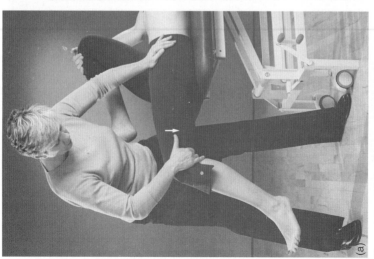

Figure 8.71 (a) Test for extensibility of iliacus. The arrow indicates the direction of motion of the femur induced by the therapist. (b) Test for extensibility of rectus femoris. The arrow indicates the direction of motion of the tibia induced by the therapist. (c) Test for extensibility of the anterior band of the tensor fascia latae. The arrow indicates the direction of motion of the tibia induced by the therapist. (Reproduced with permission from © Diane G. Lee Physiotherapist Corp.)

Iliacus, rectus femoris, tensor fascia latae, adductors
With the patient supine, lying at the end of the table, one femur is flexed and supported against the therapist's lateral thorax. The anterior aspect of the iliac crest and the ASIS of the limb being tested are palpated. With the other hand, the therapist guides the femur into extension, avoiding full knee flexion to test the length of the iliacus muscle (Fig. 8.71a) and then with the knee flexed to test the length of the rectus femoris muscle (Fig. 8.71b). Both the quantity of femoral extension and knee flexion as well as the end-feel of motion are noted. The test is repeated on, and compared to, the opposite extremity.

An inextensible iliacus muscle will restrict extension of the femur regardless of the position of the knee whereas an inextensible rectus femoris muscle will only restrict extension of the femur if the knee is flexed. According to Kendall et al (1993), in this position the thigh should reach the table and the knee should flex to 80°. If the anterior band of the tensor fascia latae muscle is tight, full femoral extension will only occur if the hip is allowed to abduct. In addition, knee flexion with femoral extension results in lateral tibial rotation when the muscle is tight. If the tibial rotation is passively blocked during the test (Fig. 8.71c), knee flexion will be restricted.

The length of the adductors is tested with femoral abduction. The short adductors are tested with the knee flexed (Fig. 8.72), the long adductors with the knee extended. Both the quantity and the end-feel of motion are noted. The test is repeated on, and compared to, the opposite extremity.

Piriformis/deep external rotators of the hip The patient is supine, the lower extremity comfortably flexed at the hip and knee. The lateral aspect of the iliac crest and the ASIS are palpated with the cranial hand, while the caudal hand flexes the femur to 90° of flexion. From this point, the femur is guided into adduction and internal rotation with the caudal hand while the cranial hand monitors the subsequent medial rotation of the innominate (Fig. 8.73). The extensibility of the piriformis muscle has been

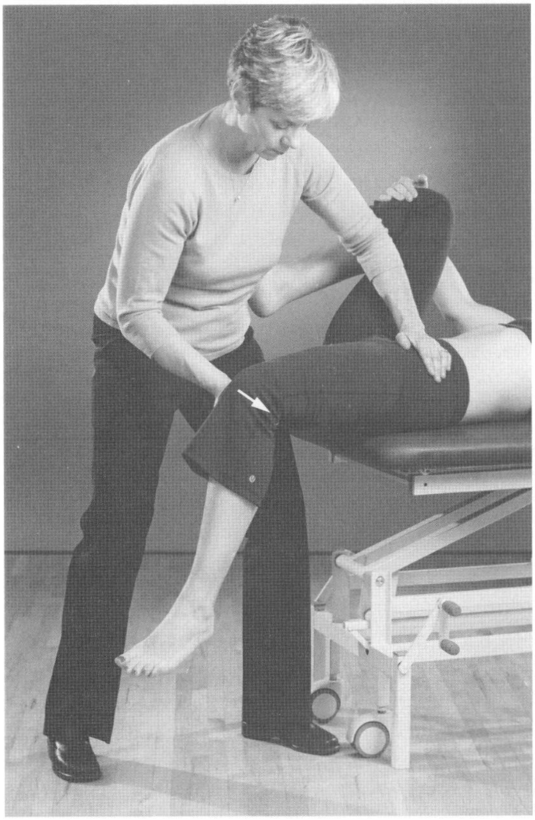

Figure 8.72 Test for extensibility of the short adductors of the thigh. The arrow indicates the direction of motion of the femur induced by the therapist. (Reproduced with permission from © Diane G. Lee Physiotherapist Corp.)

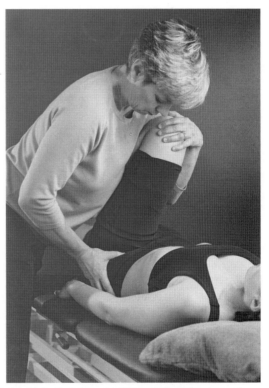

Figure 8.73 Test for extensibility of the piriformis muscle. (Reproduced with permission from © Diane G. Lee Physiotherapist Corp.)

reached when the innominate is felt to rotate medially. Both the quantity and the end-feel of this combined motion (flexion, adduction, and internal rotation) are noted. The test is repeated on, and compared to, the opposite extremity. Piriformis, together with the deep external rotators of the hip (obturator internus, externus, and quadratus femoris), can produce an anterior displacement of the femoral head (Fig. 8.41) such that adduction from the position of 90° of femoral flexion causes marked impingement pain in the groin. In addition, internal rotation from this position can be reduced to 0°. The external rotators are then specifically palpated for tender trigger points. When the ischiococcygeus is hypertonic and supersensitive, the range of motion of the femur is not affected; however, a trigger point can be palpated just inferior to the superior attachment of the inferior arcuate band of the sacrotuberous ligament (Fig. 10.43a). Hypertonicity of the obturator internus (together with piriformis) has a marked impact on the femoral head position and consequently the range of femoral motion. A tender trigger point is often found medial to the inferior attachment of the inferior arcuate band of the sacrotuberous ligament (Fig. 10.45).

Pain provocation tests: contractile lesions

The presence and the location of pain evoked during resistance testing are correlated with the muscle's strength, thus enabling the therapist to reach a diagnosis of muscle "sprain" and/or rupture. Grades 1 and 2 muscle sprains are painfully strong when resisted isometrically, as opposed to grade 3 sprains (i.e., complete ruptures), which are relatively pain-free and weak when resisted isometrically. Of course, there exists an entire spectrum of dysfunction between the two extremes. It must be remembered that contractions of muscles induce compression forces across joints and also increase tension in the various ligaments to which they attach. Therefore, a pain response may not be indicative of a muscle strain at all, but rather the pain may be coming from a joint which reacts to compression or from a ligament which is painful to stretch.

Real–time ultrasound analysis of local system function

Jackie Whittaker

Ultrasound imaging has been established as a safe, cost-effective and accessible method for visualizing and measuring the deep muscles of the trunk (Bernstein et al 1991, Hides et al 1995a, Blaney et al 1999, Bunce et al 2002, Hodges et al 2003a). The local system is comprised of muscles that lie deep inside the body; as such their contraction cannot be viewed directly from the surface. The value of ultrasound imaging is that it allows for dynamic study (real-time images) of these deep muscle groups as they contract (Hides et al 1995b). The complementary use of ultrasound imaging can enhance the clinical analysis of these muscles and has been advocated by various authors (Hides et al 1992, McKenzie et al 1994, Richardson et al 1999, Dietz et al 2001).

RTUS has been used for assessment of four of the local system muscles (McKenzie et al 1994, Hides et al 1995b, Richardson et al 1999, Dietz et al 2001). This section will outline the assessment procedures for three: transversus abdominis, the deep segmental fibers of multifidus, and the pelvic floor. All applications use a diagnostic ultrasound imaging unit set in B-mode (brilliance/brightness) and a 5 MHz curved (convex) array transducer (Fig. 8.74a, b).

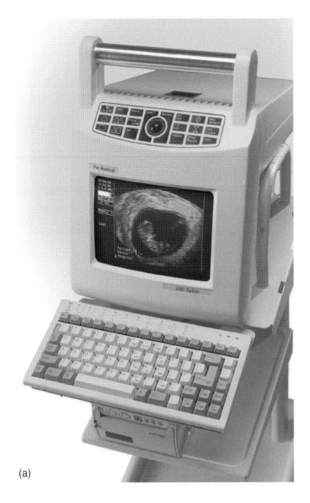

(a)

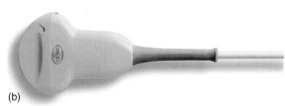

(b)

Figure 8.74 (a) Diagnostic ultrasound imaging unit (Falco model, Esaote Pie-Medical); (b) 5 cm curved array ultrasound transducer.

The use of RTUS for the assessment of the musculoskeletal system requires two steps: image generation and image interpretation (Ch. 10). As with therapeutic ultrasound, sound waves are generated within the transducer and then enter the body through a gelatinous medium. As the waves propagate they encounter and reflect off various tissues. This echo is captured by the transducer and then displayed on a digital screen. The density of the tissue and the angle at which the sound encounters it determine the amplitude of reflection and consequently the brightness of the displayed image. A medium that lacks density, such as fluid (blood, urine), creates minimal reflection and appears black on the screen (see Fig. 8.83a). Denser mediums such as internal organs, periosteum, muscle, and fascia generate greater reflection and appear as varying shades of gray to white (see Fig. 8.76a). Extremely dense mediums such as bones do not permit wave penetration, and reflect 100% of the sound waves at their interface. Consequently they appear as a very bright white outline with a black shadow behind (see Fig. 8.80a).

Despite the density of the medium, the reflection created is largely determined by the angle at which the sound waves encounter the tissue interface. The angle of the transducer, as well as knowledge of the anatomy of the structure being imaged, is critical for successful image generation. Placing the transducer perpendicular to the target tissue will optimize the reflection and enhance the quality of the image; placing the transducer parallel to the target tissue will minimize the reflection and reduce the quality of the image.

Image interpretation is unique for each muscle and will be discussed individually. Further discussion on image interpretation can be found in Chapter 10. The collective objective is to determine if the patient can produce, and maintain, an isolated, isometric, *low-level* contraction which tenses its associated fascia. This suggests that the specific motor control pathway to the target muscle is healthy. Subsequently, RTUS can be used to assess co-contraction within the local system and coordination with respiration.

It is important to understand that the amount of change seen in a muscle's architecture (thickness and length) during a contraction does not represent the intensity or amount of actual muscle activity. Hodges et al (2003a) note that, during an isometric contraction of transversus abdominis and internal oblique, the increase in thickness and decrease in length seen via RTUS has a non-linear relationship to actual muscle activity measured by indwelling electromyography. This study determined that ultrasound is sensitive for low-level contractions (less than 20–30% maximal voluntary contraction) of transversus abdominis and internal oblique. The significance of these findings is that ultrasound imaging cannot be used to discriminate between

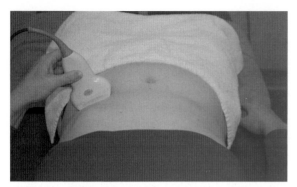

Figure 8.75   Ultrasound transducer placement for imaging the anterolateral abdominal wall.

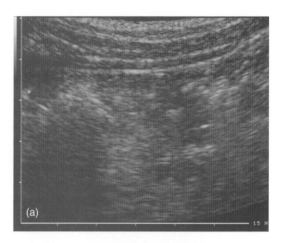

(a)

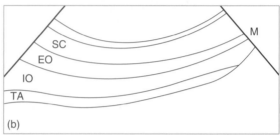

(b)

Figure 8.76   Lateral abdominal wall ultrasound imaging. (a) Resting transverse image of the anterolateral abdominal wall. (b) Labeled outline of the same image. M, midline; SC, subcutaneous tissue; EO, external oblique; IO, internal oblique; TA, transversus abdominis.

moderate and strong contractions. Comparatively, they found no relationship between muscle thickness on ultrasound and EMG activity for the external oblique.

Transversus abdominis

Goal   The primary goal is to determine if transversus abdominis can be activated in isolation from the superficial abdominal musculature (internal oblique, external oblique, and rectus abdominis) and maintained as an isometric, low-level contraction which results in fascial tensioning and co-contraction of other local system muscles (Richardson et al 1999).

Patient position   To standardize the technique and to facilitate access to the abdomen, the supine, crook lying position is used. The abdomen should be exposed from the xiphoid to below the umbilicus (preferably to the symphysis pubis). Realize that this position is not always the optimal position for training transversus abdominis (see Ch. 10).

Ultrasound transducer placement   Place the ultrasound transducer transversely just superior to the iliac crest, on the anterolateral aspect of the abdomen (Fig. 8.75). Manipulate the angle of the transducer until there is a clear transverse image of all three abdominal muscles (Fig. 8.76a, b) and the anterior midline fascial connection of transversus abdominis (Fig. 4.26a, b).

Most transducers have a light or marker on one side that corresponds with a marker on the left side of the ultrasound screen to help orient the viewer. In this application, use the marker to orient patient left (i.e., keep the marker facing the left side of the patient). Adjust the depth control to focus on the more superficial structures such that the muscle layers fill approximately 40–50% of the screen. Due to the curved shape of the ultrasound transducer, mild pressure may be needed to increase the visualized area; adequate use of ultrasound gel increases the area of contact and minimizes this need.

Ideal response   Note the movement of the muscle layers as the patient breathes quietly. Hodges & Gandvevia (2000a) note that activity of the transversus abdominis should be minimal during quiet breathing. They also note that when there is an increase in the chemical drive (increased carbon dioxide levels) or the elastic loading through the thorax (due to a thoracic joint fixation, disease process, or bracing with the global muscles), transversus abdominis is the first abdominal muscle recruited to assist expiration. A modulated contraction of transversus abdominis (or the oblique abdominals) corresponding with expiration is a likely indicator of dysfunction.

After monitoring the abdominal musculature during quiet breathing, the patient is asked to produce a transversus abdominis contraction using one of the following verbal commands:

"Slowly and gently draw your lower abdomen in."
"Slowly and gently squeeze the muscles around your urethra as if to stop your urine flow."
"Slowly and gently draw your vagina (or testicles) up into your body."
"Imagine there is a wire connecting your hips bones anteriorly [ASISs] from the left to right side. Think about generating a force which would draw these two bones together."
"Imagine there is a wire connecting your hip bones posteriorly [PSISs] from the left to right side. Think about generating a force which would draw these two bones together."

An ideal response (Fig. 8.77a) produces a slow and controlled increase in the thickness and decrease in the length of the transversus abdominis with no change in the internal oblique. It is important that the transversus abdominis corsets, or arcs in its lateral aspect, and that the tension in the midline fascia increases as the transversus abdominis slips under the internal oblique (Richardson et al 1999). Correlate the response noted on imaging with that noted on clinical palpation (see section Local system – co-contraction analysis, above).

If an isolated contraction occurs then the patient is asked to repeat the contraction and hold it while breathing normally. Concurrently, the examiner palpates for a co-contraction of the lumbosacral multifidus (Fig. 8.64). This will establish the muscle's endurance capacity, as well as its ability to coordinate and co-contract with the other muscles of the local system.

It is critical that the patient is observed and that the transversus abdominis is palpated during the RTUS assessment. There is a tendency with this technology to focus on the digital screen; RTUS is only an adjunct to the examination process.

Abnormal responses Abnormal responses of transversus abdominis can include an absent or insufficient recruitment with or without substitution of the global system (hypoactive) or an inability to contract in isolation from the global system. The response is often asymmetrical, therefore both sides of the abdomen should be imaged. It is important to note that ultrasound imaging cannot be used to make a conclusion regarding external oblique muscle activity (Hodges et al 2003a) as its thickness

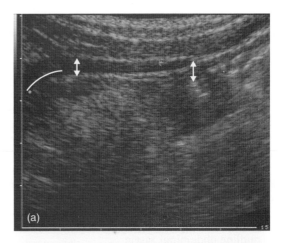

(a)

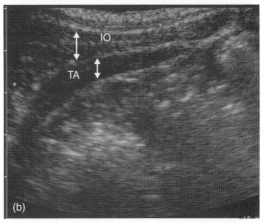

(b)

Figure 8.77 (a) Ultrasound image showing an isolated response of transversus abdominis: note the isolated increase in girth of transversus abdominis (arrows) and lateral corseting as it slides under internal oblique (curved line). (b) Ultrasound image showing a hyperactive response from the anterolateral abdominal muscles: note the increase in girth of both internal oblique (IO) and transversus abdominis (TA).

does not change consistently with muscle contraction. Consequently an increase in activity will require palpation or use of supplementary surface electromyography.

An absent or insufficient response results in ineffective force closure of the lumbopelvic region and is secondary to a deficiency of the contractile component (absent or hypoactive contraction, altered length tension or atrophy), and/or a loss of integrity of the fascial system (diastasis of the linea alba or another breakdown in the "circle of integrity"). When the contractile component is insufficient, the anterior and/or posterior fascia is not sufficiently tensed and little change will be seen between the resting and contracted images.

Co-contraction of transversus abdominis with the oblique abdominals or rectus abdominis (global system) (inability to isolate a separate contraction) results in inappropriate force closure of both the pelvis and thorax. The ultrasound image will demonstrate a concurrent phasic increase in thickness and decrease in length of the transversus abdominis and the internal oblique (Fig. 8.77b). This simultaneous contraction will not produce the slipping of the transversus abdominis and the medial fascia under the internal oblique. In addition, depression of the ribcage towards the pelvis will be observed (thoracopelvic flexion) (Fig. 8.55b).

The midline abdominal fascia

The integrity of the fascial extensions of the local muscles is critical for their function. With respect to the transversus abdominis, it is common to see a loss of the fascial integrity in the linea alba. A quick screen of the integrity of this structure can be made by placing the ultrasound transducer transversely at various sites along the linea alba (Fig. 8.78a). Initially, the width is assessed and then the structure is observed for any widening with activation of the rectus abdominis (i.e., lifting of the head) (Fig. 8.51). Sapsford et al (1998) state that above the umbilicus the width of the linea alba is between 1 and 2 cm, while below it is narrower. A normal linea alba is seen in the ultrasound image in Figure 8.78b. The medial edges of the rectus abdominis muscle come together and resemble "cat eyes." Abnormalities can be structural (loss of fascial architecture: see Fig. 8.78c), and this allows a separation greater than 2 cm between the medial edges of the rectus abdominus, or functional (a separation of the medial edges with activation of the rectus abdominis).

Multifidus

Goal   The goal is to determine if the deep fibers of the lumbar multifidus can be activated in isolation from the superficial fibers and maintained as an isometric, low-level contraction which results in fascial tensioning and co-contraction of other local system muscles.

Patient position   To standardize the technique and to optimize the patient's feedback from the ultrasound screen, the side lying position with the hips and knees comfortably flexed is used. The lumbar spine should be positioned in neutral and, if there is large discrepancy between the hip and waist

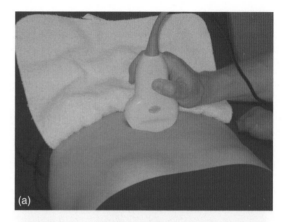

(a)

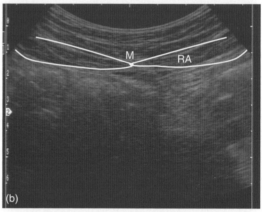

(b)

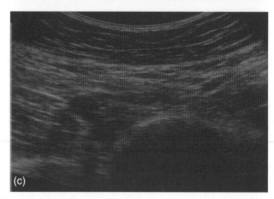

(c)

Figure 8.78   Midline rectus abdominis ultrasound imaging. (a) Ultrasound transducer placement for midline assessment of the rectus abdominis sheath. (b) Normal ultrasound image of the midline rectus abdominis sheath. RA, rectus abdominis; M, midline. (c) Ultrasound image of an abnormal rectus abdominis sheath.

circumference, a folded towel/pillow should be placed at the waist angle. The trunk should be exposed so that the abdomen, lower ribcage, and vertebral column from the mid thoracic spine to the

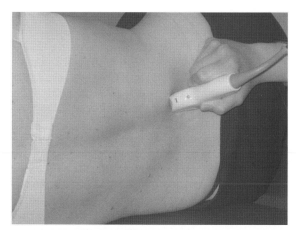

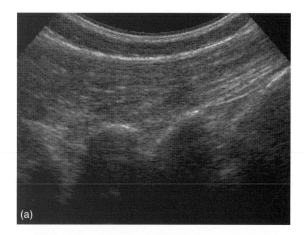

(a)

Figure 8.79 Ultrasound transducer placement for longitudinal imaging of the lumbar multifidus.

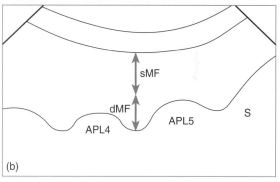

(b)

Figure 8.80 Longitudinal multifidus ultrasound imaging. (a) Longitudinal resting image of lumbar multifidus just lateral to the spinous processes and over the L3–S1 articular column. (b) Outline of the same image. APL4, articular process L4; APL5, articular process L5; S, sacrum; dMF, deep multifidus; sMF, superficial multifidus.

sacrum are visible. Realize that this position is not always the optimal position for training multifidus (see Ch. 10).

Ultrasound transducer placement Place the ultrasound transducer longitudinally just lateral to the spinous processes (over the articular pillar), angled slightly medial. Orient the marker on the transducer (indicating the left side of the screen) towards the patient's head (Fig. 8.79). Manipulate the angle of the transducer until a clear longitudinal view of the lumbar multifidus, sacrum, and articular processes of L5–S1, L4–L5, and L3–L4 is achieved (Fig. 8.80). Once the view is identified, adjust the depth control so that the multifidus and spinal column make up the majority of the image displayed on the screen. The best image of multifidus will be obtained with a linear array transducer of slightly higher frequency (7.5 MHz) (Hides et al 1995a).

The delineation between the deep (local) and superficial (global) fibers of the lumbar multifidus is not as defined as the layers of the abdominal muscles. The deep fibers of multifidus are located near the articular pillar and the superficial fibers are near the top of the screen and the subcutaneous tissue. This delineation will become more obvious as the contraction is observed.

Ideal response The patient is asked to produce a contraction of the deep segmental portion of the lumbar multifidus using one of the following verbal commands:

"Imagine there is a wire connecting your hip bones posteriorly [PSISs] from the left to right side. Think about generating a force which would draw these two bones together."

"Imagine there is a wire connecting your inner thigh (or pubic bone) to your low back [therapist presses deeply over the dysfunctional segment]. Think about generating a force which would draw these two points together."

"Slowly and gently squeeze the muscles around your urethra as if to stop your urine flow."

"Slowly and gently draw your vagina (or testicles) up into your body."

"Imagine there is a wire connecting your hips bones anteriorly [ASISs] from the left to right side. Think about generating a force which would draw these two bones together."

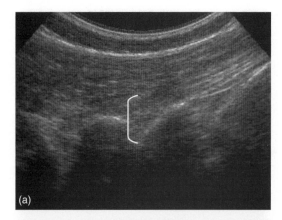

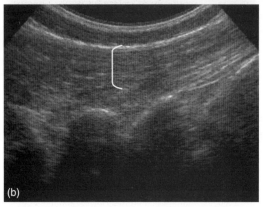

Figure 8.81 (a) Ultrasound image indicating the location for an isolated response of the deep fibers of lumbar multifidus. (b) Ultrasound image indicating the location for a hyperactive response from the superficial fibers of lumbar multifidus.

An ideal response (Fig. 8.81a) produces a slow increase in thickness of the deeper part of the muscle as the fibers increase in girth. Carefully note where the increase in muscle girth occurred (deep versus superficial) as both will increase the thickness; however, only a deep contraction is the ideal response. It is critical that the patient is observed and that the multifidus is palpated throughout the RTUS assessment. There is a tendency with this technology to focus on the digital screen; RTUS is only an adjunct to the objective examination.

If an isolated contraction occurs, then the patient is asked to repeat the contraction and hold it while breathing normally. Concurrently, the examiner palpates for a co-contraction of the transversus abdominis (Fig. 8.64). This will establish the muscle's endurance capacity, as well as its ability to coordinate and co-contract with the other muscles of the local system.

Abnormal responses Abnormal responses of multifidus can include an absent or insufficient recruitment with or without substitution of the global system (hypoactive) or an inability to contract in isolation from the global system. The response can be segmental, multisegmental, or asymmetrical (Hides et al 1994), hence imaging should be repeated at various levels bilaterally.

An absent insufficient response results in ineffective force closure of the lumbopelvic region secondary to a deficiency in the contractile component (absent or hypoactive contraction, altered length tension, or atrophy), and/or a loss of integrity of the fascial system (loss of ligamentous or fascial integrity). When the contractile component is insufficient, the thoracodorsal fascia is not sufficiently tensed and little change will be seen between the resting and contracted images.

Co-contraction of both the deep and superficial fibers of multifidus (as well as the erector spinae) (inability to isolate a separate contraction) results in inappropriate force closure of both the pelvis and thorax. The ultrasound image will demonstrate a concurrent phasic increase in thickness of the entire muscle from the subcutaneous interface to the articular pillar (Fig. 8.81b). In addition, spinal extension will occur.

The pelvic floor

Goal The primary goal is to determine if the pelvic floor muscles can be activated in isolation from the surrounding musculature (glutei, adductors, internal/external oblique, rectus abdominis) and maintained as an isometric, low-level contraction which results in fascial tensioning (capable of supporting the bladder) and co-contraction of other local system muscles.

Patient position To standardize the technique and to facilitate access to the lower abdomen, the patient is supine with the legs straight and the hips relaxed. The patient's abdomen should be exposed from the xiphoid to the symphysis pubis.

Ultrasound transducer placement Assessment of the pelvic floor muscles can be achieved through either a parasagittal or transverse abdominal view of the posteroinferior aspect of a moderately full bladder.

Parasagittal application Orient the transducer in a superolateral to inferomedial sagittal plane on the abdomen just superior to the pubic symphysis, slightly lateral to midline (Fig. 8.82a). Orient the marker on the transducer (indicating the left side of the screen) towards the patient's head. Manipulate

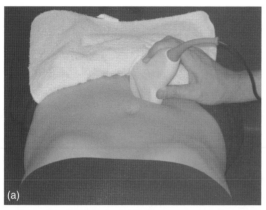
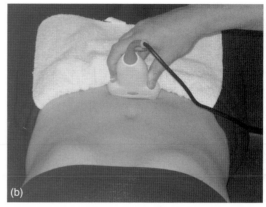

(a)   (b)

Figure 8.82   (a) Ultrasound transducer placement for parasagittal abdominal imaging of the urinary bladder. (b) Ultrasound transducer placement for transverse abdominal imaging of the urinary bladder.

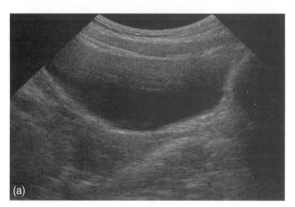
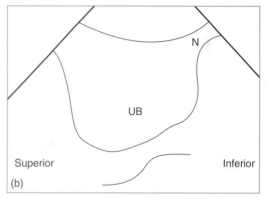

(a)   (b)

Figure 8.83   Parasagittal abdominal ultrasound imaging. (a) Resting parasagittal abdominal image of the urinary bladder. (b) Labeled outline of the same image. UB, urinary bladder; N, neck of the bladder.

the angle of the transducer, pointing it inferior and posterior to the symphysis pubis and until it produces a clear image of the urinary bladder and the urethrovesical neck (Fig. 8.83a, b) (Whittaker 2004).

Transverse application   Orient the transducer transversely across the midline just superior to the pubic symphysis and angle it approximately 60° from the vertical; aim towards the gluteal region (Fig. 8.82b). Orient the marker on the transducer towards the patient's left side. Manipulate the angle of the transducer until there is a clear image of the urinary bladder (Fig. 8.84a, b) (Whittaker 2004).

As with all abdominal imaging, gas (either between the transducer and the skin, or within the abdomen) and/or excessive adipose tissue can interfere with image generation as both scatter the sound waves and obliterate the echo. Care must be taken when generating the image (with adequate

use of gel as well as manipulating the transducer) and in its interpretation.

Ideal response   Once the appropriate image has been generated, the transducer is held steady and the patient is asked to perform a contraction of the pelvic floor muscles (squeeze the muscles around the urethra or lift the vagina/testicles). The bladder is supported by the pelvic floor muscles and the endopelvic fascia (levator plate) (Williams 1995, Ashton-Miller et al 2001). When the pelvic floor muscles contract, there is a consequential tensioning of the endopelvic fascia as well as a broadening of the levator ani muscle. This results in encroachment of the bladder wall which is seen as a slow indentation of its posteroinferior aspect and is accompanied by cranioventral motion of the bladder (Christensen et al 1995, Howard et al 2000, Bo et al 2001, Pranathi Reddy et al 2001, Whittaker 2004) (Fig. 8.85a, b).

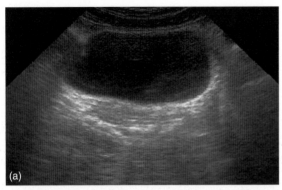
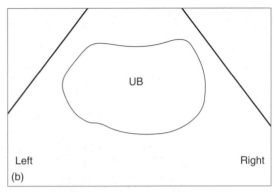

Figure 8.84 Transverse abdominal ultrasound imaging. (a) Resting transverse abdominal image of the urinary bladder. (b) Labeled outline of the same image. UB, urinary bladder.

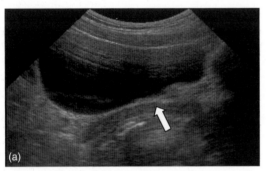
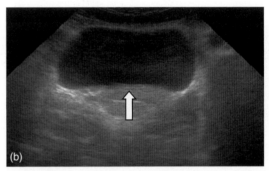

Figure 8.85 (a) Ultrasound image showing an isolated response of the pelvic floor muscles from a parasagittal abdominal view. The arrow notes where the bladder can be seen to indent with a proper pelvic floor contraction. (b) Ultrasound image showing an isolated contraction of the pelvic floor muscles as seen from a transverse abdominal view. Once again, the arrow notes where the bladder can be seen to indent with a proper pelvic floor contraction.

The indentation of the posteroinferior aspect of the bladder can be seen with both the parasagittal and transverse applications; however, Christensen et al (1995) state that the displacement is best seen in the parasagittal plane. The cranioventral motion can only be viewed using the parasagittal technique.

The value of the transverse abdominal view is that it allows for evaluation of both sides of the pelvic floor at once. This is critical as clinical experience has shown that the response is often asymmetrical and, therefore, the parasagittal image should be obtained bilaterally.

If an isolated contraction occurs then the patient is asked to repeat the contraction and hold it while breathing normally. Concurrently, the examiner palpates for a co-contraction of the transversus abdominis (Fig. 8.64). This will establish the muscle's endurance capacity, as well as its ability to coordinate and co-contract with the other muscles of the local system.

Abnormal responses An abnormal response generally involves one of two patterns – absent or insufficient recruitment (hypoactive) of the pelvic floor muscles, with or without an excessive activation of the abdominals resulting in a Valsalva (bearing-down) maneuver. Alternately, an isolated contraction may occur and then fatigue very quickly (lack of endurance). The response is often asymmetrical, therefore both sides of the abdomen should be imaged.

An absent or insufficient response results in ineffective force closure of the lumbopelvic region secondary to a deficiency in the contractile component (absent or hypoactive contraction, altered length tension, atrophy, or impaired nerve supply) and/or a loss of integrity of the fascial system. Several factors can lead to structural deficits in the endopelvic fascia: childbirth, repetitive use of a Valsalva maneuver for load transfer, and surgical procedures. For any of these clinical scenarios, the ultrasound image will be similar to the resting view.

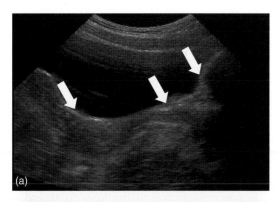

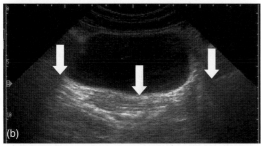

Figure 8.86   (a) Parasagittal ultrasound image of a Valsalva strategy and its influence on the bladder: arrows note motion seen in real time. (b) Transabdominal ultrasound image of a Valsalva strategy and its influence on the bladder: arrows note motion seen in real time.

When the patient uses a Valsalva maneuver (Fig. 8.57), activation of the abdominal musculature results in a caudodorsal motion of the bladder (Fig. 8.86). This may or may not be accompanied by a contraction of the pelvic floor muscles (identified by encroachment of the bladder).

Bladder stability during loading

Goal   The primary goal is to determine if the local system muscles that form the muscular boundaries of the abdomen (the transversus abdominis, the diaphragm, and the pelvic floor) can control the position of the bladder during trunk loading. The position of the patient, transducer placement, and the process of image generation are the same as described for the parasagittal pelvic floor application above. Both sides of the bladder should be assessed.

Ideal response   Once the appropriate image has been generated (Fig. 8.83a) the patient is asked to perform an ASLR (see Ch. 8). Ideally, the local system should co-contract and the bladder remain stationary. Howard et al (2000) demonstrated that some

degree of caudodorsal motion of the neck of the bladder occurs with a cough or Valsalva in both normal and patient populations. Consequently, although the bladder will remain relatively stationary, a small amount of caudodorsal motion should be considered normal.

Abnormal response   Both the literature (O'Sullivan et al 2002) and clinical experience suggest that if the local system fails to act in a coordinated fashion, the most common compensatory motor control pattern will be a Valsalva or bracing strategy. This causes significant caudodorsal motion of the bladder (Fig. 8.86).

Various loading strategies can be used in place of the ASLR: bent knee leg lift, bent knee fall out, arm elevation. In all situations, significant caudodorsal motion of the bladder is considered abnormal.

An unobtrusive method for imaging lumbopelvic muscle function in individuals with low back and pelvic pain has been presented and supported by the existing evidence. Studies are still required in both normal and patient populations to determine reliability, sensitivity, and specificity for lumbopelvic myofascial impairments. Ultimately, the use of real-time ultrasound imaging in conjunction with a vigilant history, physical, and biomechanical examination will result in a more comprehensive assessment of lumbopelvic function in individuals with low back and pelvic pain.

NEUROLOGICAL CONDUCTION AND MOBILITY TESTS

These tests examine the conductivity of the motor and sensory nerves relative to the lumbosacral plexus as well as the mobility of the dura through the intervertebral foramina. The reader is referred to Butler (2000) for a more indepth review of this topic.

Motor conduction tests

The L2 to S2 motor nerve roots are evaluated clinically via the peripheral muscles they innervate. Although there are no true peripheral myotomes in the lower quadrant (one muscle solely innervated by one nerve root), specific muscles known as *key muscles* are primarily innervated by one motor nerve and their function is a reflection of the neurological innervation. Initially, a maximal contraction is elicited from the key muscle and the quantity and quality of strength are compared to the opposite side. If the muscle tests are strong, six submaximal contractions are elicited to detect accelerated fatigability – a common finding of neurological impedance.

The motor nerves and the key muscles which are evaluated include:

L2   psoas major, adductors
L3   adductors, quadriceps
L4   quadriceps, tibialis anterior
L5   extensor hallucis, extensor digitorum, peronei
S1   hamstrings, gastrocnemius
S2   hamstrings, gluteus maximus

Sensory conduction tests

The L1–S2 sensory nerve roots are evaluated clinically via the dermatomes they innervate. Dermatome maps can be confusing since variations in dermatome distribution exist from individual to individual. Furthermore, impedance of sensory conductivity may be reflected in a range of dysesthesia from slight hyperesthesia to complete anesthesia. Detailed examination of the distal extent of the dermatome is useful in detecting early neurological interference. One of the first signs of sensory dysfunction is hyperesthesia within a specific dermatome. This sign tends to occur long before sensation becomes reduced or obliterated completely and its existence is often a surprise to the patient.

Although individual variability is recognized, the following description of dermatome distribution is one commonly seen:

L1   upper posterior buttock, anterior groin
L2   middle posterior buttock, anterior thigh to the knee
L3   lower posterior buttock, anterior thigh to the medial knee and occasionally distal to the medial malleolus
L4   lateral thigh, medial leg, dorsum of the foot to the great toe
L5   lateral leg, dorsum of the foot to toes 2, 3, 4, sole of the foot (excluding the heel) to toes 1, 2, 3
S1   posterior thigh, leg, lateral border of the foot to dorsum and sole, to toes 4 and 5
S2   posterior thigh, leg to heel
S3, S4 perineal region.

Reflex tests

The spinal reflexes are evaluated via the myotactic response to stretch of the key muscle innervated by the root in question. They include the following:

L3, L4   quadriceps (i.e., knee jerk)

L5, S1, S2   gastrocnemius (i.e., ankle jerk).

The integrity of the spinal cord is evaluated by the plantar response test.

Dural/neural mobility tests

The mobility of the dura mater surrounding the L2–S2 nerve roots is evaluated by two tests: the femoral nerve stretch test and the straight leg raise test.

Femoral nerve With the patient prone, the lower extremity is palpated above the ankle. The lower leg is passively flexed at the knee joint and the quantity and end-feel of motion are noted. When the mobility of the dura mater of the L2, L3, and/or L4 nerve roots is restricted, hip extension and knee flexion are restricted by pain felt posteriorly in the lumbar spine.

Sciatic nerve With the patient lying supine, the lower extremity is palpated above the ankle. While maintaining the knee in extension and the femur in slight adduction/medial rotation, the femur is flexed at the hip joint. The quantity and end-feel of motion are noted. When the mobility of the dura mater of the L4, L5, S1, and/or S2 nerve roots is restricted, hip flexion is limited to 30–60° by both pain and muscle spasm.

VASCULAR TESTS

These tests screen the circulatory status of the lower extremity. Careful observation of the skin color, texture, response to dependency and elevation, and the length of time for superficial wounds to heal should be noted. The femoral, popliteal, and dorsalis pedis arteries are palpated and auscultated in the femoral triangle, popliteal fossa, and dorsum of the foot respectively. If a deep vein thrombophlebitis is suspected, the response to passive dorsiflexion of the ankle should be noted (Homans sign) and the region carefully palpated for heat and/or tenderness.

ADJUNCTIVE TESTS

X-rays make good policemen but poor counselors, in that while the straight radiography may exclude serious bone disease and significant mechanical defect, it does not often provide much guidance about how to treat the patient.   (Grieve 1981)

The primary reason for obtaining the results of adjunctive tests is to rule out serious pathology and to

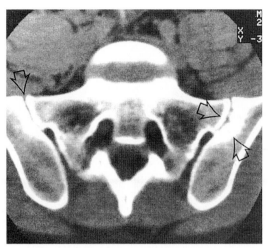

Figure 8.87   A computed tomography scan (transverse plane) of a patient with Reiter's disease. This technique clearly reveals the focal sclerosis (arrows), narrowing, and erosion of the sacroiliac joint associated with this disease. The depth of the joint is clearly visualized.

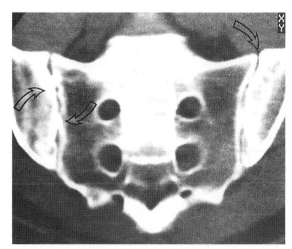

Figure 8.88   A computed tomography scan (vertical plane) of a patient with Reiter's disease illustrating narrowing, erosion, and focal sclerosis (arrows) of the articular surfaces of the sacroiliac joints.

discover the presence of anatomical anomalies prior to treatment.

The adjunctive tests available include the following:

1. radiography (X-rays)
2. diskography
3. myelography
4. radiculography
5. epidurography
6. tomography
7. transverse axial tomography
8. computed transverse axial tomography
9. radiographic stereoplotting
10. interosseous spinal venography
11. cineradiography and fluoroscopy
12. thermography
13. nerve root infiltration
14. electrodiagnosis
15. intervertebral disk manometry
16. cystometry
17. radioactive isotope studies
18. ultrasonography
19. nuclear magnetic resonance.

With respect to the SIJ, Lawson et al (1982) reported on the benefits of computed axial tomography (CT scanning techniques) as opposed to conventional radiography in the detection of mild erosions and narrowing of the joint. Because of the three-dimensional spatial orientation of the SIJ, CT scanning was superior in obtaining visualization of the

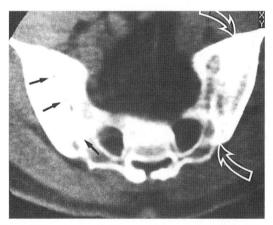

Figure 8.89   A computed tomography scan of a patient with ankylosing spondylitis. Note the total ankylosis of the right sacroiliac joint (open arrows).

joint space. Thus the diagnosis of inflammatory sacroiliitis, which is based on the identification of joint narrowing, sclerosis, ankylosis, or erosion, was facilitated. Figures 8.87–8.91 illustrate the visualization of both the synovial and the ligamentous portions of the SIJ that is possible with this adjunctive test.

CT scanning techniques can reveal congenital and/or acquired anatomical changes in the lumbar spine (Fig. 8.78). The dimensions of the central spinal canal as well as the lateral recess are clearly visualized and often confirm or deny the clinical findings of physical trespass.

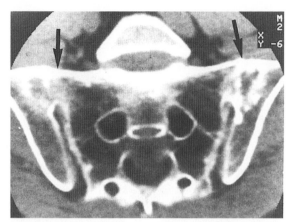

Figure 8.90 A computed tomography scan of a patient with ankylosing spondylitis. Note the bilateral bony ankylosis of the sacroiliac joints. (Figures 8.87–8.90 are reproduced with permission from Lawson et al (1982) and the publishers Raven Press.)

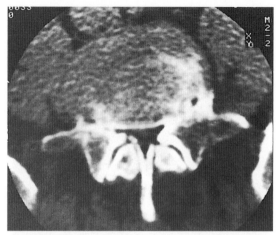

Figure 8.91 A computed tomography scan of the L5–S1 segment illustrating central stenosis secondary to enlargement of the zygapophyseal joints bilaterally. (Reproduced with permission from Kirkaldy-Willis 1983.)

The lumbosacral junction is often the site of congenital anomalies which may or may not be significant to the clinical picture. Their presence, however, should be ascertained. The anomalies which are seen at this level include:

1. asymmetry of the posterior zygapophyseal joints
2. congenital absence of a pedicle
3. accessory laminae
4. osseous bridging of the transverse processes
5. dysplasia or absence of the spinous process of the L5 or S1 vertebrae (spina bifida)
6. dysplasia of the pars interarticularis
7. spina magna of the L5 vertebra
8. trapezoidal L5 vertebra, lumbarized S1 vertebra – partial or complete
9. sacralized L5 vertebra – partial or complete
10. anomalous adventitious joint between the transverse process of the L5 vertebra and the ala of the sacrum
11. asymmetric height of the ala of the sacrum with one side higher than the other, creating a sacral tilt
12. calcified iliolumbar ligament (Grieve 1981).

The findings noted on adjunctive testing of the lumbopelvic-hip complex must be correlated with the findings noted on clinical examination if their significance is to be understood. Rarely can treatment be directed by the results of these tests alone.

Chapter 9

Defining the impairment

CHAPTER CONTENTS

CLASSIFICATION: MEDICAL MODEL

In the medical model, disorders of the low back have been classified (MacNab 1977) as visceral, vascular, neurogenic, psychogenic, sociogenic, and/or spondylogenic in origin. Disorders of the pelvic viscera can refer pain to the lumbar region and are easily confused with benign mechanical dysfunction. Insufficiency of the peripheral vascular system can secondarily give rise to backache and/or symptoms resembling sciatica. Neurogenic disorders include benign and/or malignant tumors of the central or peripheral nervous system. A central lesion at the lumbosacral junction can mimic a cauda equina compression lesion. Pure psychogenic or sociogenic backache is not often seen, although emotional states do play a significant role in the experience of pain (Holstege et al 1996, Butler & Moseley 2003, Hodges & Moseley 2003). Spondylogenic disorders have been further classified (MacNab 1977) as:

1. Pathologic soft tissue and bony
   a. Scheuermann's disease – vertebral osteochondritis
   b. Infective – pyogenic vertebral osteomyelitis
   c. Systemic inflammatory – rheumatoid arthritis, ankylosing spondylitis
   d. Metabolic – osteoporosis, Paget's disease, tuberculosis, Calvé's disease, diffuse idiopathic skeletal hyperostosis (DISH)
2. Traumatic soft tissue and bony
   a. Fractures
   b. Contusions
   c. Spondylolisthesis/spondylolysis

Table 9.1 Conditions affecting the sacroiliac joint (Bellamy et al 1983)

Inflammatory disorders
  Ankylosing spondylitis
  Reiter's syndrome
  Inflammatory bowel disease
  Psoriatic spondylitis
  Rheumatoid arthritis
  Juvenile rheumatoid arthritis
  Pustulotic arthroosteitis
  Familial Mediterranean fever
  Behçet's syndrome
  Relapsing polychondritis
  Whipple's disease

Joint infection
  Pyogenic
  Brucellosis
  Tuberculosis

Metabolic disorders
  Gout
  Calcium pyrophosphate deposition disease
  Hyperparathyroidism

Miscellaneous
  Osteitis condensans ilii
  Paget's disease
  Acroosteolysis in polyvinyl chloride workers
  Alkaptonuria
  Gaucher's disease
  Tuberous sclerosis

Table 9.2 Classification of hip disorders according to age group (Cyriax 1954)

Newborn
Congenital dislocation of the hip

Ages 4–12 years
Perthes disease
Tuberculosis
Transitory arthritis

Ages 12–17 years
Slipped femoral epiphysis
Osteochondritis dissecans

Young adults
Muscle lesions
Bursitis

Adults
Arthritis
  Osteoarthritis
  Rheumatoid arthritis
  Ankylosing spondylitis
Bursitis
Loose bodies

3. Aging, adaptation, degeneration
   a. Arthrosis of the posterior zygapophyseal joints
   b. Spondylosis of the intervertebral disk.

At the turn of this century, practitioners believed that the sacroiliac joint (SIJ) was the major source of sciatica, admitting that, as well as sciatica, "lumbago [and] backache ... were frequently caused by an abnormal amount of motion in the pelvic joints, especially the sacroiliac synchondrosis" (Meisenbach 1911). Aside from trauma, the influence of poor posture as well as lumbopelvic adaptation to extrinsic factors were recognized as being integral to the etiology of decompensation.

The etiology of the pelvic girdle dysfunction is not always clear, but there are many features of definite importance. At times, the lesion apparently represents simply an excess of a normal physiological process. At other times, trauma is a definite factor, "sitting down hard," or the "giving way" under severe strains, such

as lifting, being the two most common forms of injury. Attitudes or postures are also of importance in causing or predisposing to joint weakness or displacement.

(Goldthwait & Osgood 1905)

The causes of mechanical pelvic girdle dysfunction remain the same today. Aside from mechanical impairments, there are a number of systemic diseases which can affect the pelvic girdle. The majority of these are listed in Table 9.1 and the reader is referred to Bellamy et al (1983) for a further description of each.

In the medical model, hip disorders are commonly classified according to the age group in which they occur (Table 9.2) or, alternately, disorders have been classified as articular or non-articular (Table 9.3).

CLASSIFICATION: INTEGRATED FUNCTIONAL MODEL

The medical models of classification rarely enhance the ability of the therapist to treat the patient. Functionally, mobility of the lumbopelvic-hip region can become either restricted or poorly controlled due to either excessive or insufficient articular compression, regardless of the underlying etiology. In keeping with the integrated model of function

Table 9.3 Articular versus non-articular disorders of the hip (Adams 1973)

Articular disorders of the hip
Congenital deformities
Congenital dislocation of the hip
Arthritis
Transient arthritis of children
Pyogenic arthritis
Rheumatoid arthritis
Tuberculous arthritis
Osteoarthritis
Ankylosing spondylitis
Osteochondritis
Perthes disease (pseudocoxalgia)
Mechanical disorders
Slipped upper femoral epiphysis
Osteitis deformans (Paget's disease)
Non-articular disorders in the region of the hip
Deformities
Coxa vara
Infections
Tuberculosis of the trochanteric bursa

(Fig. 5.1), the causes for impairment can be due to dysfunction of:

- form closure (structure)
- force closure (forces produced by myofascial action/inaction)
- motor control (specific timing of muscle action/inaction during loading).

In addition, force closure and motor control can be affected by the emotional state of the patient. This chapter will consider the clinical findings from the subjective and objective examination for specific lumbar, pelvic girdle, and hip impairments according to this model. The chapter will conclude with a discussion of stress urinary incontinence; or ineffective force closure of the urethra.

EXCESSIVE ARTICULAR COMPRESSION

Excessive articular compression can result from articular pathology which:

- ultimately fuses the joint (SIJ – ankylosing spondylitis or DISH)
- causes fibrosis of the articular capsule (secondary to joint sprain) or
- fixates the joint.

In addition, the joints can be compressed by overactivation of muscles which become hypertonic (Janda 1978, Bergmark 1989, Richardson et al 1999) and are often supersensitive (Gunn 1996).

The fused joints cannot be mobilized whereas the fibrosed joints require specific mobilization. Manual therapy techniques (see Ch. 10) help to restore the articular mobility and osseous alignment; motor control retraining is necessary to retain the benefit gained. When the excessive compression is secondary to muscle hypertonicity and supersensitivity, appropriate motor control training which emphasizes optimal stabilization strategies (see Ch. 10) will be required.

THE LUMBAR SPINE

The impact of excessive compression on the structures of the low back has been described and illustrated by Kirkaldy-Willis et al (1978), Kirkaldy-Willis (1983) and Taylor & Twomey (1986, 1992) (Table 9.4). The cause for the joint restriction may be either articular, myofascial, or both and is often the result of an excessive rotation or compression force which exceeded the physiological range of the joint either suddenly (traumatic event) (Farfan 1973, Kirkaldy-Willis et al 1978, Gracovetsky et al 1981, Kirkaldy-Willis 1983, Gracovetsky & Farfan 1986, Twomey et al 1989, Taylor et al 1990, Bogduk 1997) or over time (impact of altered posture) (O'Sullivan et al 2001).

The specific anatomical changes include:

1. synovitis of the posterior zygapophyseal joints (grade 1–2 sprain)
2. minor circumferential tears of the outer layers of the annulus and the associated anterior and posterior longitudinal ligaments (Fig. 9.1)
3. minor joint subluxations (trapped intraarticular meniscoid)
4. end-plate fractures (compression overload) (Farfan 1978, Kirkaldy-Willis 1983, Bogduk 1997)
5. tears of the capsule and ligamentum flavum as well as subchondral fractures of the superior articular process (in more severe injuries) (Taylor et al 1990). These injuries were not evident on X-ray.

Subjective findings

The mode of onset may be either insidious (postural) or sudden (trauma). The pain may be unilateral or bilateral and is usually localized to the low back (region between T12/12th rib and the iliac crest) with

Table 9.4 The degenerative process of the lumbar spine (Kirkaldy-Willis 1983)

ZYGAPOPHYSEAL JOINTS			INTERVERTEBRAL DISK
Synovitis	**DYSFUNCTION**		Circumferential tears
↓			↓
Fibrillation of articular cartilage			Radial tears (herniation)
↓			↓
Capsular laxity and continued cartilage destruction	**INSTABILITY**		Internal disruption
↓			↓
Subluxation →	Lateral nerve entrapment	←	Disk resorption
↓			↓
Enlargement of articular process →	**STABILIZATION**	←	Osteophytosis
	One-level stenosis		
	↓		
	Multilevel spondylosis and stenosis occur as a result of recurrent strains		

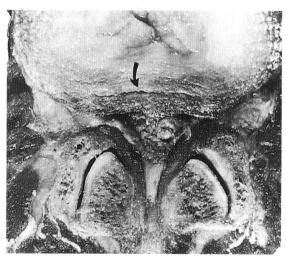

Figure 9.1 A transverse circumferential tear in the annulus fibrosus (arrow).

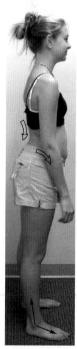

Figure 9.2 This young dancer's posture reflects her muscle imbalance. The tight calves are pulling her legs posteriorly (arrows on leg and foot) (restricting dorsiflexion at the talocrural joint); the dominant erector spinae coupled with a relatively weaker anterior abdominal wall result in an anterior pelvic tilt (arrow on pelvis) and excessive thoracolumbar lordosis (arrow posterior to the lumbar spine). (Reproduced with permission from © Diane G. Lee Physiotherapist Corp.)

occasional radiation to the buttock. Dysesthesia is not often reported. The aggravating activities include the extremes of range of motion (forward/backward bending, rotation), prolonged standing, and lifting. Rest in the supine lying position (knees over a bolster) usually affords relief.

Objective findings

Gait In the first few days after a traumatic injury (substrate phase), the acute patient presents with marked difficulty walking since pelvic rotation beneath the lumbar spine is required for optimal stride length. Once the acute pain has settled, gait may no longer be provocative unless long distances are attempted.

Posture A wide variation of postures will be noted when there is excessive compression of the

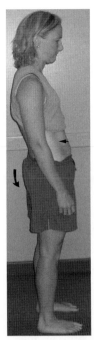

Figure 9.3 This posture reflects overactivation of the internal oblique and lengthening of the external oblique (note the vertical lateral abdominal crease: small arrow), overactivation of the upper portion of the rectus abdominis, coupled with underactivation of the transversus abdominis (depressed upper abdomen and bulging lower abdomen). Note also the lengthening of the erector spinae and the long thoracolumbar kyphosis. The pelvis is posteriorly tilted (curved arrow) and the thighs are displaced anterior to the line of gravity. (Reproduced with permission from © Diane G. Lee Physiotherapist Corp.)

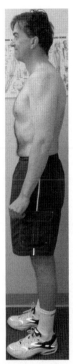

Figure 9.4 When both the abdominal wall and the erector spinae are overactive, bracing occurs. This posture dramatically increases compression through the lumbar spine. (Reproduced with permission from © Diane G. Lee Physiotherapist Corp.)

lumbar spine, pelvic girdle, or hip. In the lumbar spine, overactivation of a segmental muscle may manifest as a segmental rotation in standing which becomes magnified with motion. Regional multisegmental global muscle imbalance is more obvious on postural examination. Four common patterns are:

1. Posterior displacement of the legs relative to the foot (plantarflexion at the talocrural joint) associated with an anterior pelvic tilt and increased thoracolumbar lordosis (Fig. 9.2). Overactivation of the erector spinae coupled with underactivation of the abdominal wall occurs with this postural pattern.

2. Anterior displacement of the legs relative to the foot (dorsiflexion at the talocrural joint) associated with a posterior pelvic tilt and decreased thoracolumbar lordosis (flat back). Overactivation of the anterior abdominal wall (thoracopelvic flexors – external oblique, internal oblique, or rectus abdominis) and lengthening of the erector spinae occur with this postural pattern (Fig. 9.3).

3. Overactivation of both the anterior abdominal wall and the erector spinae (bracing). This pattern of stabilization excessively compresses the lumbar spine without a resultant displacement between the thorax and the pelvis or the lower extremity and the foot (Fig. 9.4).

4. Unilateral overactivation of either of the above muscle groups causes a multisegmental rotoscoliosis of the thoracolumbar spine coupled with a lateral shift of the thorax relative to the pelvis (Fig. 9.5a). Rarely is the asymmetry confined to the vertebral column; intrapelvic torsion of the pelvis and internal rotation of one hip and external rotation of the other are frequently seen with this postural pattern (Fig. 9.5b).

Regional movement tests In the first few days after an injury to the lumbar zygapophyseal joint, the patient with acute symptoms will present with marked restriction of all ranges of motion. The range of motion is bilaterally limited when the sprain is bilateral, and unilaterally limited when the pathology is unilateral. As the acuity of the pain subsides (4–6 days) the pattern of segmental restriction

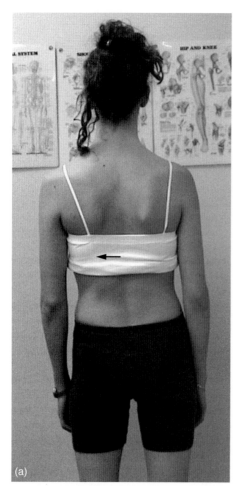
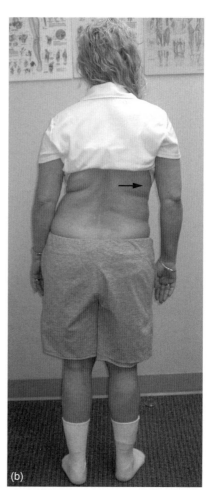

Figure 9.5 Asymmetric activation of either the abdominals and/or erector spinae causes a multisegmental rotoscoliosis of the thoracolumbar spine. This can result in a lateral shift of the thorax relative to the pelvis and lumbar spine (a). The arrow indicates a left lateral shift of the thorax relative to the pelvic girdle. (b) Note the external rotation of the right lower extremity. This is coupled with a left transverse plane rotation of the entire pelvis and right lateral shift of the thorax (arrow). (Reproduced with permission from © Diane G. Lee Physiotherapist Corp.)

becomes more evident and localized to the traumatized joint.

One-leg standing If the restriction involves the L4–L5 or L5–S1 joint, the hip flexion phase of this test may reveal asymmetry since L4 and L5 must be free to rotate to the side of the non-weight-bearing lower extremity (side of hip flexion) during this test. Load transfer during the support phase may be impacted if the pain is severe.

Form closure: positional tests/mobility/stability The severity of the pain usually restricts a detailed form closure analysis in the acute phase; however, with resolution over time, the passive physiological tests for osteokinematic mobility confirm the restricted motion. If restrictive capsular adhesions develop

(fibrotic stiff joint), the neutral zone for arthrokinematic motion of the superoanterior and/or posteroinferior glide will be reduced and the elastic zone will reveal a very firm end-feel. If the joint is compressed by overactivation of the global system (myofascially compressed joint) the neutral zone of motion will also be reduced; however, the elastic zone will feel very resistant (like pushing a boat up a river with a strong current), unlike the firm stop end-feel of a fibrotic, stiff joint. The passive tests for arthrokinetic stability are normal.

Force closure/motor control Several investigators (Hides et al 1994, Danneels et al 2000, O'Sullivan 2000, Hungerford 2002, Moseley et al 2002) have studied the response of multifidus in low back and pelvic pain patients and note that the deep fibers of multifidus become inhibited and reduced in size in these individuals. The atrophy of multifidus can be found both segmentally and multisegmentally. In addition, it is common to find a timing delay or absence of contraction of the transversus abdominis muscle (Hodges & Richardson 1997, Hodges et al 1999, Hodges 2001, 2003) either unilaterally or bilaterally. When the local stabilizing system is ineffective, the active straight leg raise (ASLR) test is positive (Figs 8.55–8.57) and lumbopelvic control is lacking. Palpation of the segmental multifidus and transversus abdominis during the active bent leg raise and also during the co-contraction response to verbal cueing (see Ch. 8) will reveal the individual's specific pattern of local system dysfunction.

A segmental restriction of the lumbar spine can be subclassified according to the position in which the vertebra is held. For example, a flexed L5 vertebra exhibits a bilateral restriction of extension, whereas an extended L5 vertebra exhibits a bilateral restriction of flexion. The unilateral lesions produce a segmental rotation of the vertebra as well as a compensatory multisegmental curve above and below. A flexed, rotated/sideflexed left (FRSL) L3 vertebra exhibits a restriction of extension and right rotation/sideflexion (and sideflexes/rotates left in extension: Fig. 9.6), whereas an extended, rotated/sideflexed left (ERSL) L3 vertebra exhibits a restriction of flexion and right rotation/sideflexion (and sideflexes/rotates left in flexion: Fig. 9.7). Note that this terminology does not identify the cause of the restriction.

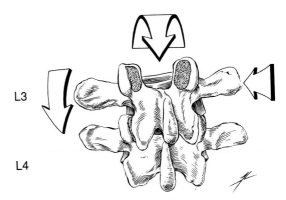

Figure 9.6 Flexed, rotated/sideflexed left L3–L4: left rotates/sideflexes at the limit of extension.

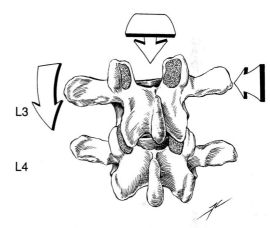

Figure 9.7 Extended, rotated/sideflexed left L3–L4: left rotates/sideflexes at the limit of flexion.

THE PELVIC GIRDLE

Excessive compression of the SIJ can result from systemic articular pathology such as ankylosing spondylitis (fusion) or from mechanical articular pathology which causes fibrosis of the capsule (fibrotic stiff joint). Excessive compression of the SIJ also occurs when there is overactivation of certain global muscles (myofascially compressed joint).

When an individual develops a stabilization strategy that uses predominantly the deep external rotators of the hip joint as well as the ischiococcygeus, the constant activation of these muscles compresses the inferior aspect of the SIJ (butt gripping: Fig. 8.40).

Subjective findings

The mode of onset for the SIJ compressed by fibrosis (stiff) is usually traumatic. The joint stiffens in

response to the joint sprain and the patient usually presents several months later complaining of pain in the opposite SIJ, lumbar spine, or groin. The fibrotic joint is rarely the current source of pain, although patients may report that their symptoms began there.

The mode of onset for the SIJ compressed by myofascia is usually altered motor control patterning. This may be secondary to sports which repetitively induce external rotation of the hip such as ballet, soccer, hockey, or a compensatory strategy which developed subsequent to loss of motor control in the local system. The location of the pain is variable and depends on which tissues are being stressed as a consequence of the altered biomechanics produced by this compression. If the pain is from the SIJ, it will be pelvic pain (within the limits of the iliac crest and gluteal fold) and may radiate down the posterolateral thigh to the knee (Fig. 7.1).

The aggravating activities include walking and any activity which requires intrapelvic torsion.

Objective findings

Gait   When the SIJ is stiff due to capsular fibrosis, the stride length for the hip joint is not affected; however, there is a noticeable lack of intrapelvic motion during gait.

When the SIJ is myofascially compressed by over-activation of the external rotators of the hip joint (Figs 8.40 and 8.41), the individual tends to walk with the legs externally rotated (Charlie Chaplin gait). Since the femoral head is held anteriorly in the acetabulum (Figs 8.41 and 9.8), flexion and extension of the hip joint is limited and the stride length (mid-stance to toe-off) is shortened. The pelvis cannot rotate transversely relative to the femoral head and the pelvis resembles a block moving through space.

Posture   The fibrotic, stiff SIJ is not evident in postural analysis; however, the myofascially compressed SIJ (secondary to overactivation of the external rotators of the hip) has a classic appearance (Fig. 8.40 and see Figs 9.10b and 9.13). Normally, the lumbopelvic region should resemble the shape of a pyramid (Fig. 9.9) with a wide pelvic base narrowing superiorly at the waist. The bilateral "butt gripper" has a buttock which resembles an inverted pyramid (Fig. 9.10a, b) and in standing, a large divot posterior to the greater trochanter can be palpated. These intrapelvic postural changes can occur in addition to the general postural changes noted in the lumbar spine section above (Figs 9.2–9.5). The bilateral "butt gripper" tends to stand with the pelvic girdle posteriorly tilted and the L4–L5 and L5–S1 joints flexed. The unilateral "butt gripper" often stands with a twisted pelvis (intrapelvic torsion) and the L4–L5 and L5–S1 joints tend to rotate away from the side of excessive compression.

Regional movement tests   In both forward and backward bending the fibrotic, stiff SIJ will create an intrapelvic torsion and the asymmetry will be consistent each time the individual moves in the sagittal plane. Axial rotation will be limited towards the side of the restriction and lateral bending will be limited away from the side of the restriction. A SIJ which is myofascially compressed unilaterally by the external rotators of the hip joint will also create the above findings; however, in addition there will be a marked limitation of anterior tilt of the pelvic girdle in forward bending. The apex of the forward-bending curve will be in the thorax (Fig. 9.11).

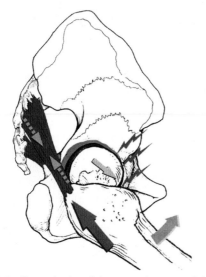

Figure 9.8   Overactivation of the external rotators of the hip joint displaces the femoral head anteriorly in the acetabulum and restricts femoral flexion and extension, as well as anterior rotation of the pelvic girdle. (Reproduced with permission from © Diane G. Lee Physiotherapist Corp.)

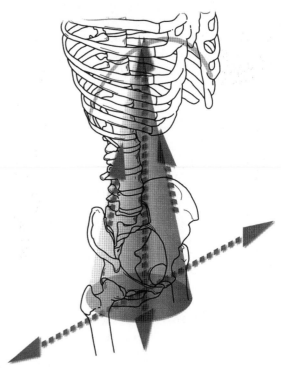

Figure 9.9   The optimal lumbopelvic pyramid. (Reproduced with permission from © Diane G. Lee Physiotherapist Corp.)

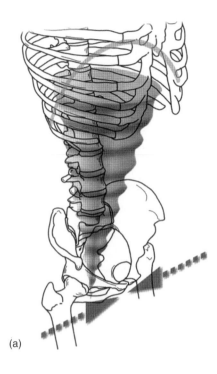

(a)

One-leg standing   In both instances the hip flexion phase of the one-leg standing test will reveal asymmetry of posterior rotation of the innominate. The individual with the fibrotic, stiff SIJ will have no difficulty transferring load through either leg during the support phase; however, the myofascially compressed SIJ may have difficulty transferring load through the hip joint due to the anterior displacement of the femoral head.

Form closure: positional tests/mobility/stability   Both the fibrotic, stiff SIJ and the unilateral myofascially compressed SIJ have a reduced neutral zone of motion (Fig. 8.10c, d) for both inferoposterior glide (anterior rotation of the innominate) and anterosuperior glide (posterior rotation of the innominate); the findings on testing the elastic zone differentiate between the two. The fibrotic, stiff joint has a consistent hard end-feel whereas the myofascially

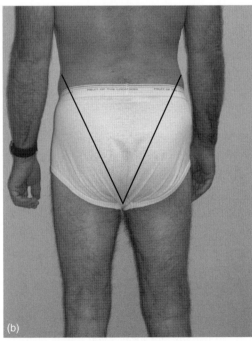

(b)

Figure 9.10   (a) The inverted pyramid. (b) The pelvis appears very compressed inferiorly and resembles the shape of an inverted pyramid. Note the flexion of the lower lumbar segments. (Reproduced with permission from © Diane G. Lee Physiotherapist Corp.)

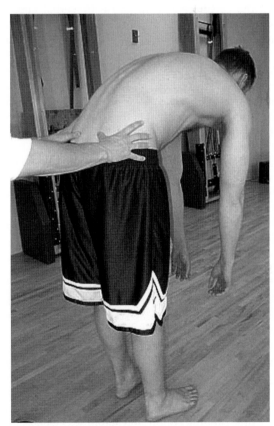

Figure 9.11   This is the pattern of forward bending commonly seen in an individual who cannot release the hip joints to allow the pelvic girdle to tilt anteriorly relative to the femoral heads (butt gripping). Note the open hip angle (minimal hip joint flexion) and the excessive thoracolumbar flexion. (Reproduced with permission from © Diane G. Lee Physiotherapist Corp.)

compressed joint has a muscular resistance feeling. The quality of the end-feel varies with the speed of the test when the compression is due to overactivation of the muscle system. The passive tests for arthrokinetic stability are normal.

Force closure/motor control Often poor motor control accompanies both the fibrotic, stiff SIJ and the myofascially compressed SIJ. The dysfunctional patterns used for lumbopelvic stabilization during the ASLR test are highly variable and may include abdominal bulging and breath-holding (Fig. 8.57), excessive oblique abdominal activation with thoracolumbar flexion and posterior pelvic tilt (Fig. 8.55), excessive erector spinae activation with thoracolumbar extension, and anterior pelvic tilt or lumbopelvic rotation (Figs 8.54 and 8.56). A lateral shift between the thorax and the pelvis may also occur. Palpation of the segmental multifidus and transversus abdominis during the active bent leg raise and also during the co-contraction response to verbal cueing (see Ch. 8) will reveal the individual's specific pattern of local system dysfunction. When the external rotators of the hip are overactive, femoral flexion and adduction combined with internal rotation are markedly limited (Fig. 9.12). Subsequent palpation of the obturator internus and piriformis is required to determine the location of the trigger point. Ischiococcygeus will also compress the SIJ but will not impact the range of motion of the femur.

Real-time ultrasound imaging often reveals the patient's inability to isolate a contraction of transversus abdominis without a co-contraction of the internal oblique (Fig. 8.77b). A marked descent of the bladder is commonly seen when the stabilization strategy is a Valsalva (Fig. 8.86a, b).

THE HIP

The hip joint degenerates secondary to traumatic disruption of the articular surfaces or as a consequence of too much compression during loading. When the hip joint functions with the femoral head anterior in the acetabulum (Fig. 8.41), the afferent input from the mechanoreceptors within the joint capsule can be disturbed. This adversely affects the perceptual component of static joint position, dynamic proprioception, and stability as well as the resting tone of the muscles about the hip joint. The patient may state that the limb feels weak and tends to give way rather than be restricted in range, particularly during athletic endeavors. If the hip is continuously loaded in this non-centered position,

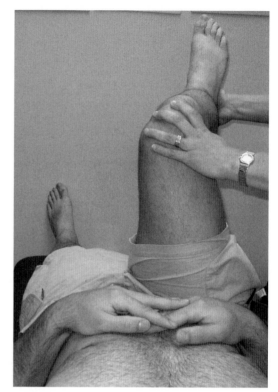

Figure 9.12 When the femoral head is held displaced anteriorly, there will be a marked limitation of femoral flexion combined with adduction and internal rotation. The femoral head impinges on the anterior structures of the hip joint and often causes groin pain. (Reproduced with permission from © Diane G. Lee Physiotherapist Corp.)

and the patient is unable to release the muscles which are holding the femoral head anterior, the range of motion becomes restricted (flexion, adduction, and internal rotation) (Fig. 9.12) and the posterior capsule can become stiff. Over time, degenerative changes of the superoanterior aspect of the joint may result. Excessive compression of the hip may initially be secondary to myofascial causes which ultimately lead to fibrosis of the capsule in the absence of any significant trauma.

Subjective findings

In the early stages, the compressed hip joint which is secondary to muscle imbalance produces symptoms which are usually not local. Even minor restrictions of femoral motion can cause compensatory hypermobility of the SIJ, the lumbosacral junction, and/or the knee/patellofemoral joint and these articulations are more commonly the source of pain. With time,

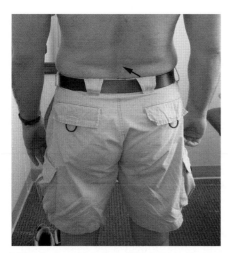

Figure 9.13   Backward bending of the trunk in the presence of restricted femoral extension. This person is butt gripping (note how his shorts go up the gluteal cleft – a sure sign of gripping!) His pelvic girdle is already posteriorly tilted relative to the femoral heads and further backward bending is occurring at the expense of his low back, which is developing a translatoric instability (arrow). (Reproduced with permission from © Diane G. Lee Physiotherapist Corp.)

Table 9.5   Pain patterns in 89 patients with osteoarthritis of the hip joint (Wroblewski 1978)

Area of pain	Number of patients
Greater trochanter	71
Medial buttock	40
Groin	47
Anterior thigh	63
Knee	70
Shin	40

the patient begins to complain of anterior groin pain and impingement with leg crossing. When trauma is not a factor, the onset of symptoms is insidious.

Compensatory pain from the SIJ and/or the lumbosacral junction is aggravated by any activity which requires excessive motion from the low back/pelvis in compensation for restrictions of the femur. For example, backward bending of the trunk often elicits pain at the lumbosacral junction when L5–S1 overextends to compensate for restricted femoral extension secondary to an anteriorly displaced femoral head. Since the pelvic girdle is already posteriorly tilted, further hip extension is not available during backward bending and the L5–S1 compensates (Fig. 9.13).

A painful, long dorsal ligament is aggravated in forward bending of the trunk when biceps femoris cannot sufficiently lengthen. The tension which develops in the sacrotuberous ligament (through the attachment of biceps femoris) prevents the sacrum from remaining nutated relative to the innominate when the pelvic girdle anteriorly tilts in forward bending.

When the hip joint itself becomes symptomatic, the location of pain can be variable. Wroblewski (1978) studied the pain patterns in 89 patients with osteoarthritis of the hip joint and the variation noted is tabulated in Table 9.5. The hip joint, being derived

from the L3 mesoderm, can refer pain anywhere within the L3 dermatome and/or sclerotome.

With moderate articular degeneration, the aggravating activities include walking, stair climbing/descent, and weight-bearing in flexion (i.e., squat). In the early stages, more demanding activities such as sport may be required to aggravate the condition.

Objective findings

Gait   Excessive compression of the hip joint results in decreased mobility and this is reflected in the patient's gait pattern. The stance phase is often shortened, creating a vertical limp. If the altered mechanoreceptor input from the articular capsule significantly alters the strength of the lateral system (stabilizers of the hip), there will be a loss of dynamic stability (force closure) compensated for by a lateral limp (compensated Trendelenburg: Fig. 6.25). The center of gravity deviates laterally in order to reduce the muscle requirements of unilateral stance.

Posture   A wide variety of postures can be found: the butt-gripping posture is very common (Figs 8.40 and 9.13, and see lumbar spine above, Figs 9.2–9.5).

Regional movement tests   When the hip joint is restricted in flexion/extension unilaterally, full forward/backward bending of the trunk produces a rotation of the pelvic girdle on top of the femoral heads as well as intrapelvic torsion. A compensatory, multisegmental rotoscoliosis of the lower lumbar spine also occurs. Lateral bending of the trunk will be restricted such that the pelvic girdle cannot translate in the coronal plane without deviation when abduction or adduction is limited. Axial rotation of the trunk is limited in both directions when the femoral head is compressed anteriorly.

One-leg standing   The hip flexion phase is not impacted unless the range of hip flexion is markedly limited, at which point posterior rotation of the innominate will occur much earlier in the range. The support phase is often positive (the innominate tends to rotate anteriorly) when the femoral head is held anterior since the weight-bearing line is affected.

Form closure: positional tests/mobility/stability   Positionally, the femoral head is easily palpated anteriorly in the groin in both standing and supine lying. The patient tends to stand with the lower extremity externally rotated and the leg rests in external rotation when supine. The passive physiological tests for osteokinematic mobility of the femur reveal the pattern of restriction. The fully established capsular pattern of restriction (Cyriax 1954) of the hip joint is:

1. 50–55° limitation of femoral abduction
2. 0° of femoral medial rotation from neutral
3. 90° limitation of femoral flexion
4. 10–30° limitation of femoral extension
5. femoral lateral rotation and adduction (in supine) is fully maintained.

However, as was previously mentioned, the degenerative process of the hip joint occurs over time such that, in the presence of early pathology, the only objective finding may be a slight limitation of medial rotation, flexion, and adduction in 90° of femoral flexion (positive combined movement test). As the pathology progresses, the full capsular pattern of restriction emerges. Arthrokinematically, the neutral zone of motion is reduced in all directions. The elastic zone analysis helps to differentiate a fibrotic, stiff joint from one which is myofascially compressed. A very hard end-feel is indicative of an articular restriction whereas a softer end-feel is usually muscular. Clinically, the two are usually seen in combination. The torque test may provoke symptoms anteriorly if these structures are painful.

According to Cyriax (1954), all major lesions or serious pathology in the buttock present with:

> an arresting pattern of physical signs that draws immediate attention to the buttock. Passive hip flexion with the knee held extended … is slightly limited and painful. Passive hip flexion, this time with the knee flexed too, is again limited and more painful. Further examination reveals a non-capsular pattern of limitation of movement at the hip joint.   (Cyriax 1954)

The end-feel of motion is empty (i.e., limited by pain) as opposed to that of articular or myofascial tissue resistance. This "sign of the buttock" should alert the examiner to the potential presence of serious pathology such as:

1. osteomyelitis of the upper femur
2. chronic septic sacroiliac arthritis
3. ischiorectal abscess
4. septic bursitis
5. rheumatic fever with bursitis
6. neoplasm at the upper femur
7. iliac neoplasm
8. fractured sacrum.

Force closure/motor control   Janda (1978, 1986) has observed that very early in the degenerative process of the hip joint certain muscle groups respond by tightening (hamstrings, rectus femoris, iliopsoas, tensor fascia latae, adductors, and piriformis) while others respond by becoming weak (gluteus maximus, medius, and minimus). This is one example of changes (lengthening/shortening) in the longitudinal and lateral global sling systems and a wide variety of patterns are observed clinically. The femoral head remains anterior during the ASLR test and posterior rotation of the innominate occurs early in the range (at approximately 50° of femoral flexion).

EXCESSIVE ARTICULAR COMPRESSION WITH AN UNDERLYING INSTABILITY

When a force is applied to the joint sufficient to attenuate the articular ligaments, the muscles will respond to prevent dislocation and further trauma to the joint. The resulting spasm holds (fixates) the joint in an abnormal resting position and marked asymmetry of the bones is present. This is an unstable joint under excessive compression (joint fixation: Fig. 8.10f). Treatment usually requires a high-velocity manipulation technique (see Ch. 10) to distract and reposition the joint. These techniques will reduce the articular compression and restore the resting position of the bones. Repeat analysis of the form closure tests will now reveal a *decrease* in stiffness compared to the opposite side (Fig. 8.10b). Restoration of the force closure mechanism through an appropriate exercise program (see Ch. 10) must follow. This is an impairment of both form and force closure in that the relationship between the articular surfaces has been disturbed and the muscle response is excessive. Treatment of this individual which focuses on exercise without first addressing the posture, position, and alignment of the joint tends to be ineffective and commonly increases symptoms. Conversely, if treatment only includes manual therapy (mobilization, manipulation, or muscle energy) for correction of posture, position, and alignment, relief tends to be temporary and dependence on the health care practitioner providing the manual correction is common. This impairment requires a combination of manual therapy, exercise, and education for a successful outcome – in other words, an integrated approach.

THE LUMBAR SPINE

An intraarticular meniscoid (Fig. 9.14) of a moderately degenerated zygapophyseal joint can become trapped during a flexion/rotation load (lift and twist) in the presence of insufficient stabilization of the joint. The resulting spasm fixates the lumbar segment in what appears to be a "locked" posture and the findings are as follows.

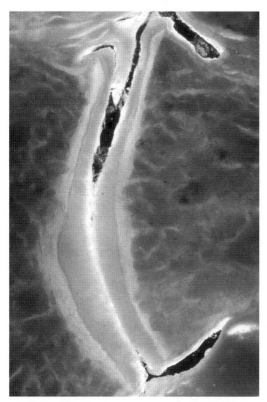

Figure 9.14   This is a coronal section through a lumbar zygapophyseal joint showing a healthy meniscoid inclusion. With degeneration, these inclusions can become thick and fibrotic and occasionally "stuck" outside the joint. The patient then presents with a flexed and laterally translated posture. This beautiful dissection is reproduced with permission from Drs. Lance Twomey and James Taylor, Curtin University.

Subjective findings

The mode of onset is usually sudden: the patient vividly recalls the precipitating event. The pain is often unilateral low back pain which is sharply aggravated by any motion which inferiorly glides the impaired zygapophyseal joint. The patient has great difficulty achieving or maintaining a neutral lumbar spine posture. Over time, the pain may radiate distally down the buttock and posterolateral thigh. Rest in the flexed, laterally translated posture (away from the side of pain) usually affords relief.

Objective findings

Gait   In the first few days after a traumatic injury (substrate phase), the acute patient presents with marked difficulty walking since pelvic rotation beneath the lumbar spine is required for optimal stride length.

Posture   The patient presents with a classic flexed and laterally translated posture. Segmentally, the impaired joint is kyphotic and rotated away from the impaired side. The pelvis is posteriorly tilted and the hip joints flexed.

Regional movement tests   Any attempt to correct the postural deformity meets with marked increase in pain. All movements are painful and limited.

One–leg standing   If the restriction involves the L4–L5 or L5–S1 joint, the hip flexion phase of this test may reveal asymmetry since L4 and L5 must be free to rotate to the side of the posteriorly rotating innominate during this test. Load transfer during the support phase may be impacted if the pain is severe.

Form closure: positional tests/mobility/stability   Positionally, the impaired joint is held in flexion and countralateral rotation (away from the side of pain). Passive osteokinematic mobility tests for extension, sideflexion, and rotation towards the impaired side are restricted. The neutral zone for arthrokinematic motion of posteroinferior gliding is completely blocked (Fig. 8.10f) and the end-feel is springy. Prior to manipulating the joint (see Ch. 10) the tests for arthrokinetic stability are normal since the joint is under excessive compression due to reactive muscle spasm.

Force closure/motor control   The ASLR is positive since further activation of the local and global systems further increases compression and pain. Augmenting the local system with specific compression of the pelvis has no impact on the patient's ability to lift the leg.

THE PELVIC GIRDLE

Subjective findings

The mode of onset is always traumatic and commonly involves a fall on the buttocks (excessive vertical load) or a lifting, twisting event (excessive horizontal load). The pain and inability to load through the pelvic girdle are immediate. The location of the pain is local to the pelvic girdle and usually unilateral (Fortin's distribution (Fortin et al 1994a, b) – within the limits of the iliac crest and gluteal fold) and may radiate down the posterolateral thigh to the knee. After a vertical load injury, the aggravating activities include any weight-bearing through the affected side (standing, walking, sitting). After a horizontal load injury, the aggravating activities include forward bending or rotation. The patient often states that no position affords relief. It is common for them to state that they have "put their hip out."

Objective findings

Gait   These impairments lead to a marked dysfunction of gait. The patient who has sustained a vertical load injury may use crutches or a cane to facilitate load transfer through the pelvis. The patient who has sustained a horizontal load injury walks in a forward-flexed, laterally shifted manner. It is readily apparent to even a casual observer that something is very wrong!

Posture   Vertical shear lesions: the pelvic girdle appears to have been sheared vertically with or without anterior or posterior rotation of the innominate. Horizontal shear lesions: the pelvic girdle appears to have been sheared horizontally with or without anterior or posterior rotation of the innominate or sacral rotation. The lumbar spine and hip joints compensate for this shear such that a multisegmental rotoscoliosis is present in the lumbar spine and the hip posture is in internal/external rotation.

Regional movement tests   In both forward and backward bending the fixated SIJ (vertical or horizontal shear lesion) will create an intrapelvic torsion and the asymmetry will be consistent each time the individual moves in the sagittal plane.

One-leg standing   The hip flexion phase of the one-leg standing test will reveal asymmetry of posterior rotation of the innominate. The fixated SIJ will not permit any posterior rotation of the innominate on the impaired side. Load transfer through

the affected side is significantly impacted in both shear lesions, thus the support phase is positive for failed load transfer.

Form closure: positional tests/mobility/stability   The positional tests differentiate the shear lesions. In the superior vertical shear lesion, the anterior and posterior superior iliac spines, iliac crest, and ischial tuberosity are all cranial on the impaired side. The inferior arcuate band (medial band) of the sacrotuberous ligament is relatively slack on the impaired side. In the horizontal shear lesion, the sacral base and inferior lateral angle are either anterior or posterior on the impaired side (anterior or posterior sacral shear lesion). The passive tests for both osteokinematic and arthrokinematic function reveal a total block to any motion analysis. It is not possible to find the joint plane for testing when the SIJ is fixated. The stability tests are negative until the joint has been decompressed with a manipulative technique. After this, the stability tests reveal an excessive neutral zone of motion in either the vertical or anteroposterior plane (or both).

Force closure/motor control   The patient has marked difficulty lifting either leg when the SIJ is fixated. Augmenting the local system via specific compression of the pelvis often makes the ASLR *more* difficult. After the joint has been manipulated and the underlying instability revealed, specific compression of the pelvis will reveal which part of the local system requires attention for stabilization of the pelvis (see below).

INSUFFICIENT ARTICULAR COMPRESSION

This situation arises when there is either inadequate or inappropriate motor control and/or ligamentous laxity such that there is insufficient articular compression during movement and loading.

THE LUMBAR SPINE

Repeated trauma to the lumbar spine can result in progressive anatomical and physiological changes leading to segmental instability (Table 9.4) (Kirkaldy-Willis 1983, Panjabi 1992a, b, Bogduk 1997). The anatomical and physiological changes include:

1. fibrillation and subsequent loss of the articular cartilage of the zygapophyseal joint(s) (Figs 9.15 and 9.16) (Taylor & Twomey 1986, Bogduk 1997)

2. laxity of the articular capsule(s) and attenuation of the iliolumbar ligament

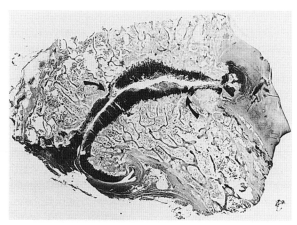

Figure 9.15 Histological section of the zygapophyseal joint. Note the thinning and fibrillation of the articular cartilage (arrows). (Reproduced with permission from Kirkaldy-Willis 1983.)

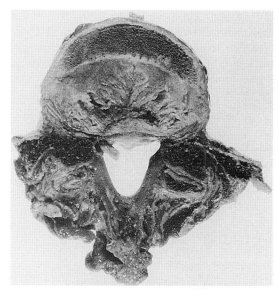

Figure 9.17 Macroscopic transverse section of the L4–L5 segment. Note the coalescence of several radial fissures and the early stages of internal disruption. (Reproduced with permission from Kirkaldy-Willis 1983.)

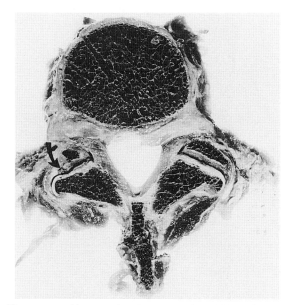

Figure 9.16 Macroscopic transverse section of the L5–S1 segment. Note the marked degeneration of the left zygapophyseal joint (arrow). (Reproduced with permission from Kirkaldy-Willis 1983.)

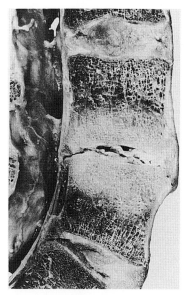

Figure 9.18 Macroscopic sagittal section of the lumbar spine. Note the sclerosis of the vertebral bodies above and below the central intervertebral disk, which is markedly resorbed. (Reproduced with permission from Kirkaldy-Willis et al 1978.)

3. fracture of the articular process with resultant strain deformation of the neural arch (Twomey et al 1989, Taylor et al 1990)

4. coalescence of the circumferential annular tears into a radial fissure (Fig. 9.17) with or without subsequent herniation of the nucleus pulposus, ultimately progressing to marked internal disruption of the disk, loss of disk height, circumferential bulging, and resorption

5. sclerosis of the adjacent vertebral bodies (Fig. 9.18).

At the lumbosacral junction, these anatomical changes allow the superior articular process of the sacrum to sublux upwards and forwards during axial rotation of the trunk (Fig. 9.19). This motion consequently narrows the lateral recess of L5–S1, potentially impeding the vascular and neurological function of the structures within the intervertebral foramen (Sunderland 1978).

With time, the posterior zygapophyseal joints enlarge to develop osteophytes, the intervertebral disk becomes fibrotic, and traction spurs may develop on the anterior and/or posterior aspect of the vertebral body, occasionally leading to spontaneous fusion (Figs 9.20 and 9.21). These changes occur during the third stage of the degenerative process, osseous stabilization, and the patient is often painfree (as well as hypomobile and no longer unstable!) (Kirkaldy-Willis 1983). The risk at this stage is the development of fixed central and/or lateral stenosis due to osseous trespass on the spinal canal and/or lateral recess with attendant peripheral symptoms of neurogenic vascular claudication (Sunderland 1978).

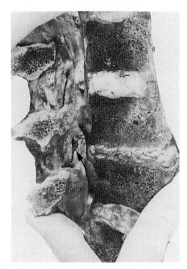

Figure 9.19 Dynamic stenosis of the lateral recess of the lumbosacral junction associated with instability. In this specimen the spinous process of the L5 vertebra has been rotated towards the observer. The zygapophyseal joint has opened (arrow), and the superior articular process has approximated the posterior aspect of the intervertebral disk, subsequently narrowing the lateral recess. (Reproduced with permission from Reilly J et al 1978.)

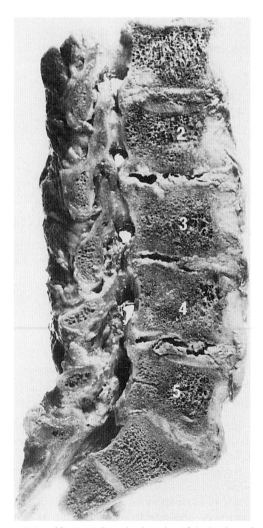

Figure 9.21 Macroscopic sagittal section of the lumbar spine illustrating multilevel spinal stenosis. (Reproduced with permission from Kirkaldy-Willis 1983.)

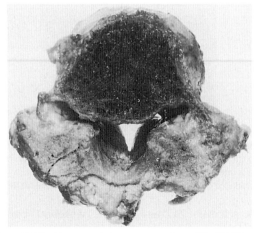

Figure 9.20 Macroscopic transverse section of the L5–S1 segment illustrating fixed central and lateral stenosis. The central and lateral canals are markedly narrowed by osteophytosis. (Reproduced with permission from Kirkaldy-Willis 1983.)

Subjective findings

Clinically, the patient with insufficient articular compression (instability) of a lumbar segment often presents with a long history of intermittent low back pain with repeat episodes of exacerbation and resolution. Alternately, this may be their first episode. The low back pain may be unilateral or bilateral and can refer as far as the distal extent of the segmental dermatome. Dysesthesia is common due to the potential for neurovascular impedance at the intervertebral foramen. The aggravating activities frequently include sustained end-range postures (flexion and/or extension of the lumbar spine with or without rotation) and those activities which induce them (prolonged standing or sitting out of neutral spine, prolonged forward or backward bending of the trunk). Rest in the supine lying position with the knees supported over a bolster usually affords relief. See Tables 9.6–9.9 for findings specific to the segmental impairment.

Objective findings

Gait Walking often relieves the pain as long as the distance attempted is not too far.

Posture/regional movement tests In addition to the general postural changes noted under excessive articular compression: lumbar spine, above (Figs 9.2–9.5), specific segmental deviations from the neutral position can be noted when instability is present in the lumbar spine. O'Sullivan (2000) has developed a very useful way of classifying these instabilities according to the posture/position they present with and the movement that is impaired (see Tables 9.6–9.9). (This is a wonderful article which "rang so true" for me and I highly recommend that every clinician obtain a copy of this paper: O'Sullivan 2000.)

Common to all patient presentations is the reported vulnerability and observed lack of movement control and related symptoms within the neutral zone. This is associated with the inability to initiate co-contraction of the local system within this zone. It appears that these patients develop compensatory movement strategies which "stabilize" the motion segment out of the neutral zone and towards an end-range position (such as flexion, lateral shift or extension). This is achieved by recruitment of global system muscles and by generating high levels of intra-abdominal pressure (bracing) during low load tasks, in what appears to be a sub-optimal attempt to preserve segmental stability.   (O'Sullivan 2000)

Table 9.6 Insufficient articular compression – clinical classification for the lumbar spine (adapted from O'Sullivan 2000)

Flexion pattern – posterior translation instability	
Onset	Flexion/rotation activities, sudden or repetitive
Aggravating activities	Sustained or repetitive flexion (shoveling, gardening, rowing, etc.)
Posture	Loss of segmental lordosis which is accentuated in sitting. Posterior pelvic tilt in sitting. Increased tone in the erector spinae in the lower thorax and upper lumbar spine
Regional movement tests	Hinging at unstable segment increases in forward bending. May require the use of the hands to forward bend and/or return to erect standing. Decreased segmental extension in backward bending Unable to achieve a neutral spine position in standing, sitting, or four-point kneeling
Form closure tests (mobility/stability)	PIVM – increased osteokinematic flexion and rotation at unstable segment PAVM – increased arthrokinetic anteroposterior translation with associated increase in the neutral zone and a softer end-feel in the elastic zone
Force closure and motor control tests	ASLR – loss of lumbopelvic control – pelvis tends to rotate to the side of elevating leg. No change in effort when compression is applied to the pelvis (to simulate the local system) unless the unstable segment is L5–S1 ABLR – palpable atrophy of multifidus bilaterally at the unstable segment Unable to co-activate transversus abdominis with multifidus Variable compensatory strategies – often tend to brace low back into flexion using external and internal obliques and erector spinae. This compresses the low thorax, preventing lateral costal expansion breathing (especially anterior)

PIVM, passive intervertebral movment; PAVM, passive accessory vertebral movement; ASLR, active straight leg raise; ABLR, active bent leg raise.

Table 9.7 Insufficient articular compression – clinical classification for the lumbar spine (adapted from O'Sullivan 2000)

Extension pattern – anterior translation instability	
Onset	Extension/rotation activities, sudden or repetitive
Aggravating activities	Sustained or repetitive extension (standing, throwing, running, dancing, swimming, etc.)
Posture	Increased segmental lordosis. Anterior pelvic tilt in standing. Increased tone in the erector spinae in the entire thoracolumbar spine
Regional movement tests	Hinging at unstable segment increases in backward bending associated with a loss of segmental extension at levels above instability. Often an obvious skin crease at unstable segment
Form closure tests (mobility/stability)	PIVM – increased osteokinematic extension and rotation at unstable segment PAVM – increased arthrokinetic posteroanterior translation with associated increase in the neutral zone and a softer end-feel in the elastic zone
Force closure and motor control tests	ASLR – loss of lumbopelvic control – pelvis tends to rotate to the side of elevating leg. No change in effort when compression is applied to the pelvis (to simulate the local system) unless the unstable segment is L5–S1 ABLR – palpable atrophy of multifidus bilaterally at the unstable segment. Unable to co-activate transversus abdominis with multifidus Variable compensatory strategies – often tend to brace low back into extension using the erector spinae. This compresses the low posterior thorax preventing lateral costal expansion breathing (especially posterior). Ribcage appears elevated when the patient lies supine

PIVM, PAVM, ASLR, active straight leg raise; ABLR, active bent leg raise.

Table 9.8 Insufficient articular compression – clinical classification for the lumbar spine (adapted from O'Sullivan 2000)

Lateral shift pattern – lateral translation instability	
Onset	Rotation injury usually in flexion
Aggravating activities	Sustained or repetitive rotation even in neutral
Posture	Loss of segmental lordosis which is accentuated in sitting. Posterior pelvic tilt in sitting with a relative lateral shift of the trunk relative to the pelvis. Increased tone in the erector spinae unilaterally
Regional movement tests	Deviation of the trunk laterally through the mid-range of forward bending Marked lateral shift of the trunk during one-leg standing
Form closure tests (mobility/stability)	PIVM – increased osteokinematic rotation at unstable segment PAVM – increased arthrokinetic lateral translation and unilateral posteroanterior translation with associated increase in the neutral zone and a softer end-feel in the elastic zone
Force closure and motor control tests	ASLR – loss of thoracopelvic control – tend to shift the thorax laterally relative to the pelvic girdle during elevation of the leg. No change in effort when compression is applied to the pelvis (to simulate the local system); however, there is often a reduction in effort when the thoracopelvic shift is manually controlled ABLR – palpable atrophy of multifidus unilaterally at the unstable segment Unable to co-activate transversus abdominis with multifidus unilateral pattern Variable compensatory strategies – often tend to brace low back into rotation and sideflexion using quadratus lumborum, superficial erector spinae on ipsilateral side of the shift

PIVM, PAVM, ASLR, active straight leg raise; ABLR, active bent leg raise.

Table 9.9 Insufficient articular compression – clinical classification for the lumbar spine (adapted from O'Sullivan 2000)

Multidirectional pattern	
Onset	Multiple recurrent episodes of trauma with increasing levels of disability after each episode
Aggravating activities	Everything – no weight-bearing position is tolerable
Posture	Vulnerable to lock in flexion, extension, or lateral shift position
Regional movement tests	All range of motion is decreased in every direction. All movement is associated with spasm and sharp pain
Form closure tests (mobility/stability)	Difficult to assess accurately – all passive movements, whether angular or translatoric, are associated with marked spasm and pain
Force closure and motor control tests	ASLR – marked difficulty lifting the leg at all, may not be able to perform test Compression often increases pain ABLR – palpable atrophy of multifidus bilaterally, often multisegmentally Unable to activate transversus abdominis or multifidus. Marked substitution with the global system Magnetic resonance imaging – often reveals excessive fatty infiltration of multifidus (Fig. 9.25)

PIVM, PAVM, ASLR, active straight leg raise; ABLR, active bent leg raise.

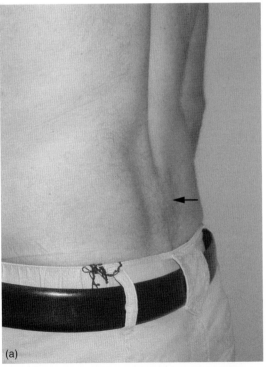 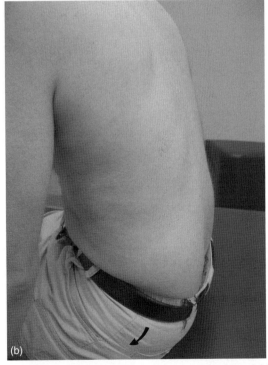

(a) (b)

Figure 9.22 A patient with a segmental flexion instability at L5–S1. Note the segmental kyphosis at L5–S1 in standing (arrow) (a) and its accentuation in sitting (b). In addition, note the posterior pelvic tilt (arrow) and loss of the lumbar lordosis in sitting.

An individual with a *flexion* instability presents with a segmental kyphosis (Fig. 9.22a) which is exaggerated in flexion (forward bending). The segmental kyphosis is also evident in sitting (Fig. 9.22b) and four-point kneeling and the individual tends to rotate the pelvis posteriorly and extend the upper lumbar and lower thoracic spine in both positions.

An individual with an *extension* instability presents with an excessive segmental lordosis which is exaggerated in extension (backward bending) (Fig. 9.23). The pelvis can be either anteriorly tilted (Fig. 9.23a, b) or posteriorly tilted (Fig. 9.13) and remain there during backward bending. The upper lumbar spine and lower thorax often remain flexed during backward bending such that the motion hinges around the unstable segment.

A unilateral flexion instability results in a segmental *lateral shift*. The segment is kyphotic and shifted laterally (Fig. 9.24). The lateral shift becomes exaggerated during the one-leg stand test and other unilateral loading tasks – see below (O'Sullivan 2000).

The segment which is unstable in multiple directions (*multidirectional instability*) is severely impaired. Excessive segmental translation is evident in all movement directions and establishing control is difficult.

When a lumbar joint is unstable, the osteokinematic motion often couples with an unphysiological arthrokinematic glide. For example, flexion is normally coupled with anterior translation. When the segment is unstable, it is not uncommon to see flexion couple with posterior translation and extension couple with anterior translation (Fig. 9.13: note the skin crease). Typically, an individual with a flexion instability forward-bends by walking the hands down the thighs (Fig. 9.25) and back up to return to erect standing. An individual with a painful extension instability backward-bends by flexing at the talocrural joints, avoiding all extension! The less painful patient may extend the low back, maintaining either an anteriorly or posteriorly tilted pelvic girdle. In this situation, a deep skin crease appears at the unstable level (usually L4 or L5).

One-leg standing The lateral shift instability becomes more evident during single-leg loading (Fig. 9.26a, b). With respect to intrapelvic motion, the hip flexion phase of this test is not often impaired or asymmetric in the presence of a lumbar segmental instability; however, the support phase is often positive. Lumbar segmental instabilities dramatically impact the function of the deep fibers of multifidus

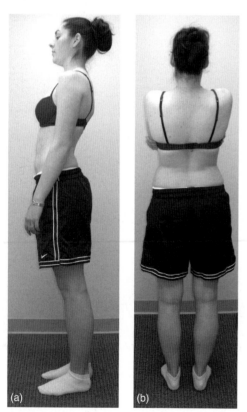

(a)   (b)

Figure 9.23   (a, b) A patient with a segmental extension instability. Note the hinging of the thorax in the mid lumbar region and the maintenance of the anterior pelvic tilt during backward bending.

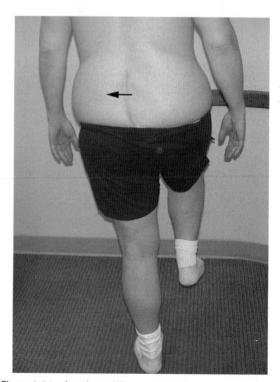

Figure 9.24   A patient with a segmental lateral translation instability to the left at L4–L5.

and this impairment is often multisegmental. If the sacral fibers of multifidus are impaired, then force closure of the posterior pelvis is reduced, leading to a loss of the self-bracing mechanism for load transfer through the pelvis (see The pelvic girdle, below).

Form closure: positional tests/mobility/stability   In the neutral resting position (lying prone) the positional fault noted in standing (posture) may or may not be evident. The passive osteokinematic tests of mobility (PIVMs) reveal the relative excessive angular motion (flexion/extension); the arthrokinematic tests reveal a relatively larger neutral zone of motion and the elastic zone is often "softer." Pain may or may not be provoked at the end of the elastic zone depending on the irritability of the local tissues. The passive tests for arthrokinetic stability reveal the direction of the translatoric instability (excessive anterior, posterior, lateral translation, or rotation).

Force closure/motor control   At the impaired segment, the atrophy of the deep fibers of multifidus is readily palpated. Figure 9.27 is a magnetic resonance

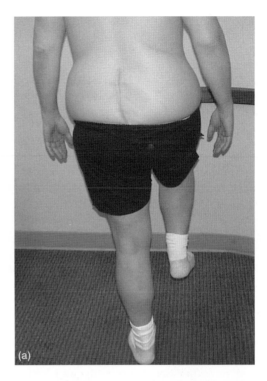

(a)

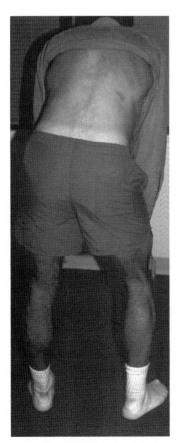

Figure 9.25   A patient with a segmental flexion instability typically forward-bends by walking the hands down the thighs.

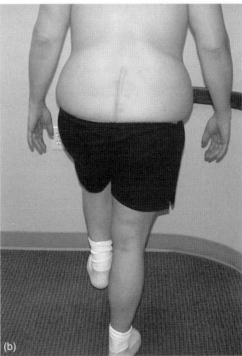

(b)

Figure 9.26   A patient with a postsurgical segmental lateral translation instability at L4–L5. Note the left lateral shift of the segment during (a) the left one-leg standing test. He is able to retain a vertical orientation of his trunk to his pelvis during (b) the right one-leg standing test.

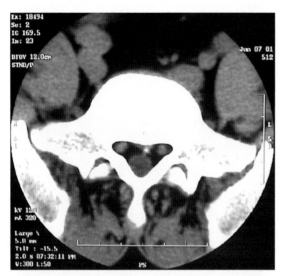

Figure 9.27 A magnetic resonance image of the lumbosacral junction. Note the dark "holes" in the deep fibers of multifidus. This is likely due to fatty infiltration of the muscle.

imaging image which shows marked fatty infiltration of the multifidus in an individual who demonstrated multidirectional instability at L5–S1. The impaired function of multifidus often coexists with a timing delay or absence of co-contraction of the transversus abdominis unilaterally or bilaterally. The ASLR test is positive and lumbopelvic control is lacking. The dysfunctional pattern used for lumbopelvic stabilization is highly variable and may include abdominal bulging and breath-holding, excessive oblique abdominal activation with thoracolumbar flexion and posterior pelvic tilt, excessive erector spinae activation with thoracolumbar extension, and anterior pelvic tilt or lumbopelvic lateral tilt and/or rotation. Palpation of the segmental multifidus and transversus abdominis during the active bent leg raise and also during the co-contraction response to verbal cueing (see Ch. 8) will reveal the individual's specific pattern of local system dysfunction. If the local system is functioning optimally and the force closure mechanism is intact, the neutral zone of motion can be stabilized (reduced to zero). If the local system is functioning optimally and the force closure mechanism is *not* intact, the neutral zone of motion will remain excessive. This is a poor prognostic sign for successful rehabilitation through exercise.

Neurological tests Impedance of neurological function (motor, sensory, reflex) and neural mobility can occur with this impairment since the translatoric instability can interfere with the dimensions of

the lateral recess. The relevant dural/neural mobility test would then be positive. The spectrum of neurological impedance is variable and depends on the degree of pathology. The patient may present with minimal motor weakness or sensory dysesthesia in the early stages, and later with a complete motor nerve block and sensory anesthesia. Careful objective evaluation is mandatory to detect the early neurological decompensation.

THE PELVIC GIRDLE

Repetitive trauma to the pelvic girdle can also result in anatomical changes which lead to instability of the SIJs and pubic symphysis. Unlike the lumbar spine, very little anatomical research has been done to document the structural changes which occur with insufficient articular compression of the pelvic joints. The consequences of the hormonal changes of pregnancy have been discussed in Chapter 6. See Tables 9.10–9.12 for findings specific to each impairment.

Subjective findings

The SIJ and/or pubic symphysis can become unstable due to pregnancy, major trauma, minor repetitive trauma, or as a consequence of compensating for hypomobility of the hip or contralateral SIJ. Consequently, the history can be quite variable. The pelvic pain is often, though not always, unilateral in Fortin's distribution (Fortin et al 1994a, b) and can refer distally to the knee. The aggravating activities frequently include unilateral weight-bearing (vertical instability), bending forward or lifting (horizontal instability), lying supine (especially if the long dorsal ligament is a pain generator), and rolling over from this position. The most comfortable position for the painful SIJ is sidelying in the semi-Fowler position with the painful side uppermost. Comfort is enhanced with a body pillow that allows the flexed hip and knee to be supported.

Objective findings

Gait The displacement of the center of gravity is exaggerated when the SIJ is unstable. The patient attempts to compensate for the lack of stability by reducing the shear forces through the SIJ. In the compensated gait pattern, the patient transfers his or her weight laterally over the involved limb (compensated Trendelenburg sign), thus reducing the vertical shear forces through the joint (Lee 1997a)

Table 9.10   Insufficient articular compression - clinical classification for the sacroiliac joint (SIJ)

Vertical pattern – craniocaudal instability – SIJ	
Onset	Sudden or repetitive vertical loading through the lower extremity or ischial tuberosity
Aggravating activities	Sustained vertical loading (sitting, walking, standing, etc.)
Posture/gait	Unequal loading through the lower extremities. Compensated or true Trendelenburg gait
Regional movement tests	Intrapelvic asymmetry produced during forward bending; however, this finding may be inconsistent when repeated. One-leg standing – hip flexion phase reveals asymmetric motion between left and right sides. Support phase – may have great difficulty weight-bearing unilaterally and when this is possible, the patient is unable to force close the SIJ such that the innominate rotates anteriorly relative to the sacrum and flexes at the hip joint
Form closure tests (mobility/stability)	PIVM – increased osteokinematic innominate rotation on side of instability PAVM – increased arthrokinetic craniocaudal translation of the SIJ with associated increase in the neutral zone and a softer end-feel in the elastic zone
Force closure and motor control tests	ASLR – loss of lumbopelvic control – tend to rotate to side of elevating leg. May have marked difficulty lifting leg off the table. Effort decreases when compression is applied to pelvic girdle, often both anterior and posterior ABLR – palpable atrophy of sacral multifidus unilaterally. Unable to co-activate transversus abdominis with multifidus. Variable local system dysfunction and variable compensatory strategies

PIVM, PAVM, ASLR, active straight leg raise; ABLR, active bent leg raise.

Table 9.11   Insufficient articular compression – clinical classification for the sacroiliac joint (SIJ)

Horizontal pattern – anteroposterior instability – SIJ	
Onset	Traumatic – lifting/twisting injury
Aggravating activities	Sustained forward bending
Posture/gait	Pelvis appears twisted – sacrum appears rotated in standing such that the inferior lateral angles are not level. Minimal intrapelvic motion during gait
Regional movement tests	Intrapelvic asymmetry produced during forward bending; however, this finding may be inconsistent when repeated. Patients tend to walk with their hands down the thighs and back up to return to standing. One-leg standing – hip flexion phase reveals asymmetric motion between left and right sides. Support phase – may have great difficulty weight-bearing unilaterally and when this is possible, the patient is unable to force close the SIJ such that the innominate rotates anteriorly relative to the sacrum and flexes at the hip joint
Form closure tests (mobility/stability)	PIVM – increased osteokinematic sacral nutation/counternutation on side of instability PAVM – increased arthrokinetic anteroposterior translation of the SIJ with associated increase in the neutral zone and a softer end-feel in the elastic zone
Force closure and motor control tests	ASLR – loss of lumbopelvic control – tend to rotate to side of elevating leg. May have marked difficulty lifting leg off the table. Effort decreases when compression is applied to pelvic girdle, often best posterior ABLR – palpable atrophy of sacral multifidus unilaterally. Unable to co-activate transversus abdominis with multifidus often unilaterally. Variable local system dysfunction and tend to compensate by activating piriformis and ischiococcygeus, which may excessively compress the joint: the underlying stability is only revealed once these muscles are released

PIVM, PAVM, ASLR, active straight leg raise; ABLR, active bent leg raise.

Table 9.12   Insufficient articular compression – clinical classification for the pubic symphysis

Vertical pattern – craniocaudal instability – pubic symphysis	
Onset	Trauma or pregnancy
Aggravating activities	Sustained vertical loading (sitting, walking, standing, etc.), or abduction/external rotation of the hip. Rolling over in bed and/or getting out of a car are two common aggravating activities
Posture/gait	Unequal loading through the lower extremities. Compensated or true Trendelenburg gait
Regional movement tests	Intrapelvic asymmetry produced during forward bending; however, this finding may be inconsistent when repeated. One-leg standing – hip flexion phase reveals symmetric motion between left and right sides. Support phase – may have great difficulty weight-bearing on either leg and when this is possible, the patient is unable to force close the pubic symphysis such that the innominate rotates anteriorly relative to the sacrum and flexes relative to the femur bilaterally
Form closure test (mobility/stability)	PIVM – increased osteokinematic innominate rotation on both innominates PAVM – increased arthrokinetic craniocaudal translation of the pubic symphysis with associated increase in the neutral zone and a softer end-feel in the elastic zone. This lesion is often associated with marked local pain
Force closure and motor control tests	ASLR – loss of lumbopelvic control – tend to rotate to side of elevating leg. May have marked difficulty lifting leg off the table. Effort decreases when compression is applied anteriorly to pelvic girdle at the level of the pubic symphysis ABLR – multifidus is often normal; however, the co-activation of the pubococcygeus and transversus abdominis is lacking. May or may not be associated with a diastasis of the linea alba

PIVM, PAVM, ASLR, active straight leg raise; ABLR, active bent leg raise.

(Fig. 6.25). In the non-compensated gait pattern, the patient tends to demonstrate a true Trendelenburg sign (Fig. 6.26). The pelvic girdle adducts excessively (on the unstable weight-bearing side). The femur abducts relative to the foot, thus bringing the center of gravity closer to the SIJ, and reduces the vertical shear force.

Posture   In standing and sitting, the patient tends to adopt a resting posture which unloads the affected SIJ.

Regional movement tests   In forward bending, inconsistent findings prevail. During one test, asymmetry (intrapelvic torsion) may be present. In the next, it may be absent and in a subsequent test the asymmetry may return. This is consistent with ineffective force closure of the pelvic girdle. If the sacrum is unable to stabilize between the innominates all movements may be inconsistently affected with or without pain.

One-leg standing   Hungerford (2002) investigated the osteokinematic and arthrokinematic motion of the innominate relative to the sacrum in both men and women who clinically manifested signs of failed load transfer through the pelvis (ineffective force closure). For inclusion in this study the subject had

to meet the following criteria:

1. unilateral pelvic pain which was aggravated by vertical loading activities
2. positive forward bending test in standing (intrapelvic torsion)
3. positive hip flexion phase of the one-leg standing test (asymmetry of motion between sides)
4. positive ASLR
5. asymmetric stiffness values for the SIJs on joint play testing.

Hungerford noted the following:

1. Hip flexion phase: posterior rotation of the innominate occurred on the non-weight-bearing side (side of hip flexion) and was associated with an anterosuperior arthrokinematic glide (Fig. 6.11). An asymmetric amount of movement occurred between the two sides and the unstable side did not always present with the greatest amount of movement in this test. This finding confirms Sturesson et al's impression (2000) that this test should not be used to determine mobility of the SIJ.

2. Support phase: *anterior* rotation of the supporting innominate occurred on the weight-bearing side

(side away from hip flexion) and was associated with an *inferior* and posterior arthrokinematic glide of the innominate relative to the sacrum (Fig. 6.14). This suggests that there was insufficient compression to effectively "lock" the SIJ during load transfer. In a previous study of normal subjects, Hungerford (2002) found that the innominate posteriorly rotated relative to the sacrum and glided posteriorly and *superiorly* during weight-bearing (see Ch. 6).

Form closure: positional tests/mobility/stability   In the absence of a fixation of the SIJ, the positional findings are often unremarkable. The passive osteokinematic tests of mobility (PIMVs) reveal asymmetric angular motion for anteroposterior rotation of the innominate and/or nutation/counternutation of the sacrum; the unstable side has relatively more motion. The arthrokinematic tests reveal asymmetry of neutral zone motion (less stiff on the unstable side). The end-feel of the elastic zone is often softer and pain may or may not be provoked depending on the irritability of the local tissues. The passive tests for arthrokinetic stability of either the SIJ or the public symphysis reveal the direction of the translatoric instability (excessive horizontal or vertical translation).

Force closure/motor control   Force closure of the pelvic girdle relies on optimal function of the deep fibers of the sacral multifidus, transversus abdominis, and the pelvic floor. Dysfunction of the local system (e.g., linea alba diastasis, atrophy of the deep fibers of multifidus, timing delay, or absence of recruitment of transversus abdominis and the pelvic floor) can be found in any combination and create subtle malalignment (Schamberger 2002) (anterior/posterior innominate rotation, inflare/outflare of the innominate, sacral torsions – forward or backward). The ASLR test is positive and lumbopelvic control is lacking. The dysfunctional pattern used for lumbopelvic stabilization is highly variable and may include abdominal bulging and breath-holding, excessive oblique abdominal activation with thoracolumbar flexion and posterior pelvic tilt, excessive erector spinae activation with thoracolumbar extension, and anterior pelvic tilt or lumbopelvic lateral tilt and/or rotation. Palpation of the segmental multifidus and transversus abdominis during the active bent leg raise and also during the co-contraction response to verbal cueing (see Ch. 8) will reveal the individual's specific pattern of local system dysfunction. If the local system is functioning optimally and the force closure

mechanism is intact, the neutral zone of motion can be stabilized (reduced to zero). If the local system is functioning optimally and the force closure mechanism is *not* intact, the neutral zone of motion will remain excessive. This is a poor prognostic sign for successful rehabilitation through exercise.

Neurological tests   It is common to see loss of function of the L5 and S1 nerve roots when the SIJ has been unstable for some time.

Table 9.13 summarizes the findings, impairment classification and subsequent treatment requirements for dysfunction according to the integrated model of function.

INSUFFICIENT URETHRAL COMPRESSION: STRESS URINARY INCONTINENCE

Urinary incontinence (UI) is defined as the involuntary leakage of urine which is objectively demonstrable. Stress urinary incontinence (SUI: leakage which occurs during physical exertion) is the most common type. Urge urinary incontinence (UUI) is defined as leakage which is precipitated by a sudden strong urge or desire to void and often occurs along with SUI (mixed or MUI). According to DeLancey (1994):

> During a cough urethral closure pressure is known to rise simultaneously with abdominal pressure to keep the urethra closed in spite of great increases in intravesical pressure. Stress urinary incontinence occurs because this normal transmission of abdominal pressure to the urethra is lost.

Essentially, ineffective force closure of the urethra and failed load transfer through the organs of the pelvis lead to SUI. How common is this? The prevalence of this condition varies according to age, study design, and definition. Ashton-Miller et al (2001) state that 8.5–38% of women experience SUI. Nygaard et al (1994) note that this condition is not limited to women bearing children and that in a study of 144 nulliparous female athletes aged 18–21 years, 28% suffered from SUI. Bo & Borgen (2001) found that 41% of elite female athletes experience SUI. Carriere quotes Fantl et al (1996) and states that incontinence affects four out of 10 women, about one out of 10 men, and about 17% of children below the age of 15.

Clearly, this is a significant problem but is it a *different* problem than a loss of effective force closure of the musculoskeletal elements of the pelvis? It is common to hear women complain of both low back

Table 9.13 Impaired lumbopelvic-hip function

	Excessive articular compression	
	Articular pathology causing capsular fibrosis – unilateral	Overactivity of global system – unilateral

Functional findings	Forward bend test – asymmetric
	One-leg standing
	  Hip flexion – asymmetric
	  Support – variable
		Forward bend test – asymmetric
		One-leg standing
		  Hip flexion – asymmetric
		  Support – improper patterning

Form closure findings	↓ Active + passive osteokinematic motion ↓ Arthrokinematic motion ↓ Neutral zone　Hard end-feel elastic zone 　　　　　　　Consistent – does not 　　　　　　　vary with speed	↓ Active + passive osteokinematic motion ↓ Arthrokinematic motion ↓ Neutral zone　Resistant elastic zone 　　　　　　　Resistance varies with 　　　　　　　speed of test
Force closure motor control findings	ASLR – effort to lift leg increases when compression applied to pelvis	ASLR – effort to lift leg increases when compression applied to pelvis
Treatment	Passive articular mobilization Sustained grade 4	Neuromyofascial release • muscle energy • functional • trigger point release • IMS acupuncture Restore local + global system function

ASLR, active straight leg raise; IMS, intramuscular stimulation.

and pelvic pain as well as UI and therapists commonly note that treating one component often impacts the other. Minimal research has been done on the correlation between the two functional impairments. In reviewing the literature, it appears that Panjabi's stability model (Fig. 5.3) can be applied to the urethra as well as to the musculoskeletal system.

URINARY CONTINENCE

In an excellent review article, Ashton-Miller et al (2001) clearly explain the mechanism by which continence is achieved during physical exertion. Essentially, continence relies on optimal function of two systems – the urethral support system and the sphincteric closure system.

Urethral support system

The structures which provide support for the urethra include:

• the passive system: this includes the endopelvic fascia which is anchored to a thick fascial band called the arcus tendineus fasciae which arises from

Table 9.13 *Cont'd*

	Insufficient articular compression	
Joint fixation	Articular pathology causing ligamentous laxity – unilateral	Underactivity of local system

Forward bend test – asymmetric
One-leg standing
  Hip flexion – asymmetric
  Support – unable to weight bear
    through affected side
	Forward bend test – inconsistent + variable
	One-leg standing
	  Hip flexion – asymmetric
	  Support – improper patterning
		Forward bend test – inconsistently variable
		One-leg standing
		  Hip flexion – varies
		  Support – varies
		Consistent finding is inconsistency

Marked positional changes ↓ Active + passive osteokinematic motion Blocked neutral zone Can't find joint plane to test elastic zone	↓ Active osteokinematic motion ↑ Passive osteokinematic motion ↑ Arthrokinematic motion ↑ Neutral zone Soft non-resistent end feel in elastic zone	↑ Active + passive osteokinematic motion ↑ Arthrokinematic motion ↑ Neutral zone Normal elastic zone
ASLR – marked difficulty to lift leg + effort dramatically increases when compression applied to pelvis	ASLR – effort to lift leg dramatically decreases when compression applied to pelvis often anywhere	ASLR – effort to lift leg decreases when compression specifically applied to pelvis to simulate where more compression is needed
Articular distraction manipulation Re-evaluation usually reveals an underlying instability (see lig laxity)	Prolotherapy and/or motor control retraining of local + global systems	Motor control retraining of local + global systems

the pubic bone anteriorly and inserts into the ischial spine (Figs 4.28 and 4.29)

- the active system for this fascial hammock or sling: this includes the levator ani muscle which contains primarily type 1 fibers and exhibits constant tone
- the control system: this includes the pudendal nerve which innervates the levator ani as well as the central control of reflex function between the detrusor muscle and the pelvic floor.

Together, the passive and active systems form a hammock of support for the urethra (Fig. 4.29) and the integrity/function of these tissues is essential if force closure of the urethra is to be effective. If this system gives way easily, it cannot provide a backstop against which the urethra can be compressed. A useful analogy (Ashton-Miller et al 2001) is to imagine a garden hose (urethra), with water running through it (urine), lying on a trampoline bed (the pelvic floor). Stepping on the hose will block the flow of water if the bed is very stiff and provides an equal and opposite counterforce (functional pelvic floor). If however, the bed is very flexible (i.e., there is loss of myofascial support), the downward pressure on the hose will cause the bed to stretch and allow the hose to indent the bed. The flow of water will continue uninterrupted.

Sphincteric closure system

In addition, the urethra is closed by a system of both intrinsic and extrinsic muscles:

- The striated muscles within the wall of the urethra (intrinsic) contract prior to any pressure received by the bladder, suggesting an anticipatory neural response mechanism (mediated by the pudendal nerve?).
- The striated urethral sphincter muscles (extrinsic compressor urethra and urethrovaginal sphincter muscles) are also comprised of type 1 fibers and are well suited to maintain constant tone.

Constantinou & Govan (1982) measured the intraurethral and intrabladder pressures in healthy continent women during the Valsalva maneuver and coughing and found that during a cough the intraurethral pressure increases before any pressure increase is detected in the bladder by approximately 250 ms. This did not occur during a Valsalva (bearing down or straining). This suggests an anticipatory reflex between the pelvic floor and urethra (the pelvic floor is active during a cough and inactive during a Valsalva). This anticipatory closure of the urethra was confirmed in a subsequent study by Thind et al (1991). They also noted that the urethral pressure remained elevated for a short time after the pressure normalized in the bladder.

Bo & Stein (1994) used needle electromyogram (EMG) to measure activity in the urethral wall during a cough and Valsalva as well as during activation of the hip adductors, abdominals, and gluteal muscles. They found that the urethral wall contracted synergistically with the pelvic floor, hip adductors, and gluteals and also during a cough. They conclude that strengthening the pelvic floor will also strengthen the urethral wall, but will it restore the anticipatory reflex mechanism?

Sapsford et al (2001) investigated the co-activation pattern of the pelvic floor and abdominals via needle EMG for the abdominal wall and surface EMG for the pelvic floor and found that the abdominals contract in response to a pelvic floor contraction command and that the pelvic floor contracts in both a "hollowing" and "bracing" abdominal command. They also found that a submaximal command of pubococcygeus elicited the *greatest* response in transversus abdominis. The results from this research suggest that the pelvic floor can be facilitated by co-activating the deep abdominals and vice versa. However, it is wrong to assume that all patients will

be able to contract the muscles of the pelvic floor through verbal commands alone, either through the abdomen or the pelvic floor. Bump et al (1991) found that only 50% of women could actually perform a pelvic floor muscle contraction with just a verbal instruction. Careful analysis (see Ch. 8) is required to ensure that the reflex connection between the transversus abdominis and the pelvic floor is intact before this strategy is used.

STRESS URINARY INCONTINENCE

SUI can result when there is loss of the integrity, or function, of the pelvic floor (muscles and fascia) secondary to a major trauma or microtrauma over prolonged periods of time. Inefficient load transfer strategies through the low back and pelvis, particularly those which excessively increase the intraabdominal pressure and result in the bladder being repetitively compressed inferiorly, can lead to incontinence. Some of these strategies have already been mentioned and include abdominal bulging and breath-holding, excessive oblique abdominal activation with thoracolumbar flexion and posterior pelvic tilt, excessive erector spinae activation with thoracolumbar extension, and anterior pelvic tilt. When the bladder is observed with real-time ultrasound imaging, it can be seen that these strategies cause the bladder to descend (Figs 8.85b and 8.86b). In a group of pelvic pain patients, O'Sullivan et al (2002) noticed via real-time ultrasound imaging that the bladder tended to descend during an ASLR test. When compression was applied to the pelvic girdle, this descent was minimized.

How much descent of the bladder is optimal, or normal, during functional activities? Peschers et al (2001b) measured the mobility of the bladder neck via perineal ultrasound during coughing and Valsalva in 39 healthy, nulliparous women. They found that the bladder neck descended a variable amount (2–32 m) in both a cough and Valsalva and questioned the long-held view that SUI was associated with urethral mobility. Like the SIJ (Buyruk et al 1995b), there appears to be a wide variation in the amount of motion possible and continence (effective force closure of the urethra) relies more on control and urethral closure rather than amplitude of motion of the urethra.

Howard et al (2000) investigated descent of the bladder neck during a cough and Valsalva in three groups of women: nulliparous continent (17 subjects), primiparous continent (18 subjects), and primiparous incontinent (23 subjects). There was no statistical difference in the amount of bladder neck mobility between the groups, again suggesting that movement of the urethra is not what determines one's continence status. When they compared the amount of bladder neck movement which occurred during a cough compared with a Valsalva, they noted that in the two continent groups there was less movement during a cough. The incontinent group conversely demonstrated no difference in the amount of movement when the subjects coughed or did a Valsalva. Clearly, something was happening during a cough in the continent women that was not happening in the incontinent group. All three groups generated the same amount of cough pressures; however, the stiffness value (pressure change divided by bladder neck mobility) was the greatest in the nulliparous continent group, next highest in the primiparous continent group, and lowest in the primiparous incontinent group. Howard et al hypothesize that the reason for these differences is a functional pelvic floor in the continent women. Thind et al (1991) noted that the amplitude of the anticipatory pressure rise in the urethra was less in women with SUI and suggest that this is due to weakness of the pelvic floor.

Allen et al (1990) investigated 96 nulliparous women both prenatally and postpartum to determine if childbirth caused damage to the pelvic floor muscles and/or its nerve supply. They showed that a vaginal delivery impairs the strength of the pelvic floor and noted that recovery had not occurred at 2 months postpartum. They also demonstrated via needle EMG that vaginal delivery caused a partial denervation of the pelvic floor in 80% of these women. Women who had a long, active second stage of labor showed the most EMG evidence of denervation. Ashton-Miller et al (2001) feel that if the nerve to the levator ani is damaged, the denervated muscles will atrophy, thus placing more stress on the passive supporting structures (endopelvic fascia) which over time will stretch and result in organ prolapse. Alternately, a paravaginal defect can occur which causes a separation in the endopelvic fascia. This effectively reduces the stiffness of the fascial layer which supports the urethra and can occur unilaterally or bilaterally. When this occurs, the pelvic floor must take over to support the organ position and provide active closure to the urethra. However, they note: "if the muscle is completely detached from the fascial tissues, then it may be able to contract; but that contraction may not be effective in elevating the urethra or stabilizing its position" (Ashton-Miller et al 2001).

Bo et al (1990) demonstrated in a randomized clinical trial that retraining the function of the pelvic floor (awareness training coupled with strength and endurance training: see Ch. 10) is effective for some women (60%) in the treatment of SUI. Their program is coupled with exercises which aim to restore force closure of the pelvic girdle (transversus abdominis and multifidus).

Summary

I believe that orthopedic manual therapists who focus on restoring function to the local system of the low back and pelvis (transversus abdominis, multifidus, and the pelvic floor) and therapists who specialize in pelvic floor dysfunction are treating the same condition – failed load transfer through the lumbopelvic region, manifested either through a loss of effective force closure of the joints of the low back and pelvis, or loss of effective force closure of the urethra. The research clearly supports that we are merging to a common understanding of both function and dysfunction of the whole pelvis and not just its parts. Treatment of the impaired lumbopelvic-hip region must focus on an integrated approach – one which considers the restoration of form closure, force closure, and motor control of all the structures contained within the region. Ultimately, function requires mobility with stability (mobile stability – not rigidity) of the joints and organs, for any endeavor the individual chooses to do.

Chapter **10**

Treating the lumbopelvic-hip dysfunction

Linda-Joy Lee Diane Lee

GENERAL PRINCIPLES

Treatment for the impaired lumbopelvic-hip region must be prescriptive since every individual has a unique clinical presentation. Rarely will only one dysfunction be present (one stiff joint or one poorly controlled joint); more commonly, multiple problems coexist such that the most effective treatment consists of a unique combination of techniques and exercises specific for each patient. However, there are some principles for treatment which help guide the therapist who is inexperienced in working with this model. The first step is to analyze the findings from the assessment (Ch. 8). Does the individual appear to be:

- primarily under *too much* compression from stiff joints (form closure) or hypertonicity of the global system (force closure/motor control)?
- primarily under *too little* compression due to loose joints (form closure), a poorly controlled neutral zone of motion, and/or insufficient recruitment and timing of the local system (force closure/motor control), or
- a combination of both *too much* and *too little* compression in different areas of the lumbopelvic-hip complex?

In the first instance, the therapist may decide to use manual techniques and exercises which decompress the joints (increase mobility) and follow this with an exercise plan that re-establishes a more optimal stabilization strategy which emphasizes stability with mobility. In the second instance, the therapist may decide to start a program which emphasizes retraining of the local system right away (increase stability) and then add decompression techniques/exercises (increase mobility) later as necessary. The most common scenario is the third, where a combination of decompression and stabilization is required. Continual assessment of form closure (mobility/stability of the joints) and force closure/motor control helps direct the therapeutic plan from treatment to treatment.

The effective management of lumbopelvic-hip pain and dysfunction requires attention to all four components – form closure, force closure, motor control, and emotions. Ultimately, the goal is to teach the patient a healthier way to live and move such that sustained compression and/or tensile forces on any one structure are avoided. The therapist uses manual skills to facilitate this process; however, the primary role is to educate and coach the patient through the recovery process since only the patient can make the changes necessary for optimal function.

If the clinical findings suggest that decompression is necessary, the treatment principles are:

1. restore the zygapophyseal, sacroiliac, and/or hip joint mobility (form closure – mobility)
2. correct the osseous alignment within and between the lumbar spine, pelvic girdle, and femur
3. restore optimal force closure and control of the neutral zone through training of the local system (force closure/motor control)
4. retrain integration of the local and global systems, including functional movements (rehearse activities of daily living, work- or sport-specific movement patterns – functional integration).

If the clinical findings suggest that more compression is necessary, the treatment principles are:

1. correct the osseous alignment within and between the lumbar spine, pelvic girdle, and femur
2. restore optimal force closure and motor control through training of the local system (force closure/motor control)
3. provide an external support (not always necessary) to augment the training being taught (sacroiliac belt, taping)
4. restore articular mobility/stability to extrinsic joints (knee, foot, thorax) since their dysfunction may be contributing to compensatory patterns that put excessive stress on the joints of the lumbopelvic-hip region (form closure – mobility).

RESTORING JOINT MOBILITY

The fibrotic stiff joint

For the stiff joint, passive articular mobilization techniques are the most effective. The technique is graded according to the irritability of the articular tissues. Long-standing fibrosis requires a sustained grade 4+ passive mobilization.

The myofascially compressed joint/region

For joints which are compressed due to overactivation of muscles (myofascially compressed) there are many neuromuscular techniques which decrease hypertonicity in the global system (reduce rigidity). For the lumbopelvic-hip region they include:

1. active mobilization or muscle energy techniques (Mitchell & Mitchell 2001, Schamberger 2002)
2. functional or craniosacral techniques
3. trigger point techniques (Travell & Rinzler 1952)
4. intramuscular stimulation (IMS – dry needling) (Gunn 1996)
5. using imagery during a combination of active mobilization, trigger point release, and exercise (Franklin 1996, Lee 2001a, Lee DG 2003, Lee LJ 2003)
6. techniques to restore an optimal breathing pattern (Chaitow et al 2002, Lee DG 2003, Lee LJ 2003)
7. exercises which encourage movement with awareness (Feldenkrais, Hanna somatics, Pilates), finding neutral spine (Lee LJ 2003) and the optimal lumbopelvic pyramid (postural re-education) (Lee 2001a).

The fixated joint

For the joint which is fixated, a passive articular manipulation technique (Hartman 1997) is necessary to restore the joint position and mobility before stabilization exercises can be prescribed.

CORRECTING ALIGNMENT

Loads are transferred more effectively through joints which are properly aligned such that the compression and tension forces induced are shared amongst all structures. Malalignment can create excessive stress on individual structures (tension or compression) which ultimately leads to tissue breakdown (inflammation and pain). Therefore, techniques which correct alignment and restore the path of the instantaneous center of rotation (PICR) for joint movement (Hall & Brody 1999, Sahrmann 2001) are necessary in most treatment plans. They include:

1. active mobilization/alignment techniques (muscle energy) (Mitchell & Mitchell 2001, Schamberger 2002)
2. movement with awareness exercises – finding neutral spine (Lee LJ 2003) and the optimal lumbopelvic pyramid (postural re-education) (Lee 2001a).

RESTORING FORCE CLOSURE AND MOTOR CONTROL

Recent research has increased our understanding of muscle and joint function and consequently changed the way exercises for back pain and dysfunction are prescribed (Bergmark 1989, Bullock-Saxton et al 1993, 1994, Hides et al 1994, 1996, Hodges & Richardson 1996, 1997, O'Sullivan et al 1997, Richardson et al 1999, Danneels et al 2000, Hodges 2000, 2003, Jull & Richardson 2000, Moseley et al 2002). New concepts of how joints are stabilized and how load is transferred through the body highlight the importance of proprioception, automatic muscle activity, and motor control for regaining optimal movement after injury. It is clear from this body of evidence (see Ch. 5) that successful rehabilitation of back pain and dysfunction requires exercises that differ from those used for conditioning and training the healthy, non-painful, non-injured population.

When planning injury rehabilitation, exercises should be prescribed as part of an integrated treatment plan, not as a stand-alone treatment. If exercise is prescribed without first restoring joint mobility (form closure), the patient's pain and dysfunction often get worse. This may lead to the conclusion that certain exercises are "bad" or "unsuccessful" for treating back pain, when it may merely be a problem of *inappropriately timed* exercise intervention.

Similarly, the *type* of exercise prescribed is of utmost importance. For back and pelvic pain, the evidence cited above supports correcting deficits in motor control rather than focusing on strength and power of individual muscles. Patients who go mindlessly through a routine of exercises will have limited success in retraining motor patterns and may get worse with exercise if poor patterns and control

are reinforced, resulting in irritation of joint structures and symptom exacerbation. The problem may not be *which* exercise was prescribed, but *how* the exercise was performed. Three people performing a squat can do so with three different movement strategies, with three different combinations of muscle recruitment and timing. Therefore, when planning exercise intervention clinicians must remember that "exercise A" does not guarantee the use of "muscle A." It is up to the clinician to observe, assess, and decide if "exercise A" is reaching the goal of training "muscle A" (with appropriate recruitment, timing, endurance, etc.) for each patient. The key to correcting dysfunctional patterns of muscle activation is teaching awareness of movement; this requires mindfulness on the part of both the therapist and the patient.

The goal of restoring force closure and motor control for the lumbopelvic-hip region is to restore stabilization strategies and movement patterns such that load transfer is optimized through all joints of the kinetic chain. Optimal load transfer occurs when there is precise modulation of force, coordination, and timing in the local and global systems, ensuring control of the neutral zone for each joint (segmental control), the orientation of the spine (spinal curvatures, thorax on pelvic girdle, pelvis in relation to the lower extremity), and the control of postural equilibrium with respect to the environment (Hodges 2003). The result, and our goal for our patients, is stability with mobility, where there is stability without rigidity of posture, without episodes of collapse, and with fluidity of movement. The exercises presented in this chapter are prescribed in the context of this goal; the focus is to balance compression and tension forces by using manual cues, imagery, and movement to address alterations in the motor control system.

Optimal coordination of the local and global systems will produce optimal stabilization strategies. These patients will have:

• the ability to find and maintain control of neutral spinal alignment both in the lumbopelvic region and in relationship to the thorax and hip
• the ability consciously to recruit and maintain a tonic, isolated contraction of the local stabilizers of the lumbopelvis to ensure segmental control (control of the neutral zone)
• the ability to move in and out of neutral spine (flex, extend, laterally bend, rotate) without segmental or regional collapse

- the ability to maintain all the above in coordination with the thorax and the extremities in functional, work-specific, and sport-specific postures and movements.

Suboptimal stabilization strategies

In the lumbopelvic region, it is common to see segmental inhibition of the local system associated with a multisegmental overactivation of the global system (Arendt-Nielsen et al 1996, Kaigle et al 1998, Richardson et al 1999, Radebold et al 2000, 2001, Comerford & Mottram 2001). Restoring motor control to the region needs to address dysfunction in both the local and global systems. Inhibition of the local system results in poor control of the neutral zone; overactivation of the global muscles produces increased compression and often results in pain, loss of range of motion, and rigidity of movement. Excessive activity and tone in the global muscles of the trunk can also inhibit the recruitment and training of the local system muscles, as well as prevent retraining of proper functional movement patterns. Multisegmentally, postural changes such as excessive lumbar lordosis, insufficient lumbar lordosis, and scoliosis are common (Figs 9.2–9.5) and usually result from dysfunctional patterns in the global system. The objective examination tests described in Chapter 8 will reveal specific levels and direction of hypermobility/instability in the lumbar spine and pelvis; these findings will direct where and how to cue the correction of segmental control during exercise. The assessment process will also reveal the patient's specific pattern of global substitution and dominance, especially during functional movements and motor control tests (one-leg standing, active straight leg raise (ASLR), active bent leg raise (ABLR)). The dominant muscles involved in the suboptimal stabilization strategies need to be monitored throughout the exercise process, especially when more difficult exercises and progressions are introduced. Janda (1986) and Sahrmann (2001) have observed common patterns of imbalance in the global system and described techniques and exercises that are useful for correcting global dysfunction. However, it should be noted that purely treating global muscle imbalance is unlikely to correct deficits in the local system. Thus, the exercise rehabilitation program for restoring force closure and motor control is multifaceted and should include:

- exercises and imagery to downtrain dysfunctional patterns in the global system
- exercises for training awareness of the neutral spine position to decrease global rigidity, facilitate postural re-education, facilitate performance of local system recruitment exercises, and facilitate balanced activity in the global system
- exercises for isolation and recruitment of the individual local system muscles
- protocols to train precision, endurance, and coordination of the local system muscles
- exercises to integrate coordination and timing of the local and global systems
- exercises to target specific global muscle weakness and imbalance
- exercises to maintain/restore global muscle length
- exercises for integration of local and global muscles into functional movements and activities.

Specific exercises for each of these components will be addressed in this chapter.

RESTORING FORM CLOSURE (MOBILITY) – LUMBAR ZYGAPOPHYSEAL JOINTS

The following section outlines the specific therapy indicated for restoring mobility of the zygapophyseal joints of the lumbar spine during each stage of repair (i.e., substrate, fibroblastic, maturation) following a traumatic joint sprain. During the first 4–6 days after injury (substrate phase), the goal of treatment is hemostasis of the wound. At home, the frequent application of ice together with rest is the treatment of choice. The resting position for the lumbar spine is supine with the hips and knees semiflexed and supported over a wedge. The surface should be firm, but not rigid. At the clinic, electrotherapeutic analgesic modalities such as transcutaneous nerve stimulation and interferential current therapy can afford relief from pain; however, the patient should not attend at this stage if the physical stresses induced are greater than the relief gained.

With the resolution of some active range of movement, the specific segmental osteokinematic restriction (extended rotated/sideflexed right (ERSR), flexed rotated sideflexed left (FRSL): see Ch. 9) becomes apparent. During the fibroblastic stage of repair (up to 4–6 weeks postinjury), the goal of treatment is to restore the segmental articular mobility, ensure optimal alignment and then restore force closure and motor control segmentally and regionally. Passive and active mobilization techniques are effective in restoring the articular kinematics. In addition, specific home exercises help to maintain the increased articular mobility gained in the treatment session. The manual therapy treatment techniques and home exercises for three specific lumbar segmental dysfunctions will be described.

L5–S1: FLEXED ROTATED/SIDEFLEXED LEFT

The individual with this segmental restriction presents with a limitation of extension, rotation/sideflexion of L5–S1 to the right (osteokinematics), and a loss of the inferoposterior glide of the right L5–S1 zygapophyseal joint (arthrokinematics). The following manual therapy techniques are used to restore mobility.

Specific traction – passive mobilization technique

This is a useful preliminary mobilization technique which can be graded according to the irritability of the joint and surrounding soft tissues. Initially, grade 2 and 3 techniques are indicated, keeping well within the range of pain and reactive muscle spasm. The large afferent fiber input from the mechanoreceptors located in the articular capsule inhibits the centripetal transmission of the small-fiber input (nociception) at the spinal cord, thus reducing the perception of pain via the spinal gating mechanism (see Ch. 4). The stimulation of these mechanoreceptors also reduces the gamma efferent discharge to the intrafusal muscle fibers of the segmentally related global muscle, which is often hypertonic.

Patient and therapist position With the patient sidelying, hips and knees slightly flexed, the interspinous space between the L4 and the L5 vertebra is palpated with the caudal hand. The thoracolumbar spine is rotated until rotation of L4–L5 occurs. The cranial hand now palpates the interspinous space between the L5 vertebra and the sacrum while the caudal hand flexes the patient's uppermost hip and knee, thus posteriorly rotating the innominate; ensure that L5–S1 remains neutral. Simultaneously, the patient should extend the lower leg to the end of the table. The foot of the upper leg is allowed to rest against the popliteal fossa of the lower leg. The therapist's lower lateral thorax contacts the patient's uppermost innominate.

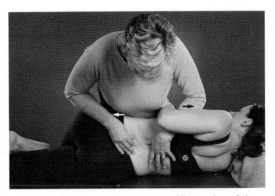

Figure 10.1 Passive mobilization – specific traction of the lumbosacral junction. The arrows indicate the direction of force applied to the patient's pelvic girdle and thorax. (Reproduced with permission from © Diane G. Lee Physiotherapist Corp.)

Correction technique – mobilization Specific traction is applied to the lumbosacral junction via a straight caudal force from the therapist's lower lateral thorax against the patient's pelvic girdle (Fig. 10.1). The therapist's cranial arm simultaneously stabilizes the patient's upper thorax. The grade of the technique is dictated by the joint/myofascial reaction.

Rotation/sideflexion – passive and active mobilization techniques

In the early stages of healing, the cause of the rotation/sideflexion restriction is usually muscular since restrictive capsular adhesions have not had time to form. A grade 2 or 3 (Grieve 1981) rotation/sideflexion passive mobilization technique can be used for a neurophysiological effect on the multisegmental muscles. The technique yields the best result when it is used in combination with the active mobilization technique (see below). If the injury is long-standing and adhesions have formed (capsular fibrosis), a grade 4+ sustained technique is the most effective.

Patient and therapist position With the patient in left sidelying, hips and knees slightly flexed, the interspinous space between the L4 and the L5 vertebra is palpated with the caudal hand. The thoracolumbar spine is rotated until rotation of L4–L5 occurs. Comfort is assured if the technique is focused and localized and full articular locking is avoided (Hartman 1997). The cranial hand now palpates the interspinous space between the L5 vertebra and the sacrum while the caudal hand flexes the patient's uppermost hip and knee, thus posteriorly rotating the innominate; ensure that L5–S1 remains

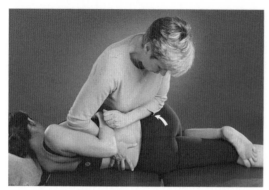

Figure 10.2   Passive mobilization for extension and right rotation/sideflexion of the lumbosacral junction (flexed rotated/sideflexed left lesion). The arrow indicates the direction of force applied by the therapist. (Reproduced with permission from © Diane G. Lee Physiotherapist Corp.)

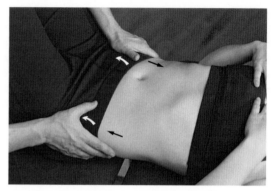

Figure 10.3   An anterior pelvic tilt (white arrows) coupled with right lateral tilting (black arrows) facilitates extension and right rotation/sideflexion of the lumbosacral junction. (Reproduced with permission from © Diane G. Lee Physiotherapist Corp.)

neutral. Simultaneously, the patient should extend the lower leg to the end of the table. The foot of the upper leg is allowed to rest against the popliteal fossa of the lower leg. The therapist's cranial arm supports the patient's thorax while the caudal arm supports the pelvic girdle.

Correction technique – passive mobilization   From this position, L5–S1 is mobilized passively into extension and right rotation/sideflexion (osteokinematic motion) through either the thorax or the pelvic girdle (Fig. 10.2). Simultaneously, the right zygapophyseal joint is mobilized inferiorly and posteriorly (arthrokinematic motion). The technique is graded according to the joint/myofascial reaction.

Correction technique – active mobilization   L5–S1 is initially mobilized passively into extension and right rotation/sideflexion. From the point of first resistance, the patient is instructed to resist further motion while the therapist applies a gentle rotation force to the pelvic girdle or the thorax. The isometric contraction is held for up to 5 s, followed by a period of complete relaxation. The joint is then passively taken to the new physiological range of extension and right rotation/sideflexion. The technique is repeated three times followed by re-evaluation of the regional movement tests, positional tests, and arthrokinematic mobility test (inferoposterior glide of the right L5–S1 zygapophyseal joint).

Home exercise   Home exercises which maintain the segmental motion regained during the treatment session are paramount to successful rehabilitation. Since wound repair occurs continuously, the orientation of the newly formed collagen fibers should be directed as often as possible (see Ch. 7).

In the early fibroblastic stage of repair, the exercises should be kept well within the painfree range. For this impairment, the patient is taught to do an anterior pelvic tilt in the supine, crook lying position (this facilitates extension). This can be coupled with lateral tilting of the pelvis beneath the lumbar spine to facilitate unilateral extension (Fig. 10.3).

L5–S1: EXTENDED ROTATED/SIDEFLEXED RIGHT

Specific traction – passive mobilization technique

As with the FRSL lesion, specific traction is a useful preliminary mobilization technique which can be graded according to the irritability of the joint. The details and the intent of this technique are identical to those described above.

Rotation/sideflexion – passive and active mobilization technique

Patient and therapist position   With the patient in right sidelying, hips and knees slightly flexed, the interspinous space between the L4 and the L5 vertebra is palpated with the caudal hand. The thoracolumbar spine is rotated until rotation of L4–L5 occurs. Comfort is assured if the technique is focused and localized and full articular locking is avoided (Hartman 1997). The cranial hand now palpates the interspinous space between the L5 vertebra and the sacrum while the caudal hand flexes the patient's uppermost hip and knee, thus posteriorly rotating the innominate; ensure that L5–S1 remains neutral. Simultaneously, the patient should extend

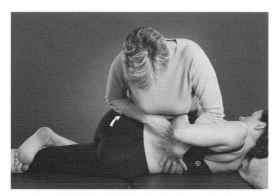

Figure 10.4   Passive mobilization for flexion and left rotation/sideflexion of the lumbosacral junction (extended rotated/sideflexed right lesion). The right zygapophyseal joint is mobilized superoanteriorly with this technique. The arrow indicates the direction of force applied by the therapist. (Reproduced with permission from © Diane G. Lee Physiotherapist Corp.)

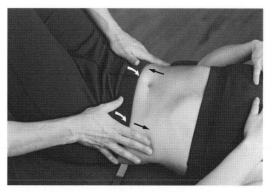

Figure 10.5   A posterior pelvic tilt (white arrows) coupled with left lateral tilting (black arrows) facilitates flexion and left rotation/sideflexion of the lumbosacral junction. (Reproduced with permission from © Diane G. Lee Physiotherapist Corp.)

the lower leg to the end of the table. The foot of the upper leg is allowed to rest against the popliteal fossa of the lower leg. The therapist's cranial arm supports the patient's thorax while the caudal arm supports the pelvic girdle.

Correction technique – passive mobilization   From this position, L5–S1 is mobilized passively into flexion and left rotation/sideflexion (osteokinematic motion) through either the thorax or the pelvic girdle (Fig. 10.4). Simultaneously, the right zygapophyseal joint is mobilized superiorly and anteriorly (arthrokinematic motion). The technique is graded according to the joint/myofascial reaction.

Correction technique – active mobilization   L5–S1 is initially mobilized passively into flexion and left rotation/sideflexion. From the point of first resistance, the patient is instructed to resist further motion while the therapist applies a gentle rotation force to the pelvic girdle or the thorax. The isometric contraction is held for up to 5 s followed by a period of complete relaxation. The joint is then passively taken to the new physiological range of flexion and left rotation/sideflexion. The technique is repeated three times followed by re-evaluation of the regional movement tests, positional tests, and arthrokinematic mobility test (superoanterior glide of the right L5–S1 zygapophyseal joint).

Home exercise   Home exercises which maintain the segmental motion regained during the treatment session are paramount to successful rehabilitation. Since wound repair occurs continuously, the orientation of the newly formed collagen fibers should be directed as often as possible (see Ch. 7).

In the early fibroblastic stage of repair, the exercises should be kept well within the painfree range. For this impairment, the patient is taught to do a posterior pelvic tilt in the supine, crook lying position (this facilitates flexion). This can be coupled with left lateral tilting of the pelvis beneath the lumbar spine to facilitate unilateral flexion on the right (Fig. 10.5).

L4–L5: ZYGAPOPHYSEAL JOINT FIXATION – LEFT

Distraction manipulation

An intraarticular meniscoid of a moderately degenerated zygapophyseal joint can become entrapped during a flexion/rotation load in the presence of insufficient stabilization of the joint. The following distraction manipulation is useful for relocating the meniscoid. Segmental neuromuscular retraining (see below) must follow if recurrences are to be prevented.

Patient and therapist position   With the patient in right sidelying, hips and knees slightly flexed, the interspinous space between the L3 and the L4 vertebra is palpated with the caudal hand. The thoracolumbar spine is rotated until rotation of L3–L4 occurs. The cranial hand now palpates the interspinous space at L4–L5 while the caudal hand flexes the patient's uppermost hip and knee, thus posteriorly rotating the innominate and flexing L5–S1; L4–L5 should remain in neutral. Simultaneously, the patient should extend the lower leg to the end of the table. The foot of the upper leg is allowed to rest against the popliteal fossa of the lower leg.

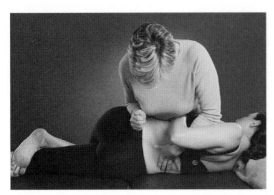

Figure 10.6 Distraction manipulation to reduce a fixation of the left zygapophyseal joint at L4–L5. The force is pure axial rotation of the pelvic girdle and L5 beneath the L4 vertebra. (Reproduced with permission from © Diane G. Lee Physiotherapist Corp.)

The therapist's cranial arm supports the patient's thorax while the caudal arm supports the pelvic girdle. The cranial hand/thumb fixes the spinous process of L4 firmly.

Correction technique – manipulation From this position, the sagittal component of the left zygapophyseal joint at L4–L5 is distracted with a high-velocity, low-amplitude thrust by applying a pure axial rotation force through the pelvic girdle with L5–S1 stabilized in flexion (Fig. 10.6). The regional movement tests confirm the success of the technique since the range of motion is often dramatically restored. However, the underlying articular instability (insufficient articular compression) and the lack of force closure/motor control become evident on subsequent retesting.

RESTORING FORM CLOSURE (MOBILITY) – SACROILIAC JOINT

This section describes the specific therapy indicated for restoring mobility of the sacroiliac joint (SIJ) during each stage of repair (i.e., substrate, fibroblastic, maturation) following a traumatic joint sprain. During the first 4–6 days after injury to the SIJ (substrate phase), the goal of treatment is hemostasis of the wound. At home, the frequent application of ice together with rest is the treatment of choice. The resting position for the painful SIJ is sidelying with the painful side uppermost and the hip and knee supported on a pillow. At the clinic, electrotherapeutic analgesic modalities such as transcutaneous nerve stimulation and interferential current therapy can afford relief from pain; however, the patient

should not attend at this stage if the physical stresses induced are greater than the relief gained. Weight-bearing activities such as walking, standing, and sitting should be minimized during the first few days. Using a cane can help to reduce the loading through the pelvis when vertical.

With the resolution of some active range of movement, the specific osteokinematic restriction (usually posterior rotation of the innominate/nutation of the sacrum) becomes apparent. During the fibroblastic stage of repair (up to 4–6 weeks postinjury), the goal of treatment is to restore the articular mobility, ensure optimal alignment, and then to restore force closure and motor control of the entire pelvic girdle. Passive and active mobilization techniques are used to restore the articular kinematics. In addition, specific home exercises help to maintain the increased articular mobility gained in the treatment session. If the injury is long-standing and adhesions have formed (capsular fibrosis), a grade 4+ sustained technique is the most effective.

SIJ: ANTERIORLY ROTATED RIGHT INNOMINATE/COUNTERNUTATED RIGHT SACRUM

The individual with this restriction presents with a limitation of posterior rotation of the right innominate (nutation of the sacrum) (osteokinematics) and a loss of the anterosuperior glide of the right SIJ (described as the innominate moving on the sacrum). The following manual therapy techniques are used to restore mobility.

Distraction of the SIJ – passive mobilization technique

This is a useful preliminary mobilization technique which can be graded according to the irritability of the joint and surrounding soft tissues. Initially, grade 2 or 3 techniques are indicated, keeping well within the range of pain and reactive muscle spasm. The large afferent fiber input from the mechanoreceptors located in the articular capsule inhibits the centripetal transmission of the small-fiber input (nociception) at the spinal cord, thus reducing the perception of pain via the spinal gating mechanism (see Ch. 4). The stimulation of these mechanoreceptors also reduces the gamma efferent discharge to the intrafusal muscle fibers of the related hypertonic muscles.

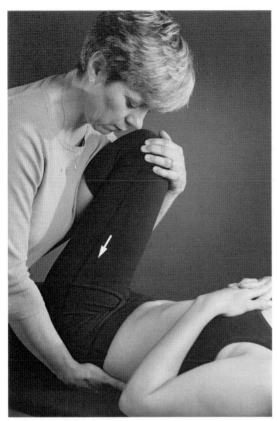

Figure 10.7   Passive mobilization for distraction of the left sacroiliac joint (SIJ) in the neutral SIJ position. The arrow indicates the direction of force applied by the therapist. (Reproduced with permission from © Diane G. Lee Physiotherapist Corp.)

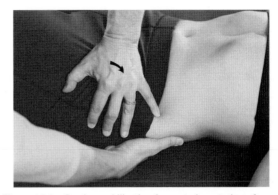

Figure 10.8   Passive mobilization for posterior rotation of the right innominate. The arrow indicates the direction of force applied by the therapist. (Reproduced with permission from © Diane G. Lee Physiotherapist Corp.)

Posterior rotation of the innominate or nutation of the sacrum – passive and active mobilization techniques

In the early stages of healing, the cause of the posterior rotation restriction of the SIJ is usually myofascial since restrictive capsular adhesions have not had time to form. A grade 2 or 3 (Grieve 1981) passive mobilization technique can be utilized for a neurophysiological effect on the myofascia. The technique yields the best result when it is used in combination with the active mobilization technique. If the injury is long-standing and adhesions have formed (capsular fibrosis), a grade 4+ sustained technique is the most effective.

Patient and therapist position   The patient is supine, with the hips and knees flexed. With the long and ring finger of one hand, palpate the sacral sulcus just medial to the PSIS (Fig. 8.28). With the other hand, palpate the ipsilateral anterior superior iliac spine (ASIS) and the iliac crest.

Correction technique – passive mobilization   A grade 2–4 posterior rotation force is applied to the right innominate to produce an anterosuperior glide at the SIJ (Fig. 10.8). This glide is also associated with nutation of the sacrum. If the joint is stiff, the force is sustained (grade 4+) for up to 3 min, during which time the connective tissue can be felt to give and subsequent arthrokinematic mobility testing confirms the restoration of articular motion. The SIJ can be mobilized through the sacrum by applying a grade 2–4 nutation force unilaterally to the right sacral base (Fig. 10.9).

Correction technique – active mobilization   The patient is supine, with the hips and knees flexed. With the long and ring finger of one hand, palpate

Patient and therapist position   The patient is supine, with the hips and knees flexed. With the long and ring finger of one hand, palpate the sacral sulcus just medial to the posterior superior iliac spine (PSIS) (Fig. 8.28). The flexed hip and knee are supported against the therapist's shoulder and arm. The femur is flexed, adducted, and internally rotated to the motion barrier of the hip joint. Distraction can be applied from either the neutral SIJ position or from the limit of posterior rotation of the innominate. This is reached by passively flexing the femur until the motion barrier for posterior rotation of the innominate is perceived.

Correction technique – passive mobilization   From this position, distraction of the SIJ is achieved by applying a dorsolateral force along the length of the femur (Fig. 10.7). The SIJ can be felt to distract posteriorly. The degree of force applied is dictated by the joint/myofascial reaction.

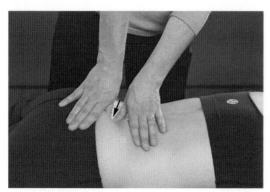

Figure 10.9   Passive mobilization for nutation of the right sacral base. The arrow indicates the direction of force applied by the therapist. (Reproduced with permission from © Diane G. Lee Physiotherapist Corp.)

the sacral sulcus just medial to the PSIS (Fig. 8.28). The limit of posterior rotation of the innominate is reached by passively flexing the femur until the motion barrier for posterior rotation of the innominate is perceived (Fig. 10.10). From this position, the patient is instructed to resist further hip flexion, which is gently increased by the therapist. The isometric contraction is held for up to 5 s, followed by a period of complete relaxation. The innominate is then passively taken to the new barrier of posterior rotation. The technique is repeated three times followed by re-evaluation of the regional movement tests, positional tests, and arthrokinematic mobility test (anterosuperior joint glide) of the SIJ.

Home exercise   This exercise can be taught as a self-active mobilization technique using a towel. The patient engages the motion barrier of posterior rotation of the innominate by flexing the femur and then gently contracts the hip extensors against the resistance of the towel (Fig. 10.11). The contraction is held for up to 5 s followed by a period of complete relaxation. The femur is then flexed further thus taking the innominate to the new motion barrier of posterior rotation.

SIJ: POSTERIORLY ROTATED RIGHT INNOMINATE/NUTATED RIGHT SACRUM

The individual with this restriction presents with a limitation of anterior rotation of the right innominate (osteokinematics) and a loss of the inferoposterior glide of the right SIJ. This is not a common articular restriction since the injured SIJ usually postures, and subsequently stiffens, in anterior rotation. However, it is common to find the innominate held posteriorly

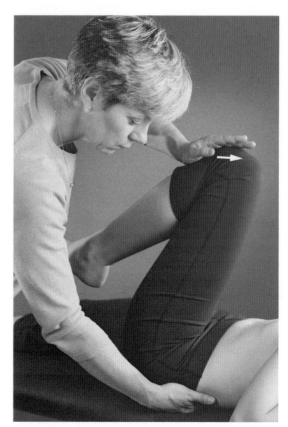

Figure 10.10   Active mobilization for posterior rotation of the right innominate. The arrow indicates the direction of gentle force applied by the therapist which the patient is to resist. (Reproduced with permission from © Diane G. Lee Physiotherapist Corp.)

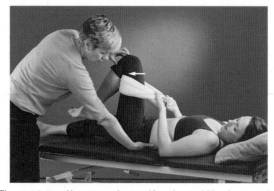

Figure 10.11   Home exercise – self-active mobilization exercise to maintain the range of motion (posterior rotation of the innominate) gained in the treatment session. The patient engages the motion barrier of posterior rotation of the innominate by flexing the femur and then gently contracts the hip extensors against the resistance of the towel. The new motion barrier for posterior rotation of the innominate is engaged after a period of relaxation. The arrow indicates the direction of gentle force applied by the patient. (Reproduced with permission from © Diane G. Lee Physiotherapist Corp.)

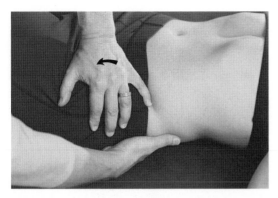

Figure 10.12   Passive mobilization for anterior rotation of the right innominate. The arrow indicates the direction of force applied by the therapist. (Reproduced with permission from © Diane G. Lee Physiotherapist Corp.)

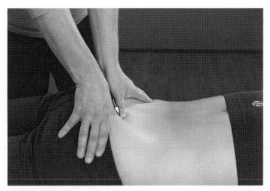

Figure 10.13   Passive mobilization for counternutation of the right sacral base. The arrow indicates the direction of force applied by the therapist. (Reproduced with permission from © Diane G. Lee Physiotherapist Corp.)

rotated by an imbalance in the global system (see Techniques to correct alignment: Intrapelvic torsions: Posterior rotation innominate, below).

Anterior rotation of the innominate or counternutation of the sacrum – passive and active mobilization techniques

Patient and therapist position   The patient is supine, with the hips and knees flexed. With the long and ring finger of one hand, palpate the sacral sulcus just medial to the PSIS (Fig. 8.28). With the other hand, palpate the ipsilateral ASIS and the iliac crest.

Correction technique – passive mobilization   A grade 2–4 anterior rotation force is applied to the innominate to produce an inferoposterior glide at the SIJ (Fig. 10.12). This glide is also associated with counternutation of the sacrum. If the joint is stiff, the force is sustained (grade 4+) for up to 3 min, during which time the connective tissue can be felt to give and subsequent arthrokinematic mobility testing confirms the restoration of articular motion. The SIJ can be mobilized through the sacrum by applying a grade 2–4 counternutation force unilaterally to the inferior lateral angle of the sacrum (Fig. 10.13).

Correction technique – active mobilization   With the patient prone, lying close to the edge of the table, the anterior aspect of the distal thigh is palpated with the caudal hand, while the PSIS of the innominate is palpated with the heel of the cranial hand. The limit of anterior rotation of the innominate is reached by passively extending the femur with the caudal hand and applying an anterior rotation force to the innominate with the cranial hand (Fig. 10.14). From this position, the patient is

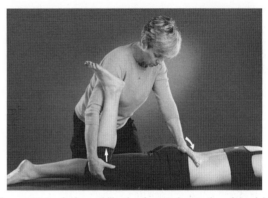

Figure 10.14   Active mobilization for anterior rotation of the right innominate. From the motion barrier, the therapist applies a gentle extension force which the patient resists. The arrows indicate the direction of force applied by the therapist. (Reproduced with permission from © Diane G. Lee Physiotherapist Corp.)

instructed to resist further hip extension which is gently increased by the therapist. The isometric contraction is held for up to 5 s followed by a period of complete relaxation. The innominate is then passively taken to the new barrier of anterior rotation. The technique is repeated three times followed by re-evaluation of the regional movement tests, positional tests, and arthrokinematic mobility test (inferoposterior joint glide) of the SIJ.

Home exercise   A modified unilateral lunge with the anterior leg resting on a foot stool or chair and the other correctly aligned (neither internally nor externally rotated at the hip joint) in extension will facilitate anterior rotation of the innominate on the extended side (Fig. 10.15). Ensure that the patient does not posteriorly tilt the pelvis by "butt gripping" on the extended leg side.

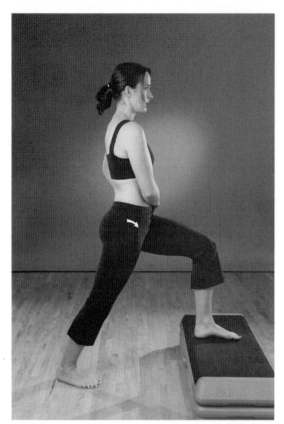

Figure 10.15 Home exercise – specific unilateral hip extension exercise to facilitate anterior rotation (arrow) of the innominate. (Reproduced with permission from © Diane G. Lee Physiotherapist Corp.)

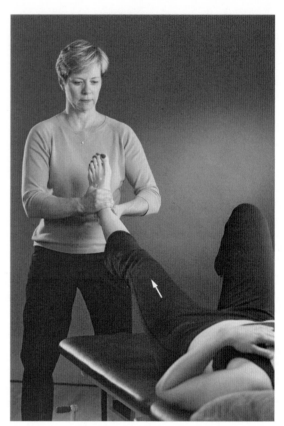

Figure 10.16 Manipulation to decompress a vertical shear fixation of the left innominate in posterior rotation. The arrow indicates the direction of force applied by the therapist. (Reproduced with permission from © Diane G. Lee Physiotherapist Corp.)

SIJ: SUPERIOR SHEAR FIXATION – INNOMINATE

When a force is applied to the SIJ sufficient to attenuate the articular ligaments (fall on the buttocks or a lift/twist injury), the muscles will respond to prevent dislocation and further trauma to the joint. The resulting spasm may fix the joint in an abnormal resting position and marked asymmetry of the pelvic girdle (innominate and/or sacrum) can be present. This is an unstable joint under excessive compression (Fig. 8.10f) and decompression as well as alignment correction is required before stabilization exercises are given.

A superior shear fixation of the SIJ can occur when a vertical force through the pelvic girdle (a fall on the inferior pelvis) exceeds the ability of the SIJ to resist. On positional testing, the ASIS, PSIS, and ischial tuberosity are superior on the impaired side (the sacrum is relatively inferior). In addition, the innominate may be either anteriorly or posteriorly rotated. If the innominate is anteriorly rotated and superior, the ipsilateral sacrotuberous ligament will be slack. The neutral zone of motion of the SIJ cannot be located for testing until after the joint is decompressed.

Inferior distraction of the SIJ – passive manipulation

Patient and therapist position If the innominate is anteriorly rotated and superiorly fixated, the patient is prone. If the innominate is posteriorly rotated and superiorly fixated, the patient is supine. The lower leg is grasped proximal to the talocrural joint. The hip joint is extended (if the innominate is anteriorly rotated) or flexed (if innominate is posteriorly rotated) and medially rotated. The manipulation barrier is reached by applying a longitudinal pull through the leg (Fig. 10.16).

Correction technique – manipulation A high-velocity, low-amplitude tug is applied through the leg to distract the inferior aspect of the SIJ. After the fixation is reduced, the arthrokinetic stability test of the SIJ will reveal an increased neutral zone of motion in the craniocaudal direction. Any residual malalignment between the innominate and sacrum should be corrected (see Techniques to correct alignment, below), following which the pelvic girdle is supported with a proper belt (see below) or taped. Treatment to restore force closure/motor control (stabilization exercise therapy) then follows.

SIJ: ANTERIOR SHEAR FIXATION – INNOMINATE

An anterior shear fixation of the innominate at the SIJ can occur when a posteroanterior force through the pelvic girdle (a fall on the posterior pelvis) exceeds the ability of the SIJ to resist. On positional testing, the ASIS and pubis are *anterior* on the impaired side (the pelvis feels like it has been torqued into a rhomboid shape). In addition, the innominate may be either anteriorly or posteriorly rotated. The neutral zone of motion of the SIJ cannot be located for testing until after the joint is decompressed.

Posterior distraction of the SIJ – passive manipulation

Patient and therapist position The patient is supine, with the hips and knees flexed. With the long and ring finger of one hand, palpate the sacral sulcus just medial to the PSIS (Fig. 8.28). The flexed hip and knee are supported by the therapist's shoulder and arm. The femur is flexed, adducted, and internally rotated to the motion barrier of the hip joint. The manipulation barrier for distraction of the posterior aspect of the SIJ is reached by applying a dorsolateral force along the length of the femur.

Correction technique – manipulation A high-velocity, low-amplitude dorsolateral thrust (Fig. 10.17) is applied through the femur to the SIJ. After the fixation is reduced, the arthrokinetic stability test of the SIJ will reveal an increased neutral zone of motion in the anteroposterior direction. Any residual malalignment between the innominate and sacrum should be corrected (see Techniques to correct alignment, below), following which the pelvic girdle is supported with a proper belt (see below) or taped.

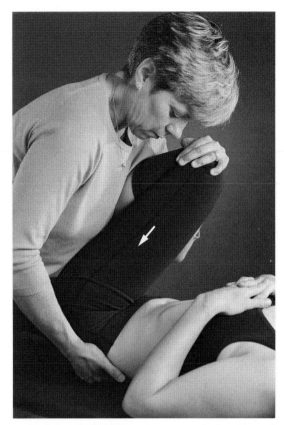

Figure 10.17 Manipulation to decompress a horizontal anterior shear fixation of the right innominate (posterior sacroiliac joint distraction in neutral rotation). The arrow indicates the direction of force applied by the therapist. (Reproduced with permission from © Diane G. Lee Physiotherapist Corp.)

Treatment to restore force closure/motor control (stabilization exercise therapy) then follows.

SIJ: POSTERIOR ROTATION FIXATION – INNOMINATE

This fixation usually occurs in a young, athletic individual. The mode of onset is usually traumatic, commonly a rotary force through the leg. An over-zealous kick against a missed target is a common cause. When the innominate is fixated in posterior rotation, the ASIS is superior, the PSIS is inferior, the ischial tuberosity is ventral but level in the craniocaudal plane, and the sacrotuberous ligament is under marked tension on the side of the fixation. The L5 vertebra as well as the sacrum tends to be rotated towards the side of the dysfunction. The neutral zone of motion of the SIJ cannot be located for testing until after the joint is decompressed.

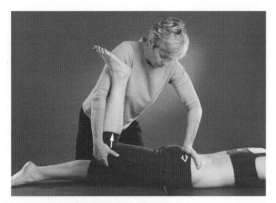

Figure 10.18 Manipulation to decompress a posterior rotation fixation of the right innominate. The arrows indicate the direction of force applied by the therapist. (Reproduced with permission from © Diane G. Lee Physiotherapist Corp.)

Posterior distraction/anterior rotation of the SIJ – passive manipulation

Patient and therapist position With the patient prone, lying close to the edge of the table, the anterior aspect of the distal thigh is palpated with the caudal hand, while the PSIS of the innominate is palpated with the heel of the cranial hand. The manipulation barrier for anterior rotation of the innominate is reached by passively extending the femur with the caudal hand and applying an anterolateral force to the innominate with the cranial hand (Fig. 10.18).

Correction technique – manipulation A high-velocity, low-amplitude thrust is applied through the innominate in an anterolateral direction while the other hand simultaneously extends the femur, thus anteriorly rotating the innominate. The lateral pressure on the PSIS distracts the posterior aspect of the SIJ. After the fixation is reduced, the arthrokinetic stability test of the SIJ will reveal an increased neutral zone of motion in the anteroposterior direction. Any residual malalignment between the innominate and sacrum should be corrected, following which the pelvic girdle is supported with a proper belt (see below) or taped. Treatment to restore force closure/motor control (stabilization exercise therapy) then follows.

SIJ: ANTERIOR ROTATION FIXATION – INNOMINATE

The mechanism of injury is traumatic, with hyperextension of the leg being a significant factor. On positional testing, the ASIS is inferior, PSIS superior, ischial tuberosity is dorsal but level in the craniocaudal

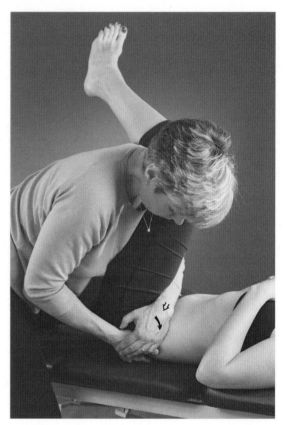

Figure 10.19 Manipulation to decompress an anterior rotation fixation of the right innominate (posterior rotation and distraction of the sacroiliac joint). The arrows indicate the direction of force applied by the therapist. (Reproduced with permission from © Diane G. Lee Physiotherapist Corp.)

plane, and the sacrotuberous ligament, although still palpable, is less taut than normal on the side of the dysfunction. The L5 vertebra and the sacrum tend to rotate away from the affected side. The neutral zone of motion of the SIJ cannot be located for testing until after the joint is decompressed.

Posterior distraction/posterior rotation of the SIJ – passive manipulation

Patient and therapist position The patient is supine, with the hips and knees flexed. With the long and ring finger of one hand, palpate the sacral sulcus just medial to the PSIS (Fig. 8.28). The flexed hip and knee are supported over the therapist's shoulder and arm. The femur is flexed and adducted to the motion barrier of the hip joint. The manipulation barrier for distraction of the posterior aspect of the SIJ is reached by applying a dorsolateral force coupled with posterior rotation of the innominate (Fig. 10.19).

Correction technique – manipulation A high-velocity, low-amplitude dorsolateral thrust is applied through the innominate to distract the sacroiliac joint. After the fixation is reduced, the arthrokinetic stability test of the SIJ will reveal an increased neutral zone of motion in the anteroposterior direction. Any residual malalignment between the innominate and sacrum should be corrected, following which the pelvic girdle is supported with a proper belt (see below) or taped. Treatment to restore force closure/motor control (stabilization exercise therapy) then follows.

SIJ: HORIZONTAL SHEAR FIXATION (ANTERIOR OR POSTERIOR) – RIGHT SIDE OF SACRUM

The mode of onset is commonly a lifting, twisting injury. The patient often reports hearing and feeling a pop and a sharp pain localized to the SIJ at the time of the injury. On positional testing, the sacral base and the inferior lateral angle (ILA) are either anterior or posterior on the side of the articular restriction and this displacement persists in all positions of the trunk – hyperflexion, neutral, and hyperextension. The neutral zone of motion of the SIJ cannot be located for testing until after the joint is decompressed.

Posterior distraction of the SIJ passive manipulation

Patient and therapist position With the patient in left sidelying and the lower leg extended and the upper hip and knee flexed, the thoracolumbar spine is rotated until L5–S1 is felt to be fully rotated to the right. The L5 vertebra is firmly stabilized with one hand to maintain the rotation at the lumbosacral junction. With the other hand, the right innominate is internally rotated *about a pure vertical axis through the pelvic girdle* to gap or distract the posterior aspect of the SIJ (Fig. 10.20). The technique can be focused to the S1, S2, or S3 segment.

Correction technique – manipulation From this position, a high-velocity, low-amplitude thrust is applied through the right innominate to distract the posterior aspect of the SIJ. This technique is effective for either an anterior or posterior shear fixation of the sacrum. After the fixation is reduced, the arthrokinetic stability test for the SIJ will reveal an increased neutral zone of motion in the anteroposterior direction. Any residual malalignment between the innominate and sacrum should be corrected (see below) or taped. Treatment to restore force

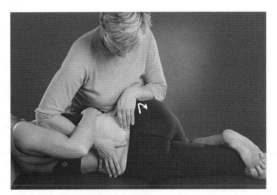

Figure 10.20 Manipulation to decompress a horizontal sacral shear fixation of the right sacroiliac joint. The arrow indicates the direction of force applied by the therapist. (Reproduced with permission from © Diane G. Lee Physiotherapist Corp.)

closure/motor control (stabilization exercise therapy) then follows.

RESTORING FORM CLOSURE (MOBILITY) – HIP JOINT

Limited range of motion of the hip is extremely common and often painless. It can lead to secondary hypermobility of the sacroiliac and/or lumbar joints which then become painful. The hip joint can also be malaligned by muscle imbalance of the global muscle slings (Fig. 8.41). Both the stiff joint and the malaligned (non-centered) joint will have significant consequences for mobility. The following passive mobilization techniques are used to restore the articular kinematics when the joint is stiff. Specific home exercises help to maintain the increased mobility gained in the treatment session. See Restoring force closure and motor control, below, for techniques to realign the femoral head and release the "butt gripper."

THE FIBROTIC HIP JOINT

Lateral distraction of the hip – passive and active mobilization

This is a useful preliminary mobilization technique which can be graded according to the irritability of the joint and surrounding soft tissues. A grade 2 or 3 technique is indicated for the painful joint. If the joint is stiff, a grade 4+ technique sustained for up to 3 min is indicated.

Patient and therapist position With the patient lying supine, hip and knee flexed, a mobilization

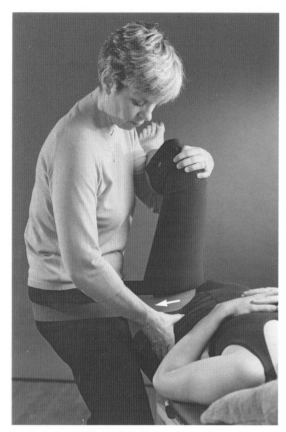

Figure 10.21 Passive mobilization for distraction of the hip joint. The arrow indicates the direction of force applied by the therapist. (Reproduced with permission from © Diane G. Lee Physiotherapist Corp.)

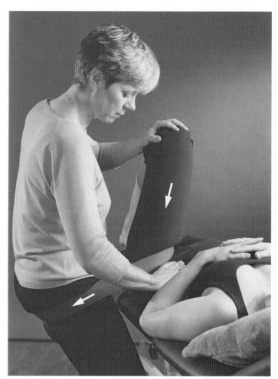

Figure 10.22 Passive mobilization for posterior glide of the femoral head in flexion. Encourage relaxation of the external rotators of the hip by telling the patient to imagine the femur is sinking into soft soil (arrow on femur). The femur is dorsally glided through the mobilization belt as the therapist bends the knees; distraction of the hip joint can be added to this technique. The arrow on the patient's femur reflects the "sinking femur" and the arrow on the mobilization belt indicates the direction of force applied by the therapist. (Reproduced with permission from © Diane G. Lee Physiotherapist Corp.)

belt is placed around the proximal thigh and secured around the therapist's pelvis (Fig. 10.21).

Correction technique – passive mobilization The hip joint is distracted by applying a lateral force parallel to the neck of the femur. The posteroanterior orientation of the applied force will vary and depends on the degree of femoral anteversion present. The technique is graded according to the joint/myofascial reaction.

Correction technique – Mulligan mobilization An active mobilization with movement technique (Mulligan) can be added by maintaining the lateral distraction described above and having the patient actively move into the direction of the restriction (flexion, extension, abduction, adduction, internal, or external rotation).

Home exercise Range of motion exercises (general flexion, extension, abduction, adduction, internal rotation, external rotation) which maintain the movement gained in the treatment session should be taught.

Posterior glide of the femoral head – in femoral flexion

Sustained overactivation of the external rotators of the hip can cause the posterior capsule to tighten. The following technique can be used *after* the deep external rotators have been released (see Reducing rigidity – downtraining the global system, below).

Patient and therapist position With the patient lying supine, hip and knee flexed, a mobilization belt is placed around the proximal thigh and secured around the therapist's pelvis. Flex/adduct the femur to the motion barrier without impinging the anterior aspect of the joint.

Correction technique – passive mobilization The motion barrier of femoral flexion and adduction is maintained and an anteroposterior glide of the femoral head is applied through the mobilization belt by slightly bending your knees (Fig. 10.22).

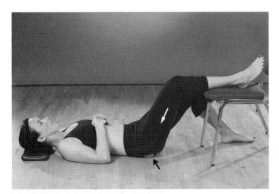

Figure 10.23   Home exercise to reseat the femoral head posteriorly. The ball (note the small black arrow) provides pressure to the muscles of the posterior buttock. With a conscious release of the posterior buttock muscles, gravity allows the femur to "sink" dorsally (large white arrow) thus reseating the femoral head and applying a gentle stretch to the posterior capsule of the hip joint. (Reproduced with permission from © Diane G. Lee Physiotherapist Corp.)

Therapist facilitation – verbal cues   Instruct the patient to imagine the femur as a telephone pole sinking into soft soil or mud and to try to allow the femoral head to *release* posterior into the acetabulum. This image will facilitate further relaxation of the external rotators of the hip and allow a deeper posterior capsular stretch. Lateral distraction of the joint can be added to this technique.

Home exercise   The patient is lying on the floor with the affected leg supported on a foot stool or the foot supported on the wall. A small ball can be placed posteriorly just behind the greater trochanter or over a tender trigger point (Fig. 10.23). The exercise is to relax the posterior buttock (let the ball sink into the muscles of the buttock) and allow gravity to take the leg dorsally such that the femoral head disengages from the anterior acetabulum and provides a stretch to the posterior capsule. Patients often find that the image of the telephone pole sinking into mud is helpful to facilitate this relaxation and stretch. A four-point kneeling rock (Fig. 10.24) or rock'n'roll on a gym ball (Fig. 10.25) are also useful exercises for this.

Posterior glide of the femoral head – in femoral extension

The following technique is useful for reseating the femoral head in extension, which is a requirement of the terminal stance phase of gait.

Patient and therapist position   With the patient lying prone with the knee flexed, palpate the distal end of the femur with one hand and the posterior aspect of the greater trochanter with the other.

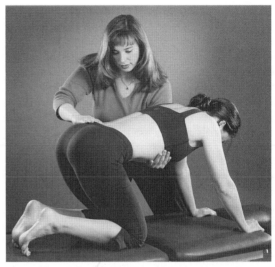

Figure 10.24   Hip rock in the four-point kneeling position. The patient is taught to position the thoracolumbar spine in a neutral position with the pelvic girdle anteriorly tilted 90°. While maintaining this position, the patient is instructed to rock directly posterior, thus increasing the angle of hip flexion. The tendency will be to tilt the pelvis posteriorly (flex the hips) and lose the lumbar lordosis. The therapist supports the ribcage to assist in the maintenance of the thoracic kyphosis while one hand cues lengthening in the lumbar spine to maintain the lordosis. (Reproduced with permission from © Diane G. Lee Physiotherapist Corp.)

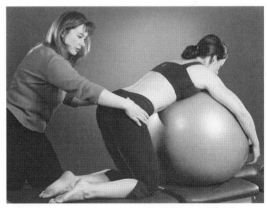

Figure 10.25   Rock'n'roll on a gym ball. The ball supports the primary thoracic curve, the therapist ensures that the lumbar lordosis and anterior pelvic tilt are maintained as the patient rocks backwards and then rolls forwards. The tendency will be for the patient to tilt the pelvis posteriorly and flex the lumbar spine during the backward rock and remain flexed and posteriorly tilted during the forward roll. The pelvis can be rocked diagonally backwards to incorporate rotation with hip flexion. (Reproduced with permission from © Diane G. Lee Physiotherapist Corp.)

Correction technique – passive mobilization The motion barrier of femoral extension/internal rotation is maintained with the caudal hand and an anteroposterior glide of the femoral head is applied by gliding the greater trochanter anteriorly and medially.

Therapist facilitation – verbal cues Instruct the patient to relax the hip to allow the femoral head to seat posteriorly into the acetabulum.

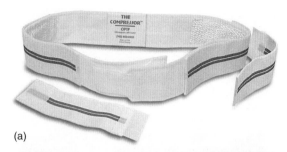

(a)

SACROILIAC BELTS AND TAPING

Subsequent to manipulating a SIJ fixation, the underlying increase in neutral zone motion becomes apparent. At this time an external support can help to control the excessive translation until such time as force closure and motor control can be restored. The external support (taping or a belt) is used only as an adjunct to the restoration of force closure. Damen et al (2002c, d) were able to show using Doppler imaging that the stiffness of the SIJ increases when a belt is applied to the pelvis. There are many sacroiliac belts on the market and most will be effective in providing some degree of compression (Vleeming et al 1992c). However, patients sometimes require more or less compression than a general belt can supply and often it is difficult to specify the location of the compression (bilateral anterior, bilateral posterior, unilateral anterior, and/or unilateral posterior). This led to the development of a new sacroiliac belt – the *Compressor*™ (Lee 2002) (Fig. 10.26a, b). Essentially this belt consists of a light fabric material which is wrapped around the pelvic girdle and secured with Velcro. The compression straps are then attached to the belt specifying the location of compression. The straps can be overlapped (doubled up) to increase the amount of compression at that location. Four straps of two different lengths are included with the belt. The ASLR test (Ch. 8) is used to determine exactly where and how much compression is needed. If bilateral anterior compression of the pelvis (approximate the ASISs: Fig. 8.58) allows the patient to lift the leg with less effort, then two straps are applied by anchoring each band laterally and pulling them to the anterior midline (pubic symphysis). One band is applied at a time. If bilateral posterior compression of the pelvis (approximate the PSISs: Fig. 8.59) allows the patient to lift the leg with less effort, then two straps are applied by anchoring each band laterally and pulling them to the posterior midline.

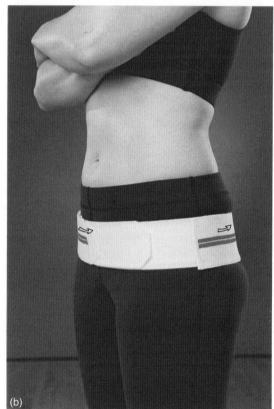

(b)

Figure 10.26 (a) The *Compressor*™ is a belt designed for the pelvic girdle which allows for specifying both the amount and location of the compression by varying the number and location of the compression straps. (b) In this application, the compression straps are applied to compress the right anterior pelvis and the left posterior pelvis. (Reproduced with permission from © Diane G. Lee Physiotherapist Corp.)

One band is applied at a time. If unilateral anterior compression and unilateral posterior compression are the most effective, then one band is applied anteriorly and one band posteriorly (Fig. 10.26b). Once the bands are applied, the ASLR is repeated. The patient should notice a marked difference in the ability to transfer load through the pelvic girdle through a reduction in the effort required to lift the leg when either supine or in standing. The same principles and tests are applied if tape is used instead of the *Compressor*™.

Initially, the pelvis should be taped or supported by a belt whenever the patient is vertical (i.e., standing, sitting, or during any activity of daily living). As force closure returns, the patient should wean off the belt by reducing the amount of compression (loosen the tension in the compression straps) and finally removing the belt altogether for short periods of time (begin with 30 min). Ultimately, the patient should be able to eliminate the need for any external support.

PROLOTHERAPY

Prolotherapy (Dorman 1994, 1997) is indicated when there has been a loss of form closure (articular instability) and the local system cannot supply sufficient compression to compensate and force close the joint under load. When the force closure mechanism is effective, co-contraction of the muscles of the local system should compress the joint and thereby increase its stiffness. The neutral zone of motion is subsequently reduced to zero. If the local system is contracting appropriately and yet is unable to increase the stiffness (stability) of the joint, then the active force closure mechanism is ineffective for controlling shear. This is a poor prognostic sign for successful rehabilitation with exercise and the primary indication for prolotherapy. In prolotherapy, the ligaments of the unstable joint are injected with an irritant solution which creates an inflammatory reaction. The subsequent migration of fibroblasts into the inflamed tissue promotes the production of collagen which increases the stiffness of the ligament. Typically, the ligaments are injected every 2 weeks and the treatment is repeated for four to six sessions. The role of the therapist during this process is to ensure that the joint is stabilized with an external support or tape to prevent excessive shearing of the joint and to ensure that optimal alignment is maintained through the use of active mobilization techniques. Since prolotherapy is often painful, the therapist should be prepared to provide emotional support during this process. Once the force closure mechanism begins to affect the neutral zone of motion (the joint glide can be reduced by a co-contraction of the local system), biomechanical recovery has begun. Force closure and motor control retraining can now begin.

RESTORING FORCE CLOSURE AND MOTOR CONTROL

Before specific exercises can be described, it is important to discuss some key considerations for developing the program. The therapist should:

• Educate the patient as to the importance of a new approach to exercise. Discuss what happens to the brain's programming of muscle coordination with pain and injury (Ch. 5) and the importance of practice, mindful movement, and incorporation into daily activities. It is helpful to remind patients that this is not really exercise but rather "changing the way you live in your body."

• Remind the patient that "practice makes permanent, not perfect" to reinforce the importance of *quality* of movement, rather than *quantity* of exercise.

• Ensure that the exercise program is specific to the patient's needs and not generic. This requires that faulty movement patterns are identified. The therapist should have identified:

– the levels of poor control (Ch. 8: Regional movement tests)
– the direction(s) of poor control (Ch. 8: Regional movement tests and form closure analysis)
– the levels or regions of restricted mobility (Ch. 8: Form closure analysis)
– the overactive/dominant global muscles or slings of muscles (Ch. 8: Force closure/motor control analysis)
– the inactive/underrecruited muscles (local stabilizers) or slings of muscles (global muscles) (Ch. 8: Force closure/motor control analysis)
– any specific muscle length/strength imbalances (Ch. 8: Force closure/motor control analysis).

• Design and modify the exercise program based on tissue health, tissue irritability, and stage of healing (Ch. 7). Speed of progression will depend on a number of factors, including the capacity of the patient for learning new tasks.

Strength, endurance, and power of the global trunk muscles are important components of muscle function that should be assessed and treated when identified as deficits. However, it is not the intent of this chapter to cover exercises or protocols for these components as several sources exist on these topics (McArdle et al 1991, Farrell et al 1994, Brukner & Khan

2002, McGill 2002). Instead, the focus of the exercises presented is the restoration of motor control whereby underrecruited muscles are reactivated through mind–body awareness and imagery. This connection and activation of underrecruited local and global muscles is essential prior to prescribing exercises for strength, as unless the brain is using the muscle, exercises for strengthening that muscle will only serve to strengthen alternate muscles being substituted for the action (e.g., hip extension exercises for gluteus maximus can be performed using the hamstrings). Thus, the focus of the exercises here is control of movement, with optimum technique, and with an awareness of the segments and areas of poor control that need to be corrected. Once the brain has "found" the muscle, protocols for endurance, strength, and power can be used if needed for patient-specific goals. Following the presentation of the lumbopelvic stabilization program, exercises for strengthening specific muscles commonly affected in patients with lumbopelvic-hip dysfunction are presented.

Altered muscle length has implications for strength (due to length–tension relationships) and for restriction of mobility. Assessment of the underlying cause of altered muscle length is crucial for correcting the dysfunction in the muscle. It is rarely a matter of simply stretching a tight muscle. Chapter 8 described tests for common patterns of muscle length restrictions (see Global system slings: length analysis). These test positions can be adapted into therapist-assisted stretching techniques or home exercises. Often, a technique that incorporates activation of neural pathways is more effective for releasing the muscle; these include active mobilization or muscle energy, reciprocal inhibition, and IMS. It is beneficial to follow these techniques with home exercises that maintain extensibility in the released muscles. Some examples of these exercises are presented later in this chapter. The reader is referred to other sources (Kendall et al 1993, Stark 1997, Hall & Brody 1999) for a more comprehensive covering of stretching and flexibility exercises.

REDUCING RIGIDITY – DOWNTRAINING THE GLOBAL SYSTEM

POSTURAL RE-EDUCATION, NEUTRAL SPINE, AND RELEASING THE "BUTT GRIPPER"

This section will introduce exercises that emphasize movement with awareness in finding neutral spine,

correcting breathing patterns, and releasing the hip. Sapsford et al (2001) investigated spinal position and the effect of position on abdominal muscle recruitment during "hollowing" (aimed to recruit primarily transversus abdominis (TA) and internal oblique (IO)), and "bracing" (a contraction of all the abdominal muscles) maneuvers. The spinal position found to produce the greatest increase in TA activity was the neutral spine position. In the flexed position the external oblique (EO) muscle had the greatest increase in activity. Although the study was performed with a small number of subjects, the findings are consistent with what we observe in the clinical setting. Notably, a common substitution strategy for patients with lumbopelvic dysfunction is a "butt gripping" (Fig. 8.40) or an abdominal bracing (Fig. 9.4) strategy to transfer load. These patterns of activation result in a posterior pelvic tilt, a flexed lumbar spine, and a braced hip joint. Attempting to teach exercises that isolate the local muscles (TA, deep fibers of multifidus) without first correcting the spinal position can often lead to frustration for both the therapist and the patient.

Two methods for postural correction can be used:

1. positioning the patient passively into a neutral spine position and then teaching the patient how to perform self-positioning at home (see sidelying position below) or
2. teaching the patient to find neutral spine with an active exercise but *without excessive global activity, especially in the erector spinae and superficial multifidus muscles.*

It has been our clinical experience that by addressing spinal position, cues for recruitment and isolation of the local muscles are more effective and efficient. Usually both passive positioning for exercises as well as active exercises to learn neutral spine are included in a patient's program; however, initially they may be separate exercises performed in two different positions. For example, a patient who lies in a posterior pelvic tilt in crook lying may be given the roll-up–roll-down exercise (see below) to learn how to find the neutral spine position and release holding in the global muscles of the trunk and hip. This may take a fair amount of mental concentration; the patient's spinal position will improve with practice of the exercise and with the concurrent manual release and mobilization techniques being performed by the therapist. If the patient cannot fully release into neutral spine in this exercise (i.e., remains in some posterior pelvic tilt but to a less degree), the addition of cues to recruit TA in this position will still bias recruitment of the EO. Thus, recruitment and isolation of TA are taught in a different position. By changing the position for practicing TA isolation exercises, the brain is given a short concentration break, which is important with exercises that retrain motor learning. The alternate position chosen is the one where the patient can easily find neutral and thus will have the easiest time recruiting TA. Sidelying or prone are the most common alternate positions for patients who have difficulty moving out of posterior pelvic tilt (see below).

It should be noted that there are other benefits and effects of neutral spine exercises. Notably, by using active exercise to retrain neutral spine, the patient is learning a new place to live in the body, which then reinforces new stabilization strategies as they are learned. Correcting asymmetries in the spinal curves and in thoracopelvic alignment facilitates more symmetrical activity in the global slings and places restricted portions of the global slings on continuous stretch. Furthermore, a key rehabilitation goal is to progress the stabilization exercise program to upright, functional positions and activities. When performing exercises in the standing position the patient often reverts to a habitual poor posture or an overerect posture that simply increases already dominant global muscle activity, moves through existing hypermobilities, and avoids movement through typically stiff joints. In the initial stages of rehabilitation, it is often difficult for the patient to assume a neutral spinal position in standing, even with verbal and tactile cueing. Supine and four-point kneeling over a ball are less loaded positions where this skill can be developed and then applied to more upright positions as the exercise program is progressed. Thus, training of neutral spine is an essential part of the postural re-education process and addressing dysfunction in both the local and global systems.

The neutral spine position is defined as the position where the normal spinal curves are present and the thorax is centered over the pelvis. In each different body position (supine, four-point kneeling, sitting, standing), the same spinal orientation is desired: gradual, even curves with a neutral pelvic tilt (ASISs and pubic symphysis in the same coronal plane), lumbar lordosis, thoracic kyphosis, and cervical lordosis. Kendall et al (1993) provide a foundation from which to classify different postures; however, often a more specific segmental analysis and specific palpation are needed. In each region,

we are not only looking for an increase or decrease in the normal curve, but also for specific levels of abnormal curvature. A common presentation is excessive lordosis in the upper lumbar levels, the thoracolumbar junction, and lower thoracic spine, while the lower lumbar spine has a loss of lordosis (L4–L5 and L5–L1 levels remain flexed) with a posterior pelvic tilt (Fig. 9.22a). The patient with a spondylolisthesis often has a decreased lordosis or flexed segments above and below the level of excessive anterior shear. Thus, a segmental analysis of spinal posture/curves is required during assessment, and levels of excessive flexion or extension should be targeted for correction with manual and verbal cues during the exercises below.

Neutral spine – passive positioning sidelying

Patient and therapist position   The patient is sidelying facing the therapist with the knees bent. Stand facing the patient with your body at the level of the patient's lumbar spine. With your cranial hand, palpate the lumbar curve. Identify levels of excessive flexion or extension. The caudal hand slides under the patient's ankles and the weight of the legs is supported by the therapist's caudal thigh (Fig. 10.27).

Correction technique   The legs are passively moved into flexion and extension as the lumbar spine is palpated for changes in the curve. When a gentle, even lordosis is achieved, place the legs on the plinth at that position. Note the position of the feet relative to the rest of the body. The neutral spinal position is often obtained where the soles of the feet lie in the same plane as the trunk. Instruct the patient how to find this position at home. The idea of pretending to lie against a wall with the soles of the feet and

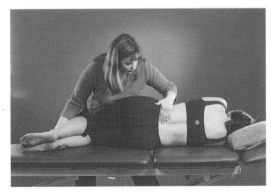

Figure 10.27   Neutral spine: sidelying, passive positioning. (Reproduced with permission from © Diane G. Lee Physiotherapist Corp.)

the back both touching the wall is a helpful cue. Have the patient palpate the lumbar spinal curve both in the habitual sidelying position and in the new position. Ensure that the patient can find the neutral position without your assistance.

Neutral spine – crook lying roll-up–roll-down

Patient and therapist position The patient is supine with the hips and knees comfortably flexed. Stand at the patient's side. Slide one hand under the lumbar spine, spreading the fingers to allow palpation of several interspinous spaces. Make note of the resting lumbar spine orientation. Observe the ribcage and look for a lifted sternum or space under the lower thoracic spine. While in this position, use your fingers to give tactile feedback as you educate the patient about the goal of the exercise ("your low back is very flat/the curve is uneven here, this is where we need to change the curve"). In order to help the patient learn the exercise movement, the patient's hands are placed on the upper and lower

sternum, and the therapist's hands are placed so that one hand palpates at one hip, and the other hand palpates in the lower abdomen (Fig. 10.28a). During the exercise and in subsequent repetitions of the movement the therapist's hands will move to palpate and facilitate at several key points of control, depending on the correction needed for optimal exercise execution.

Correction technique – verbal and manual cues The patient is asked to draw the lower abdomen to the bed, then to push through the feet and lift the hips off the bed, rolling the spine gently into a "C" (posterior pelvic tilt and spinal flexion), lifting up to the level of the lower thoracic spine (Fig. 10.28b). How high the hips and lumbar spine are lifted depends on the patient's ability to maintain a flexed spine. Lifting is not permitted beyond a point where spinal extension and/or activity in the erector spinae muscles occur. Next, ask the patient to lie the spine back down on the bed, starting from the ribcage. The thorax is kept heavy on the bed to maintain the thoracic kyphosis, and the vertebrae

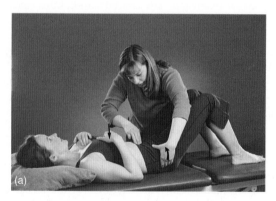
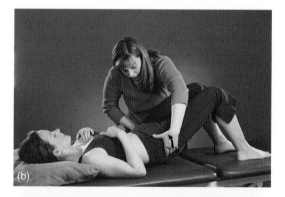
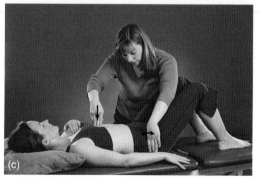

Figure 10.28 Neutral spine: crook lying roll-up–roll-down. (a) The patient palpates the sternum to self-cue a heavy, relaxed thorax (vertical arrow) during the movement. No lifting of the sternum is permitted. The therapist palpates at the lower abdomen to cue a gentle drawing-in of the lower abdomen and around the hip to facilitate a posterior tilt (curved arrow) of the pelvis and flexion of the lumbar spine (arrow). (b) The hips and pelvis are lifted off the bed to continue the flexion movement into the upper lumbar and lower thoracic levels. The hips are lifted only to the point that spinal flexion can be maintained; in this example the lift is stopped at the thoracolumbar junction. (c) Release into lumbar lordosis. The therapist provides gentle posterior pressure on the lower sternum (vertical arrow) to prevent thoracolumbar extension as the pelvis falls forward into an anterior tilt. The therapist's left hand is providing a cue to release the anterior hip as well as drawing the pelvis anteriorly and inferiorly (curved arrow). On subsequent repetitions of the exercise the therapist can palpate the lumbar spine to facilitate the lordosis and ensure that the superficial multifidus and erector spinae remain relaxed during the roll-up and at the final release into neutral lordosis. (Reproduced with permission from © Diane G. Lee Physiotherapist Corp.)

are unrolled one segment at a time. Once the lumbar spine is flat on the bed, ask the patient to "let the tailbone fall to the bed" or "let the pelvis roll forward" and *allow* a small curve in the low back to occur (Fig. 10.28c). Observe and palpate for where the lordosis occurs – watch for a sternal lift (thoracic extension) and feel for excessive segmental lordosis (e.g., L3). The goal is a lumbar lordosis shared by all lumbar segments. Have the patient repeat the movement several times, each time using your hands and cues to improve the end released position. Do not let the patient force the spine into lumbar extension. This active movement will cause a strong thoracic erector spinae contraction or superficial multifidus contraction (parts of the global slings), and will inhibit recruitment of the deep local stabilizing muscles (as well as potentially increasing back pain and soreness due to excessive compression).

Key points of control for hands:

- Fingers can provide proprioception at levels that need to lengthen into a lordosis – glide your fingers along the spinous processes in a vertical line.
- Hand on sternum to prevent lifting of chest – keep "heavy."
- Hands in hip creases to facilitate "folding" of hips and "opening" of pelvis (anterior tilt) (Fig. 10.28c).
- Use small wiggles (gentle rotation) of the ribcage, pelvis, and/or hips to facilitate decreased global muscle contraction and rigidity.

Verbal/visual cues:

- "Relax your buttocks, and let your sitz bones go wide as the tailbone falls to the bed."
- "Let your hips go heavy as they sink to the bed."
- "Let your low back lengthen as you let your pelvis fall forward."
- "Imagine a line between the bottom of the sternum and the pubic bone; the line should get longer during the release phase; the length comes from the pubic bone falling forward, while the sternum point stays still."
- "Keep the chest heavy, relax the back."

Ideal response   As the roll-up portion is performed, there is a relaxation of the lumbar and thoracic extensor muscles and segmental flexion occurs from the pelvis to the lower thorax. At the end of

the roll-down component, the thorax remains in a flexed position as the lumbar spine passively falls into a lordosis. The anterior and posterior hip muscles are relatively relaxed (no areas of marked hypertonicity).

Progressions/other considerations   Support the legs at the knees with a bolster if the patient cannot relax the buttocks and perform the exercise through a smaller range of motion.

Postural re-education of neutral spine in sitting – setting the optimal pyramid base

Patient and therapist position   The patient sits on a chair or plinth. The therapist stands or kneels beside the patient on the same side as the "butt gripping" hip. Place one hand under the ischial tuberosity, and the other hand along the top of the iliac crest (Fig. 10.29).

Correction technique – verbal and manual cues   Ask the patient to focus on the amount of weight on each buttock, and to decide if the weight is evenly distributed between the left and right sides. Instruct the patient to lean away from you slightly, taking

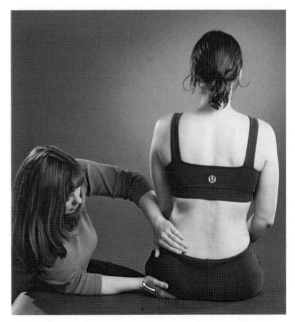

Figure 10.29   Neutral spine in sitting: setting the optimal pyramid base. Here, the patient leans to the right while the therapist resets the left innominate position (arrow). The force used is determined by how much "butt gripping" is present. The final position should reveal a level pelvis and equal weight-bearing through the left and right buttocks. (Reproduced with permission from © Diane G. Lee Physiotherapist Corp.)

the weight off the affected buttock. Now, lift and pull the ischial tuberosity laterally and posteriorly, and apply a gentle medial counterforce to the iliac crest as the patient slowly returns the buttock back down to the chair. Use the cue, "As you lower your buttock, think of letting the sitz bone on this side go wide and open behind you." In the new position, the patient should feel more equal weight distribution between the two ischial tuberosities; this provides the wide, stable base of the optimal pyramid.

Ideal response In the new position, the pelvis should be in a neutral rotation in the transverse plane and the iliac crests should be level. Compared to the initial sitting position (precorrection), lateral bending and rotation curves in the lumbar spine are often less pronounced or completely corrected. The anterior and posterior hip muscles on the affected side are softer and more equal in tone to the other hip, and the femoral head seats more posteriorly in the acetabulum (there will be a deeper crease in the anterior hip).

Progressions/other considerations The patient can be taught how to set the pyramid base independently for exercises and functional activities in sitting. The patient's ipsilateral hand is used to pull the ischial tuberosity out and back as the weight is shifted and replaced. The patient may need to perform a few repetitions of this movement to get an equal placement of the ischial tuberosities. Exercises and techniques to release the posterior hip muscles should be concurrently performed, with the eventual goal that the patient can assume the wide pyramid base position without needing manual self-correction. Patients with limited hip flexion should initially sit on a higher chair or stool for this exercise so that the pelvis can move anteriorly over the femoral heads into a neutral tilt position.

Postural re-education of neutral spine in sitting – setting the spinal position

Patient and therapist position The patient sits on a chair or a ball, with the optimal pyramid base (see above). If the patient has limited hip flexion either unilaterally or bilaterally, increase the height of the sitting surface so that the pelvis is able to move anteriorly over the femurs (to allow the creation of a neutral lordosis in the lumbar spine). The therapist stands or kneels beside the patient (Fig. 10.30). Hand placement will depend on which levels of the spine need correction (see verbal and manual cues). Correct the thoracic curve first, then the lumbar curve, and finally the head/cervical position.

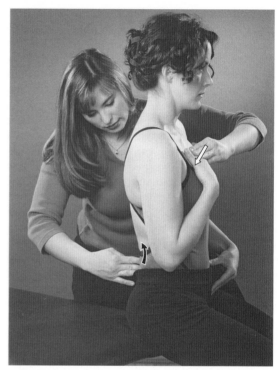

Figure 10.30 Neutral spine in sitting: setting the spinal position. In this example the therapist is correcting a flattened thoracic kyphosis and a decreased lumbar lordosis at L5 and L4. The therapist's left hand helps the patient create a "sinking" or "heaviness" on the sternum to facilitate an increase in the thoracic kyphosis in the upper thoracic spine and bring the ribcage posteriorly over the pelvis. The therapist's right hand produces a gentle cranial and anterior pressure through the lumbar spinous processes to facilitate a lifting of the sacrum, gentle lumbar lordosis, and tilting of the pelvis forward and under the ribcage. (Reproduced with permission from © Diane G. Lee Physiotherapist Corp.)

Correction technique – verbal and manual cues For areas of decreased thoracic kyphosis (usually accompanied by excessive erector spinae activity):

"Let the chest sink" or "go heavy under my hand."

"As your chest sinks, imagine your back opening between your shoulder blades."

"Imagine that the distance from your sternum to your belly button is decreasing as you let the chest go heavy."

For areas of increased thoracic kyphosis:

"Imagine a string attached to your back (palpate at level of increased curve); the string is gently being pulled up to heaven."

"Imagine that your sternum is being gently lifted."

For a decreased lumbar lordosis (flexed lumbar spine):

"Imagine a string attached to your tailbone, and someone else is gently pulling the string up to heaven."
"Grow tall from the tailbone."
"Let your pelvis fall forward as you grow tall from my fingers."
"Imagine that your pelvis is a bowl, and that it is tipping forward as you let your sitz bones go wide."
"Let your buttocks go wide, let your hips fold."
"Allow the ball to roll underneath you as the pelvis rocks forward."

For an increased lumbar lordosis (hyperextended lumbar spine at one or multilevels):

"Relax and let your back round out, then as you grow tall, think of lengthening your low back."
"Rather than arching your back, think of the spine being long and tall, with a gentle even curve."

Manual cues and options for therapist hand placement (points of control):

- upper sternum (for loss of upper thoracic kyphosis)
- lower sternum (for loss of lower thoracic kyphosis and/or anteriorly shifted ribcage)
- posterior thorax/ribcage (for excessive thoracic kyphosis)
- lumbar spine spinous processes (at level where more lordosis is required or where lordosis is excessive)
- manubriosternal symphysis and superior pubic bone (to cue vertical alignment of these points)
- bilaterally around the anterolateral or posterolateral lower ribcage (to draw the thorax as a whole posteriorly, anteriorly, or vertically)
- iliac crests and hip folds (to facilitate anterior pelvic tilt over hips).

As the verbal cues are given, the therapist uses the points of control to create the ideal curvatures. To facilitate increased thoracic kyphosis, the hand on the sternum creates an inferior and posterior pressure. To decrease an excessive kyphosis, the hands lift the ribcage from the sides or give a superior and slightly anterior pressure at the levels of excessive curve. To correct a flat lumbar spine, the fingers push gently anterior and superior, creating a lifting sensation. For an excessive lumbar lordosis at one or two segments, focus on facilitating a lordosis at levels above or below that are flexed, and then lengthening or stretching the curve at the hyper-extended segment(s) by spreading the fingers and applying a vertical pressure.

Ideal response   The creation of the lumbar lordosis should be a release into an optimum curve, not a forced effort with contraction of the erector spinae. As sitting is an upright position, there will be some tone in the erector spinae and superficial multifidus, but it should be symmetrical and not excessive. Rigidity between the thorax and pelvis (inability to dissociate the thorax from the pelvis) is a sign of excessive erector spinae activity (palpate for tone and check lateral mobility of the ribcage – see Rib wiggle, below). Once the thoracic curve has been corrected, as the lumbar lordosis is facilitated the sternal hand should not move superior or anterior (the thoracic kyphosis should be maintained). The goal is to create a gentle, even kyphosis in the thoracic spine, a gentle, even lordosis in the lumbar spine, and a gentle lordosis in the cervical spine; palpate and observe to ensure that one or two segments do not remain excessively flexed or extended. The patient's weight should be centered equally over the ischial tuberosities (the optimal pyramid base), the pubic symphysis and the ASISs should be in the same plane, and the manubriosternal symphysis should be vertically in line with the pubic symphysis. If the ribcage is shifted anterior or posterior to the pelvis (i.e., the manubriosternal symphysis is anterior or posterior to the pubic symphysis), use these two points as patient palpation points for learning and correcting thoracopelvic alignment. The therapist uses a combination of the above points of control to maintain correct thoracic position as the pelvis is brought under the ribcage or maintain the optimal pyramid base as the thorax is moved into alignment over the pelvis.

Progressions/other considerations   The breath can be used to facilitate the proper curves. "Breathe deeply and allow the air to fill the space":

- between your shoulder blades (if mid-thorax is lordotic)
- beneath your sternum (if mid-thorax is kyphotic)
- between your lowest ribs
  - posteriorly (if lordotic)
  - anteriorly (if kyphotic).

Once the spinal curves have been corrected in the sagittal plane, corrections can then be made to any rotation and/or sidebending faults. These asymmetries will correlate with imbalances of length and recruitment in the global slings, especially in those that control thoracopelvic alignment. Scapular position and the muscle balance relationships of the scapulothoracic muscles can also impact thoraco-pelvic alignment. Correction techniques include:

- Bilaterally palpating the ribcage at the levels of rotation and sidebend to correct the asymmetry manually while providing gentle traction through the thorax (this allows the patient to relax). For example, if the thorax is right-rotated and right lat-erally bent, the therapist provides a posterior and inferior force to the left lower ribcage while provid-ing an anterior and superior force to the right lower ribcage.
- A "dumped" scapula (depressed and down-wardly rotated) can contribute to thoracolumbar lateral bending to the same side. Manual or tape support to the scapula will assist in spinal position correction.
- Verbal cues such as "open the ribcage in the front on the right side" and "imagine the space between your ribcage and pelvis on the right side increasing or lengthening" provide the patient with images to self-correct the asymmetry.
- Lateral costal expansion and breathing pat-terns will be asymmetrical; use retraining of lateral costal expansion (see below) unilaterally to release tone in muscles contributing to the asymmetrical spinal position.

Once you have facilitated a neutral spine position, ask the patient to maintain the new position and breathe normally. Observe what happens to spinal position with breathing (apical breathing often causes excessive thoracolumbar extension); use re-education of the breathing pattern (lateral costal expansion, see below) to facilitate maintenance of neutral spine position. Note that small deviations of trunk and lower-limb position will occur in sync with the breathing cycle (Hodges 2003) but these should not be excessive nor result in high levels of global muscle activity and postural rigidity. Check internal and external rotation mobility of the hips; if the patient is unable to move the hips actively or allow passive rotation this is an indication of exces-sive global muscle activity and "butt gripping" (see checkpoints for global rigidity below).

A common exercise technique for finding neutral is some form of pelvic rock. The patient sits on a ball or chair, and is taught to roll the pelvis into an ante-rior tilt, then a posterior tilt, and then resume a "comfortable position halfway between the two positions." Care must be taken with this kind of exercise if given without specific manual or verbal cues. In a population with lumbopelvic dysfunc-tion, the "comfortable" position will be one that avoids restrictions and moves into areas of already excessive movement or poor control. It cannot be assumed that this is true neutral spine. It is essential that segmental palpation and observation of substi-tution patterns are performed by the therapist while giving this exercise. However, with specific correc-tions, the pelvic rock can be a useful method for teaching thoracopelvic movement dissociation and facilitate awareness of where the center of gravity falls in relation to the sitz bones. In a posterior pelvic tilt the patient can be made aware that the center of gravity falls behind the sitz bones, and in an anterior pelvic tilt the patient can be made aware that the center of gravity falls in front of the sitz bones. The goal is that the center of gravity falls in line with the sitz bones, and this awareness can be used as a self-check for the patient when practicing the exercise independently.

Neutral spine in four-point kneeling

Patient and therapist position The patient is four-point kneeling on the floor or on a plinth, shoulders over the hands, hips over the knees. If there is a uni-lateral or bilateral restriction of hip flexion, the hips should be allowed to rock forward of the knees (otherwise the patient will be unable to attain a lumbar lordosis). The therapist kneels or stands beside the patient. Therapist hand placement and facilitation will depend on the areas of thoracic and lumbar curvature that need correction (Fig. 10.31).

Correction technique – verbal and manual cues Verbal cues for decreased thoracic kyphosis:

"Let me have your ribcage; let your back open as I lift your chest."
"Take a breath and bring the air into your back."

For decreased lumbar lordosis:

"Keep your upper back open as you lengthen under my fingers."
"Let your buttocks go wide and the low back fall into a gentle arch."
"Stay supported and open in your ribcage as you let the pelvis fall forward towards the floor, letting the hips fold."

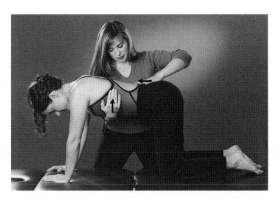

Figure 10.31   Neutral spine: four-point kneeling. In this example, the therapist uses the cranial arm under the ribcage to restore the thoracic kyphosis and bring the ribcage in line with the pelvis (vertical arrow). The caudal hand facilitates the lumbar lordosis with a cranial and anterior pressure (horizontal arrow) while verbal cues are given. (Reproduced with permission from © Diane G. Lee Physiotherapist Corp.)

For increased thoracic kyphosis:

"Lengthen your spine under my hands as you
      let your ribs fall to the floor."

For increased lumbar lordosis:

"Round out your back to the ceiling (reverse the
      curve into flexion). Now let the low back arch
      again but think long and gentle (manual cueing
      is important here; see below)."

Key points of control and options for therapist
hand placement:

- manubriosternal symphysis (for loss of upper
  thoracic kyphosis)
- support under lower ribcage (for loss of lower
  thoracic kyphosis)
- posterior thorax along the spinous processes
  (for excessive thoracic kyphosis)
- lumbar spinous processes (at level(s) where
  more lordosis is required or where the curve
  needs lengthening)
- iliac crests (to facilitate more symmetrical
  lumbar lordosis/lengthening through spine,
  anterior pelvic tilt over hips)
- hip creases (to facilitate hip folding and
  widening of buttocks).

As the verbal cues are given, the therapist uses the points of control to create the ideal curvatures. To facilitate an increased thoracic kyphosis, the fingers under the sternum can press gently posteriorly

(up to the ceiling), or the whole arm can support the ribcage and lift it posteriorly to open up the posterior thorax. To decrease an excessive kyphosis, one hand on the posterior thorax produces an anterior and slightly cranial pressure while the other hand on the sacrum provides an inferior distraction to create a sensation of lengthening to go with the verbal cue. To correct a flat lumbar spine, the fingers push gently anterior and superior, creating a lengthening sensation as the pelvis falls forward but the thoracic spine stays supported into a neutral kyphosis. For an excessive lumbar lordosis at one or two segments, have the patient reverse the entire lumbar curve into flexion, then focus on facilitating a lordosis at levels above or below the excessive lordosis as the patient returns into a lordosis. Use a light "wiggle" through the iliac crests with a caudal pull to create the sensation of lengthening or stretching the curve at the hyperextended segment(s). The head and neck position are corrected after releasing the support for the trunk. Note that asymmetries are common and that manual and verbal cues may need to be focused more to one side to create the optimal neutral spine position. For example, when one hip is "butt gripping," rotation and lateral bending will be induced in the pelvis and spine. When cueing the neutral spine position, direct the patient's attention to release the specific hip involved and lengthen between the ribcage and pelvis on the affected side.

Ideal response   As you release your manual support, the patient should be able to maintain the new position of gentle thoracic kyphosis and lumbar lordosis, without excessive bracing with the abdominals or breath-holding. Ask the patient to maintain the position and breathe normally. If there is an anterior collapse of the upper thorax, loss of control through the scapulae, loss of the lumbar lordosis, or bracing and breath-holding (the entire trunk becomes stiff), the patient is not ready for exercises in this position.

Progressions/other considerations   Have the patient breathe in, breathe out, then gently connect to the deep lumbopelvic stabilizers (see below). Gradually release your support as you ask the patient to hold the new position. Ask the patient to come out of the position into kneeling, then go back into four-point kneeling and see if the patient can find the optimal position independently. Repeat the manual/verbal cueing as needed, but reduce the manual support to train the patient to find the correct position without assistance.

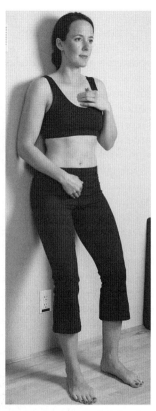

Figure 10.32 Neutral spine: supported standing. The patient is using self-palpation points to perform correction of spinal posture independently. The cranial hand palpates the manubriosternal junction and the caudal hand palpates the pubic symphysis. When practicing setting neutral spine in this position, the patient aims to have the two hands in the same vertical line. (Reproduced with permission from © Diane G. Lee Physiotherapist Corp.)

Neutral spine in supported standing

Patient and therapist position The patient stands with the back against a wall, feet approximately 15–30 cm (6–12 in.) away from the wall. The knees are bent and the primary point of contact and support is the posterior pelvis (Fig. 10.32). The head should be positioned over the thorax, not resting against the wall, as this usually results in poor cervicothoracic position. The therapist stands beside the patient and palpates the lumbar curve and sternum, or other key points of control as described above, depending on where the curves need correcting.

Correction technique – verbal and manual cues The cues described above for the sitting position can be used in this position. Again, correct the thoracic curve first, and then the lumbar curve.

Ideal response As per sitting, the goal is a gentle lumbar lordosis and thoracic kyphosis without excessive erector spinae or superficial multifidus muscle activity. It is important to palpate the lumbar curve as well as the muscle tone in the lumbar spine and thoracolumbar junction. There should be no butt gripping and the hips should remain free to move.

Progressions/other considerations The lumbar spine can be flattened against the wall and then released into a lordosis by cueing, "Relax the buttocks and let the pubic bone fall forward." Teach the patient how to palpate the lumbar curve so that the new correct position is achieved independently. Direct the patient's attention to the pressure of the buttocks against the wall and ensure that the pressure remains equal between the right and left sides; similarly, there should be equal pressure of the posterior ribcage on the wall. Unequal pressure will occur when rotational asymmetries in thoracopelvic alignment have not been corrected. Use internal and external rotation of the hips (see Checkpoints for global muscle rigidity, below rigidity) to check for "butt gripping."

Releasing the hip (the "butt gripper") in supine

Overactivation of the piriformis (piriformis syndrome) and ischiococcygeus results in excessive compression of the SIJ. In addition, overactivation of the obturator internus and externus, gemelli, and quadratus femoris increases compression of the posterior aspect of the hip joint. The following technique is useful for releasing the muscles and decompressing the hip and SIJ.

Patient and therapist position The patient is supine with the hips and knees comfortably flexed. With the cranial hand, palpate the iliac crest as well as the transversus abdominis or multifidus. This choice will be based on the findings from the force closure/motor control analysis; palpate the muscle the patient had the most difficulty isolating. With the caudal hand, palpate the muscle(s) in the posterior pelvic wall or the external rotator of the hip which is overactive (look for a tender trigger point).

Correction technique – verbal and manual cues Instruct the patient to breathe in and on the breath out lightly and gently to contract the TA or multifidus (see isolation and awareness training for the local muscle system for useful verbal cues). Have the patient maintain a very low level of contraction of TA and multifidus and on the next breath out focus attention on to the trigger point you are

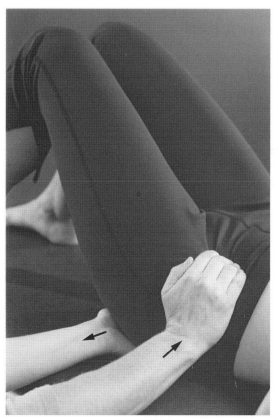

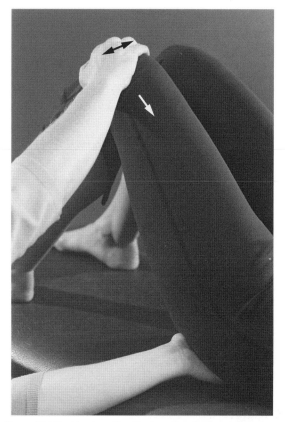

Figure 10.33 Releasing the muscles of the posterior pelvic wall and the external rotators of the hip. In this example, the therapist's right hand is monitoring the contraction of transversus abdominis and applying a very gentle medial force (arrow on the right forearm) to the ilium (proprioceptive cue) while the left hand is monitoring the trigger point in the posterior pelvic floor/wall and applying a gentle lateral force (arrow on the left hand) to the ischial tuberosity. (Reproduced with permission from © Diane G. Lee Physiotherapist Corp.)

Figure 10.34 Hand position for reseating the femoral head. A very gentle force is applied parallel to the length of the femur (white arrow on femur) to facilitate the relaxation of the external rotators of the hip. If the technique is successful, internal and external rotation of the hip (black arrow) will feel very free and easy (no resistance). (Reproduced with permission from © Diane G. Lee Physiotherapist Corp.)

palpating (gently apply pressure to the point). On the next breath out, provide the cue, "Allow the sitz bones to relax and move apart." "Focus on making the muscle under my fingers melt." Very gently, apply a medial pressure to the ilium superiorly and a lateral pressure to the ischium inferiorly (abduct the innominate) (Fig. 10.33). Monitor the muscle response; do not force the innominate or evoke a reflexive muscle contraction, merely provide a proprioceptive cue to the nervous system as to the direction of release you are looking for. Repeat this for three to four breaths, ensuring that the TA and multifidus remain engaged throughout the breath. Then, move your caudal hand to the distal femur (Fig. 10.34). Apply a very gentle force parallel to the

length of the femur (again to add a proprioceptive input into the nervous system) and on the next breath out ask the patient to imagine the femur as a telephone pole slowly sinking into mud. Cue, "Allow the weight of the leg to take the femur back into the pelvis." If the patient has been successful in following your verbal cues and has released the muscles of the posterior pelvic wall and external rotators of the hip, internal and external rotation of the hip in this position will feel very free and easy. If this motion still meets with resistance, the butt is still gripping!

Releasing the hip ("butt gripper") in standing, postural re-education

Patient and therapist position In standing, the patient palpates the posterior aspect of the greater

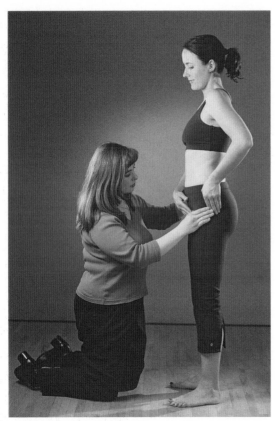

Figure 10.35 Releasing the "butt gripper" in standing. The therapist instructs the patient how to palpate the position of the femoral head anteriorly in the groin and posteriorly behind the greater trochanter. The therapist provides an image that facilitates relaxation and opening of the posterior buttock and a deepening of the anterior hip fold. (Reproduced with permission from © Diane G. Lee Physiotherapist Corp.)

trochanter in the deepest part of the "divot." The other hand palpates the anterior hip at midpoint along the inguinal ligament. Kneel in front of the patient and palpate the affected hip and the contralateral side of the pelvis (Fig. 10.35).

Correction technique – verbal and manual cues "Focus on the muscle under your fingers and my fingers. Feel the tension there, and imagine the muscle melting as your hip opens at the back. Feel your hip coming back into your fingers. Imagine the groove in the front of your hip is getting deeper and softening as the hip moves backwards." Use your hands on the patient's hips to provide a gentle force backwards and facilitate moving the pelvis underneath the thorax.

Ideal response The divot should become less palpable (less deep). The innominate should be vertically aligned over the femur and the pelvis

aligned under the thorax such that the pubic symphysis is vertically aligned under the manubriosternal junction (Fig. 8.1). If the hip has released but the pelvis is still not fully under the thorax, the alternate palpation points at the pubic symphysis and the manubriosternal junction can be used to correct the alignment further (Fig. 10.32). If further correction of the spinal curves is necessary, the cues previously described above can be used; at this point in the postural education process, the cues that are most effective for the patient will have been identified in other positions and simply need to be applied in the standing position.

RESTORATION OF BREATHING PATTERNS

The diaphragm has multiple functions including maintaining respiration while contributing to increased intraabdominal pressure for segmental spinal stabilization (see Ch. 5). Altered breathing patterns are commonly seen in patients with lumbopelvic dysfunction, resulting in compromised efficiency of both respiration and spinal stabilization. By assessing and retraining suboptimal breathing patterns, several goals can be addressed simultaneously. First, there is improved function of the diaphragm. Second, unwanted excessive global muscle activity (rigidity) can be reduced, especially in the superficial abdominals (obliques, rectus abdominis), erector spinae, and hip muscles. Finally, since respiration is a primary drive for survival, the need for spinal stability will be a secondary priority to breathing. By first retraining breathing, the stage is set for successful recruitment and endurance training in the other local system muscles (TA, deep fibers of multifidus, and pelvic floor).

When the respiratory muscles are working optimally, there is three-dimensional movement of the ribcage. Optimal diaphragmatic breathing involves both abdominal and lower ribcage expansion during inspiration (DeTroyer 1989). The most common component lost in patients with lumbopelvic dysfunction is lateral and posterolateral costal expansion. When lateral/posterolateral expansion is absent, excessive excursion occurs in the abdomen (making it difficult to attain a functional TA contraction) or in the upper chest (associated with excessive accessory respiratory muscle activity). Several factors can contribute to the loss of lateral/posterolateral expansion. These include, but are not limited to, joint restrictions in the thorax (spinal or costal), hypertonicity of the thoracic portions of the erector spinae, serratus posterior inferior and/or oblique abdominal muscles, and excessive recruitment of these global muscles during the respiratory cycle. During the objective assessment the articular restrictions and muscular hypertonicity should be noted. Abdominal muscle recruitment during respiration should also be assessed (described below). If the abdominal muscles are recruited during inspiration, ribcage expansion will be restricted to the apical region. Expiration in the supine position during relaxed breathing should be a passive event, with no activity in the superficial abdominal muscles. It is crucial that the clinician identifies and corrects these patterns prior to teaching a voluntary exercise to isolate TA. An isolated contraction of TA cannot occur if excessive abdominal muscle activity persists; furthermore, using this pattern during progressions of the exercise program prevents the optimal anticipatory contraction of TA (inappropriate timing occurs).

Observation and facilitation of lateral costal expansion

Patient and therapist position The patient is supine with the legs straight or in crook lying (whichever is more comfortable for the patient). The abdomen and lower ribcage should be exposed as much as possible. Stand at the patient's side. Before placing your hands on the patient, first observe the chest, lateral ribcage, and abdomen over several inspiratory and expiratory phases. Look for movement in the upper chest (apical breathing), the lateral lower ribcage (lateral costal expansion), and the abdomen (upper and lower abdomen). Note the area where most movement occurs. Next, place your hands on the lateral aspect of the lower ribcage to monitor movement. Check for the amount of movement and the symmetry between the left and right sides. Make note of any expiratory abdominal activation. Keep your hands on the lateral aspect of the lower ribcage and give the patient an image to redirect the inspiration (Fig. 10.36). If posterolateral excursion is the most restricted movement, move your hands more posteriorly on the ribcage. For a unilateral restriction, stand on the same side as the restriction. Place one hand posteriorly under the ribcage, and the other on the anterior ribcage at the same level (Fig. 10.37).

Correction technique – verbal and manual cues "As you breathe in, imagine bringing the air into my hands." "Imagine your ribs are like an umbrella, and

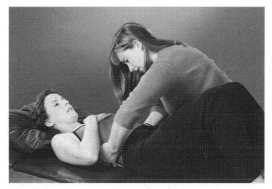

Figure 10.36   Facilitation of lateral costal expansion in supine. The therapist's hands provide awareness of where the patient needs to redirect inspiration. Further facilitation can be added with rib springing. In this example the patient uses one hand to monitor for excessive apical chest movement. (Reproduced with permission from © Diane G. Lee Physiotherapist Corp.)

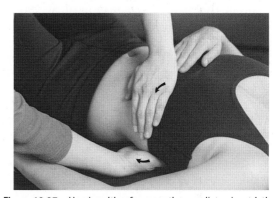

Figure 10.37   Hand position for correcting a unilateral restriction of costal expansion. On inspiration draw the posterior ribs laterally (bottom arrow); on expiration provide a posterolateral pressure to the anterior thorax (top arrow). (Reproduced with permission from © Diane G. Lee Physiotherapist Corp.)

when you breathe in the bottom of the umbrella is opening up." "With each breath open your ribs into my hands." With both hands, apply a slow, gentle, inward pressure at the end of expiration and release this pressure slightly after the start of the inspiration phase (rib springing). Allow your hands to follow the ribcage opening and then apply the gentle pressure again at the end of expiration. With the unilateral restriction, provide gentle pressure into the erector spinae and draw the ribs laterally with the posterior hand as you cue opening into your hand with inspiration. As the patient exhales, apply a posterior pressure to simulate a heavy feeling with your anterior hand (to facilitate thoracic flexion).

For muscle activity on expiration: "As you breathe out, let the air fall out of you and relax your stomach."

"Imagine I am slowly pulling the air out of you." "Sigh as you breathe out – ahhhhh." "Let your chest and sternum go heavy to the floor as you exhale." "Let your ribcage sink into my hand(s) as you breathe out." Gently wiggle the ribcage a small amount to release the muscle, holding as the patient expires.

Progressions/other considerations The patient should perform focused breathing pattern retraining two to three times a day, using both normal and deeper breaths, for several minutes. The patient uses his or her own hands on the sides of the ribcage to provide self-feedback. Alternately, resistive exercise band (e.g., Theraband) can be used around the lower ribcage for proprioceptive feedback (Fig. 10.38a); use the lowest resistance of band to allow flexibility and ribcage expansion. This technique is especially helpful for patients with decreased posterolateral expansion, excessive erector spinae activity, and excessive thoracolumbar extension. Alternate positions should be assessed as optimal breathing patterns may be easier for patients to perform in different positions. To facilitate posterolateral costal expansion, the prayer position can be used (Fig. 10.38b). The patient kneels with the elbows bent on the floor, the hips resting back over the heels, and the head resting over the hands. This flexed spinal position opens the posterior ribcage and helps release excessive erector spinae tone, while inhibiting excessive lower abdominal breathing. For patients with a large abdomen, breathing exercises in supine are often uncomfortable; moving to the sidelying position allows for greater ease and success. To encourage the transfer of the new breathing pattern into a more automatic strategy, have patients "check-in" on their pattern at different points throughout the day, in different postures and during different activities (sitting, standing, walking, etc.).

Breathing, posterolateral costal expansion and erector spinae release

Patient and therapist position The patient is supine with the legs straight or in crook lying (whichever is more comfortable for the patient). Stand at the patient's side. Scoop your hands bilaterally underneath the trunk and ribcage and palpate for hypertonic areas in the thoracic erector spinae muscles. Start at L2 and the thoracolumbar junction and move up into the middle/upper thoracic spine to find the most hypertonic area. If there is primarily a unilateral restriction, use the unilateral hand position as shown in Figure 10.37.

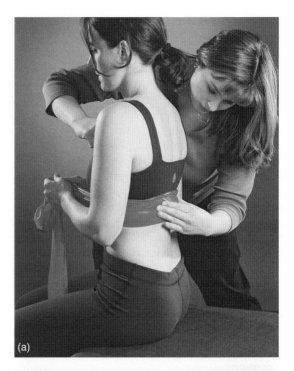
(a)

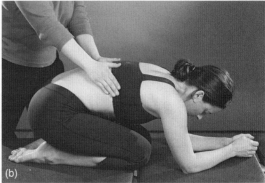
(b)

Figure 10.38 Techniques to facilitate posterolateral costal expansion. (a) Use of a resistive exercise band for proprioceptive feedback laterally and posterolaterally. With every breath in, the patient thinks of opening the ribcage into the band. In this example the therapist cues the patient to open the ribs posteriorly. (b) Prayer position. The therapist's hands give a gentle pressure on the posterior ribcage, cueing the patient to breathe in and "open the ribcage in the back." (Reproduced with permission from © Diane G. Lee Physiotherapist Corp.)

Correction technique – verbal and manual cues While using the breathing techniques described above, provide a deep sinking pressure into the hypertonic muscles as the patient exhales and then add the following verbal cue: "Imagine that your back is an ink blot that has been dropped on the floor. Imagine that with every exhale the ink blot is spreading on the floor and getting bigger and bigger." As the patient exhales, apply pressure to the trigger point in the muscles with your finger pads as you use the whole hand to draw the ribcage laterally, as if opening the posterior ribcage. If using the unilateral hand position, use posterior pressure with your anterior hand to simulate the heavy feeling as the patient exhales.

CHECKPOINTS FOR GLOBAL MUSCLE RIGIDITY

Throughout the rehabilitation process our goal is to reduce rigidity and promote stability with mobility. There are several areas to observe in the patient with lumbopelvic-hip dysfunction. As discussed previously, excessive activity in the global system will reduce ribcage mobility, lateral costal expansion, spinal mobility, and hip mobility. The following are techniques to use at any time during treatment and exercise instruction to monitor for excessive global muscle activation.

Rib wiggle

Place your hands bilaterally on the lateral aspect of the ribcage. With one hand, apply a gentle lateral translation force in one direction followed by an opposite lateral translation force with the other hand. Repeat several oscillatory translations to the left and right and note the amount of resistance to the applied force. There should be a symmetrical amount of lateral movement with only a small amount of force. A loss of this lateral joint play is an indication of a restriction of movement.

Breathing pattern

Observe the ribcage during respiration. If there is excessive global muscle activity there will be a non-optimal pattern of ribcage expansion, bilaterally or unilaterally.

Internal/external rotation of the hip

A decrease in the range of internal or external rotation of the hip can be an indication of excessive global muscle activity. When the local system is recruited there should be no change in the ease of hip rotation. Thus, in many exercises hip rotation can be used to ensure that the global system is not being overly recruited. This test can be easily performed in supine, crook lying, sitting, supported standing, and other functional positions. The therapist lightly grasps the patient's lower thigh and attempts to move the hip passively into internal rotation and then external rotation with a gentle force. Alternately, the patient can perform a self-check by attempting to move the hips actively into internal and external rotation (see the chicken exercise Maintaining neutral spine with loading: trunk and leg dissociation – supported standing, below).

Toe wiggle

As the exercises are progressed to an upright, weight-bearing position, alignment of the lower extremity and activation of the global slings of muscles must be considered. Gripping the toes into flexion indicates an imbalance in global sling activation in the lower leg; asking the patient to "keep the toes relaxed" during exercises and to "wiggle the toes" between exercise repetitions is an effective strategy to correct foot rigidity.

TECHNIQUES TO CORRECT ALIGNMENT

Once the joints of the lumbar spine, pelvic girdle, and hip have been decompressed, the osseous alignment should be addressed. Often, the decompression techniques restore the alignment; however, if malalignment persists, the following techniques can balance the tension forces in the slings of the global systems. The following techniques are used to correct a multisegmental rotoscoliosis in the lumbar spine and intrapelvic torsions (innominate rotations/flares and sacral torsions). Subsequently, exercises are required to maintain optimal alignment and prevent relapse into the old habitual patterns.

Multisegmental rotoscoliosis lumbar spine – sideflexed left/rotated right

Patient and therapist position   The patient is sitting with the arms crossed to opposite shoulders and the feet supported on the floor. The therapist sits on the patient's left side. With the dorsal hand, palpate the lumbar spine at the apex of the sideflexion curve. The ventral hand is placed on the contralateral shoulder. The motion barrier is localized by sideflexing the lumbar spine to the right and rotating the lumbar spine to the left (Fig. 10.39).

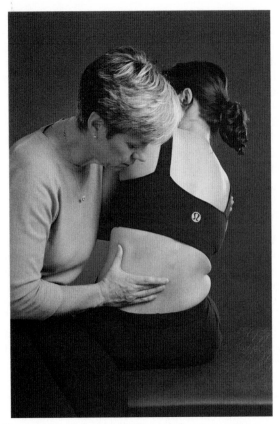

Figure 10.39 Active mobilization technique to correct a multisegmental rotoscoliosis of the lumbar spine which is sideflexed left and rotated right. (Reproduced with permission from © Diane G. Lee Physiotherapist Corp.)

Correction technique – active mobilization From this position, the patient is instructed to hold still while the therapist applies gentle resistance to right rotation of the trunk. The isometric contraction is held for up to 5 s, following which the patient is instructed to relax completely. The new sideflexion/rotation barrier is localized and the mobilization repeated three times.

Intrapelvic torsions – anterior rotation innominate

Patient and therapist position The patient is supine, with the hips and knees flexed. With the long and ring finger of one hand, palpate the sacral sulcus just medial to the PSIS. The flexed hip and knee are supported against the therapist's shoulder and arm. The femur is flexed, adducted, and internally rotated to the motion barrier of the hip joint. The limit of posterior rotation of the innominate is reached by passively flexing the adducted and internally rotated femur until the motion barrier for posterior rotation of the innominate is perceived (Fig. 10.10).

Correction technique – active mobilization From this position, the patient is instructed to resist further hip flexion which is gently increased by the therapist. The isometric contraction is held for up to 5 s, followed by a period of complete relaxation. The innominate is then passively taken to the new barrier of posterior rotation and the technique is repeated three times.

Intrapelvic torsions – posterior rotation innominate

Patient and therapist position With the patient prone, lying close to the edge of the table, the anterior aspect of the distal thigh is palpated with the caudal hand, while the PSIS of the innominate is palpated with the heel of the cranial hand. The limit of anterior rotation of the innominate is reached by passively extending the femur with the caudal hand and applying an anterior rotation force to the innominate with the cranial hand (Fig. 10.14).

Correction technique – active mobilization From this position, the patient is instructed to resist further hip extension which is gently increased by the therapist. The isometric contraction is held for up to 5 s followed by a period of complete relaxation. The innominate is then passively taken to the new barrier of anterior rotation and the technique is repeated three times.

Inflares (internal rotation) and outflares (external rotation) of the innominate reflect a loss of function of the multifidus and TA muscles and are corrected by restoring the balance and function of these two muscles of the local system (see below). Sacral torsions (forward L/L, R/R, backward R/L, L/R) reflect a loss of function of the pelvic floor and multifidus and are corrected by restoring the balance between these two muscles.

DECOMPRESSION VIA INTRAMUSCULAR STIMULATION

IMS or dry needling is a technique developed by Dr. Chan Gunn (Gunn 1996) and is extremely effective for releasing hypertonic global muscles. According to Gunn (1996), "Shortening in muscles acting across

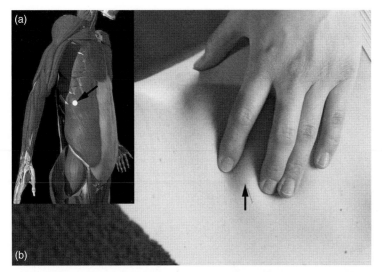

Figure 10.40   (a, b) An intramuscular stimulation point (arrows) for releasing one hypertonic fascicle of the external oblique muscle directly over the anterior aspect of the rib. Note how the therapist ensures that the needle stays anterior to the rib by fixing the rib between the fingers. Clinically, control of the needle is maintained at all times with the other hand and has only been released here for illustration purposes. ((a) Reproduced with permission from Primal Pictures © 2003. (b) Reproduced with permission from © Diane G. Lee Physiotherapist Corp.)

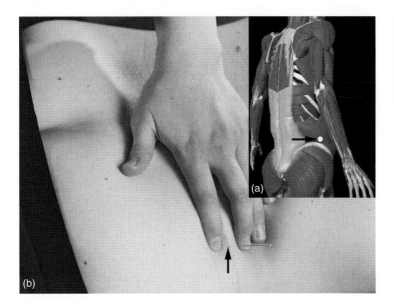

Figure 10.41   (a, b) An intramuscular stimulation point for releasing one hypertonic fascicle of the internal oblique muscle along the iliac crest. ((a) Reproduced with permission from Primal Pictures © 2003. (b) Reproduced with permission from © Diane G. Lee Physiotherapist Corp.)

a joint increases joint pressure, upsets alignment, and can precipitate pain in the joint, i.e. arthralgia." Dry needling of the shortened muscle band causes an immediate relaxation which is palpable. A sense of release and increased range of motion is often experienced by the patient. When used in conjunction with neuromuscular retraining of the local and global systems, the release obtained from IMS can be long-lasting.

Dr. Gunn advocates treating both the spinal segment of innervation for the affected muscle as well as the hypertonic trigger points within the muscle. When decompressing the lumbopelvic–hip region,

the following muscles (and their related spinal segments) can be treated with IMS:

1. external oblique – segmental innervation T7–T12 (Fig. 10.40a, b)
2. internal oblique – segmental innervation T7–L1 (Fig. 10.41a, b)
3. erector spinae – dorsal rami all spinal segments (Fig. 10.42a, b)
4. superficial multifidus over the sacrum – dorsal rami all spinal segments (Fig. 10.43a, b)
5. ischiococcygeus – sacral plexus S3, S4 (Fig. 10.43a, c)

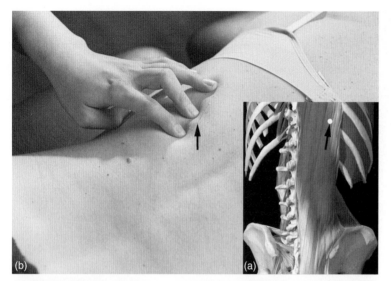

Figure 10.42 (a, b) An intramuscular stimulation point for releasing one hypertonic fascicle of the iliocostalis lumborum over the posterior aspect of the rib. Note how the therapist ensures that the needle stays posterior to the rib by fixing the rib between the fingers. Clinically, control of the needle is maintained at all times with the other hand and has only been released here for illustration purposes. ((a) Reproduced with permission from Primal Pictures © 2003. (b) Reproduced with permission from © Diane G. Lee Physiotherapist Corp.)

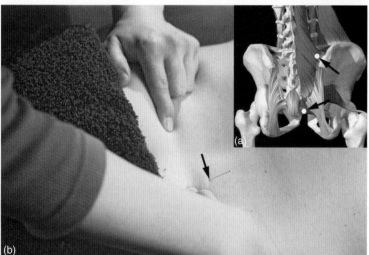

Figure 10.43 (a) Intramuscular stimulation points for releasing one hypertonic fascicle of the superficial (lateral) sacral multifidus and ischiococcygeus. (Reproduced with permission from Primal Pictures © 2003.) (b) Superficial multifidus. (c) Ischiococcygeus. ((b, c) Reproduced with permission from © Diane G. Lee Physiotherapist Corp.)

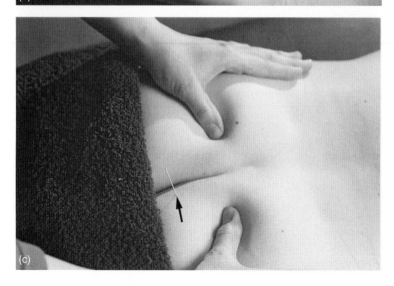

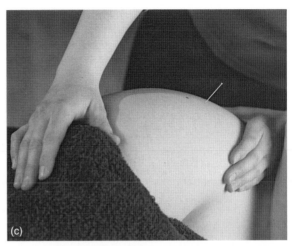

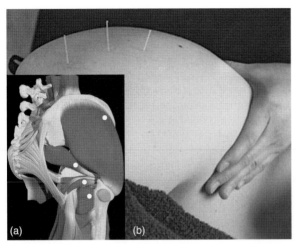

Figure 10.44   (a) Intramuscular stimulation points for releasing hypertonic fascicles within the piriformis, the deep external rotators of the hip, and gluteus medius. (Reproduced with permission from Primal Pictures © 2000.) (b) Piriformis, obturator internus/gemelli, and quadratus femoris. (c) Gluteus medius. ((b, c) Reproduced with permission from © Diane G. Lee Physiotherapist Corp.)

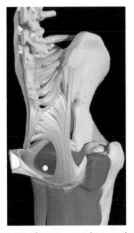

Figure 10.45   A common trigger point and therefore an effective intramuscular stimulation point for obturator internus. (Reproduced with permission from Primal Pictures © 2000.)

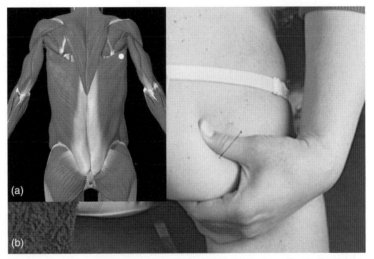

Figure 10.46   (a, b) Latissimus dorsi is a powerful compressor of both the thorax and low back. This is an effective release point with intramuscular stimulation. ((a) Reproduced with permission from Primal Pictures © 2003. (b) Reproduced with permission from © Diane G. Lee Physiotherapist Corp.)

6. piriformis, gemelli, obturator internus, quadratus femoris, and gluteus medius – ventral rami L4, L5, S1 (Fig. 10.44a–c)
7. obturator internus – L5, S1, S2 (Fig. 10.45)
8. latissimus dorsi – C6, C7, C8 (Fig. 10.46a, b)
9. gluteus maximus – L5, S1 S2 (Fig. 10.47a, b)
10. tensor fascia latae – L4, L5 (Fig. 10.48a, b).

ISOLATION AND AWARENESS TRAINING FOR THE LOCAL SYSTEM

In order to retrain the local system, patients are first taught to isolate and maintain a tonic contraction of the deep muscles, separate from the global muscles. This is artificial since in normal function the local muscles work in conjunction with the global muscles.

However, although both muscle systems work together in functional movements, the central nervous system controls the local system independently of the global system. In dysfunction, this independent control is lost; in order to address the change in motor control strategy the local system must be trained separately. This protocol of isolation, training tonic holding ability, training co-contraction of the local muscles, and then integration with global muscles and into functional activities is an effective means of retraining the coordinated function of the local system (Hides et al 1996, 2001, O'Sullivan et al 1997, Richardson et al 1999).

The assessment of co-contraction of the local system described in Chapter 8 includes instructions and images that should activate the local muscles in the healthy motor system. In the patient with dysfunction these cues alone are often inadequate to facilitate recruitment of the desired muscles, resulting in:

- no activation of one or more of the local muscles (TA, deep fibers of the multifidus, pelvic floor muscles) and/or
- asymmetrical activation (in timing or amount of response) of one or more of the local muscles and/or
- phasic activity in one or more of the local muscles and/or
- proper activation but an inability to maintain a proper diaphragmatic breathing pattern during the contraction and/or
- any of the above combined with a pattern of excessive global muscle activity.

These incorrect activation patterns are evident during palpation, observation, and real-time ultrasound imaging (Ch. 8). Any deficiencies in the local system need to be addressed in treatment; however,

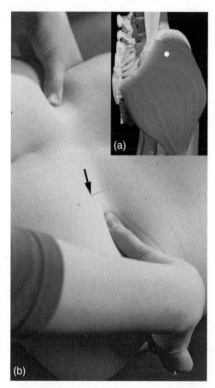

Figure 10.47 (a, b) An intramuscular stimulation point for releasing a hypertonic fascicle in gluteus maximus. ((a) Reproduced with permission from Primal Pictures © 2000. (b) Reproduced with permission from © Diane G. Lee Physiotherapist Corp.)

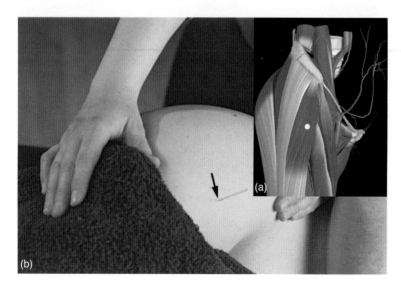

Figure 10.48 (a, b) An intramuscular stimulation point for releasing a hypertonic fascicle in tensor fascia latae. ((a) Reproduced with permission from Primal Pictures © 2000. (b) Reproduced with permission from © Diane G. Lee Physiotherapist Corp.)

as there is often dysfunction in more than one of the local system muscles, the clinician needs to decide which muscle to start with first. Clinically, we have found that the pattern of manual compression that maximally changes the ease of the ASLR test (Ch. 8) indicates which of the local muscles should be trained first. These muscles will have the most significant impact on functional tests such as the support phase of the one-leg standing test (Ch. 8). It is important that the ASLR and manual compressions be retested at each treatment session as the pattern often changes depending on the amount and location of compression from the global system and the improvement in function of the local system.

The first step in teaching recruitment of the local system involves educating the patient about the anatomy, location, and function of the muscles. Once the patient understands the difference between exercises for the local muscles (the dysfunction is in the way the brain uses the muscle, so we use cues for the brain), versus exercises for strength and power (using weights and movements), training for recruitment of the dysfunctional muscle(s) can begin.

Techniques to retrain the diaphragm have been covered above. Specific facilitation cues and techniques for the pelvic floor muscles, TA, and deep fibers of multifidus will be covered below. However, there are some general guidelines that apply to training any of the local muscles.

- The goal is a symmetrical contraction and co-contraction of the local muscles while maintaining an optimal breathing pattern.
- Encourage a *minimal* contraction, that is, 10–15% of maximal voluntary contraction. Often simply asking the patient to perform *less* of a contraction can produce the desired result.
- There should be no activity in the global system.
- There should be no spinal or pelvic movement with the contraction.
- Encourage the patient to contract the muscle as slowly as possible; speaking your cues slowly and providing slow tactile cues will facilitate the proper speed of contraction. This is a key modification whenever a phasic response is present or if activity in the global system is observed.
- Choose the position that best relaxes the global muscles, facilitates an optimal breathing pattern, and facilitates a neutral spine position.
- Use images and mental intent instead of movement to re-establish the brain–body connection: *think* instead of *do*.

- Palpate the muscles bilaterally in order to detect asymmetries in activity; encourage the patient to use a small amount of extra palpation pressure and extra mental energy for the dysfunctional side. Note that the position chosen for exercise practice can have a marked effect on the patient's ability to recruit the dysfunctional side (e.g., left sidelying versus right sidelying).

THE PELVIC FLOOR

Sapsford et al (2001) have shown that activation of the abdominal muscles should accompany contraction of the pelvic floor muscles and vice versa. Images and explanations that involve contraction of the anterior pelvic floor (pubococcygeus) are useful facilitation techniques for obtaining an isolated TA contraction and are described below. This research supports using a *submaximal* contraction of the pelvic floor in a position of neutral pelvic tilt to facilitate best contraction of TA. Palpation of the abdominal wall is a useful indicator of pelvic floor function; the presence of a bulging or bracing contraction is consistent with depression of the levator plate (functional pelvic floor) on ultrasound (O'Sullivan et al 2003). However, if a successful isolated TA contraction occurs with verbal cueing of the pelvic floor, it cannot be guaranteed that a proper contraction of the pelvic floor muscles has occurred. Bump et al (1991) found that only 49% of female patients presenting in a gynecological and urodynamic laboratory could perform a correct pelvic floor contraction when given verbal or written instructions. Dysfunction in the pelvic floor muscles can exist in patients with SIJ dysfunction (O'Sullivan et al 2002) as well as in patients with lumbosacral dysfunction (O'Sullivan et al 2003). Thus, specific assessment of the function of the pelvic floor muscles is necessary.

A non-invasive method to assess the function of the pelvic floor using real-time ultrasound imaging has been described in Chapter 8. In both transverse and parasagittal views of the bladder, contraction of the pelvic floor muscles results in a slow indentation and encroachment of the bladder wall (Fig. 10.49a, b). When the contraction is absent or a Valsalva response is observed with real-time ultrasound, the patient is given different cues to try and facilitate a proper response on the screen. To retrain the tonic stabilizing function of the pelvic floor muscles, the focus is on obtaining a slow, gentle, submaximal contraction, with concentration on a

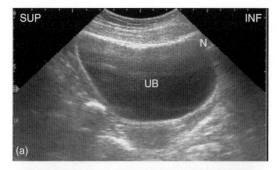

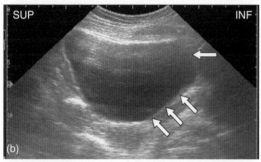

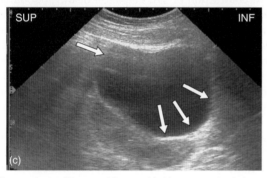

Figure 10.49 Ultrasound Images: bladder, parasagittal view. (a) Image at rest. UB, urinary bladder; N, neck of the bladder; SUP, superior; INF, inferior. If there is an inability to produce a pelvic floor contraction, the image will not change; no lift or indentation of the bladder wall is seen. (b) Recruitment of the pelvic floor muscles results in a slow indentation of the posteroinferior aspect of the bladder (arrows) and a cranioventral shift. (c) A Valsalva maneuver results in a deformation of the bladder shape and a caudodorsal shift (arrows). (Reproduced with permission from © Diane G. Lee Physiotherapist Corp.)

more anterior (vaginal or urethral) than posterior (rectal) activation. It is important that the patient understands that the final goal is a 10 s contraction, repeated 10 times, but that the duration and number of contractions performed correctly on a given day may vary. This information allows the patient to self-progress the exercise protocol. Certain subgroups of patients with stress urinary incontinence

may need to couple the protocols for training the tonic holding ability of the pelvic floor muscles with those for strength training and hypertrophy (Bó et al 1990). The approach presented here is designed to address the impairment in motor control and stabilizing function of the pelvic floor muscles, both in isolation and in conjunction with the other local muscles.

Real-time ultrasound imaging can be used in conjunction with abdominal wall palpation and observation to assess the function of the pelvic floor muscles. Common clinical patterns of abnormal responses are listed below with facilitation and correction strategies.

Ultrasound image – no indentation of the bladder, no lift observed

The bladder shape does not change at the posteroinferior aspect and there is no cranioventral motion on the parasagittal view (Fig. 10.49a). Some movement may be evident during the breathing cycle, but there is no change when the patient thinks of squeezing the urethra or lifting the vagina/testicles.

Palpation of abdominal wall   There is usually no change in the abdominal wall tension. The fingers can sink into the softness of the abdomen.

Observation   There may be concurrent breath-holding with the effort to recruit the pelvic floor or superficial abdominal muscle activity on expiration but usually no other activity in the superficial abdominal muscles is evident on an attempt to perform a contraction.

Correction technique – verbal cues   In this case the patient does not have an intact neural pathway between *thinking* about a contraction and the contraction occurring. In order to obtain a contraction, different cues are used and the response noted on ultrasound. Verbal cue examples:

- For women: "Instead of thinking of squeezing, imagine that you are lifting a tampon."
- For men: "Imagine that you are slowly walking into a cold lake, and the water is starting to come up between your inner thighs."
- "Connect a string between your pubic bone and your tailbone, then between your right and left sitz bones. Now draw the string up into the center like a drawstring."
- Alternatively, cues for TA or deep fibers of multifidus (listed below) can be used to produce a contraction.

- If incorrect breathing patterns are noted, then it is essential to teach correct diaphragmatic breathing; restoring the function of the pelvic floor muscles is closely linked with the function of the diaphragm and its effects on intraabdominal pressure.

An absent response may also result from nerve damage, insufficiency in the fascial connections of the pelvic floor muscles, or hypertonicity of the pelvic floor muscles. If no response is observed after the above cues and corrections in breathing pattern have been tried, biofeedback tools such as the Pelvic Floor Educator (www.neenhealth.com) can be used. These tools provide some proprioceptive feedback and allow patients to practice contractions with the assurance that they are performing the correct activation. Pelvic floor function can then be reassessed with real-time ultrasound in 1–2 weeks. If there is still no change evident, a referral to a therapist specializing in pelvic floor dysfunction and manual assessment of the floor is recommended.

Ultrasound image – no indentation of the bladder, caudodorsal movement (Valsalva) observed

In the parasagittal view the bladder may move caudodorsally (Fig. 10.49c). In the transverse abdominal view, the dorsal component will be observed and any asymmetry will be apparent.

Palpation of abdominal wall A bulge and/or bracing tension occurs; it may develop slowly or quickly.

Observation Activity in the superficial abdominal muscles is noted, especially in the IO and EO muscles. Flexion of the ribcage may occur if there is no co-contraction of the thoracic portions of the erector spinae muscle to counteract the flexion moment of the oblique abdominals. The abdomen may bulge with concurrent narrowing of the ribcage.

Correction technique – verbal cues The goal in this scenario is to reduce the global muscle activity that is causing the Valsalva maneuver and then train a proper lift of the pelvic floor muscles. Draw the patient's attention to the screen, and point out the movement and deformation of the bladder shape that occurs when a contraction is attempted. Cue proper breathing with a special focus on abdominal relaxation during exhalation. Palpate the inner thighs bilaterally to focus the patient's attention away from the abdomen. The same cues can be used, with some modifications. Verbal cue examples:

- "Imagine a tension that is coming up from your inner thighs into the front of your pelvic floor and then lifting your pelvic floor."

- "Really focus low down in your pelvic floor. Now imagine slowly and gently lifting a tampon."
- When a Valsalva is present it is essential to encourage a slower contraction ("This time contract at 10% of the speed of the last contraction.") and a lighter contraction ("This time I want you to think of contracting only 10% of the last contraction.").
- Cues for TA or deep fibers of multifidus can be used.

Often after the first session the patient will go home with an image to practice that ensures no Valsalva but only produces minimal or no lift. The patient is taught to palpate bilaterally in the abdomen (just medial to the ASISs) to ensure that no bulge is felt. At subsequent training sessions the lift component can then be effectively trained.

Ultrasound image – indentation and lift of the bladder, followed by a Valsalva

An ideal response of the bladder wall is observed but then quickly followed by a caudodorsal movement of the bladder. The Valsalva may also occur slowly as the patient attempts to maintain a tonic contraction.

Palpation of abdominal wall A tension in the abdominal wall consistent with a TA contraction is followed by a bulge and/or bracing.

Observation A small flattening of the lower abdominal wall is followed by activity in the superficial abdominal muscles, especially in the IO and EO muscles. Flexion of the ribcage may occur if there is no co-contraction of the thoracic portions of the erector spinae muscle to counteract the flexion moment of the oblique abdominals. A bulge in the lower abdomen is usually present; there may be concurrent narrowing of the ribcage.

Correction technique This response is best corrected by cues that focus on decreasing the speed and effort of the contraction (see verbal cues as above). The correct neural pathway exists but is overridden by the incorrect Valsalva. It is very effective to have the patient observe the screen and to learn to stop the contraction before the Valsalva occurs and pushes the bladder caudodorsally. Before the patient goes home to practice the exercise, it is important to have the patient try several contractions without watching the screen while stopping before the Valsalva. This ensures internalization of the new motor strategy. It is also important to assess how long the patient can hold a contraction before a Valsalva starts to occur. Note the number of seconds the isolated contraction is maintained. Teach the patient to palpate the abdominal wall to monitor for bulging; the patient is instructed to practice holding the correct contraction as long as possible without the Valsalva occurring.

Ultrasound image – indentation and lift of the bladder, slow release of contraction when attempting to increase the duration of hold (decreased endurance)

Palpation of abdominal wall A tension in the abdominal wall consistent with a TA contraction occurs but slowly releases as the patient attempts to maintain the contraction.

Observation A small flattening of the lower abdominal wall occurs but releases as the patient attempts to maintain the contraction.

Correction technique Often the patient *thinks* that they are maintaining a contraction but it is evident from the ultrasound image and palpation of the abdominal wall that the contraction has been released. The key in this case is to make the patient aware of when the contraction is truly occurring and the point at which it starts to let go. Teaching the patient to palpate the abdomen while watching the screen and then repeating contractions without watching the screen will internalize the new awareness.

Ultrasound image – asymmetrical activation

An asymmetrical activation is usually corrected by having the patient direct extra focus and attention to the side of the abnormal response. However, if there are neural, fascial, or muscle tone impairments then retraining of symmetrical function is facilitated by referral to a therapist who specializes in internal palpation and treatment of the pelvic floor.

TRANSVERSUS ABDOMINIS

Patient and therapist position

The initial position chosen to teach this exercise will depend on which position encourages relaxation of the global muscles while ideally providing some stretch on the abdominal wall for proprioceptive feedback. The best position for each patient will vary depending on their substitution strategies. For example, supine crook lying is most supportive and allows relaxation of global muscles such as the

erector spinae; however, there is little stretch on the abdominal wall to provide feedback for the patient of where the "drawing-in" action of TA should occur. The sidelying position provides more stretch on the abdominal wall due to the pull of gravity on the abdomen. When a rolled towel is placed under the waist and a pillow inserted between the knees, the sidelying position can be supportive to allow global muscle relaxation. The four-point kneeling position provides the greatest amount of pull on the abdomen and is a good starting place to help the patient understand the feeling of "drawing-in" the lower abdomen. However, it is not often the easiest position to perform an isolated contraction. Substitution strategies occur due to the greater loading and postural challenge in this position, and are often more easily identified in this position. A more supported position for training an isolated contraction can then be chosen based on the global substitution pattern observed. Ideally, a neutral position for the lumbar spine should be attained since this position is known (Sapsford et al 2001) to facilitate the isolation of TA, especially in patients exhibiting a dominance of the oblique abdominal muscles (avoid a flexed, flat lumbar spine and posterior pelvic tilt).

Palpate the abdomen 2.5 cm (1 in.) medial to and slightly inferior to the ASIS bilaterally (Fig. 10.50). The patient should be taught how to palpate here for a proper contraction. In sidelying, the therapist

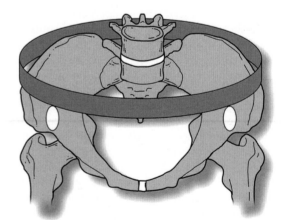

Figure 10.50 The oval circles just medial to the anterior superior iliac spine on each side indicate the points for palpating a contraction of transversus abdominis. An isolated contraction will be felt as a slow, gentle flattening and tensioning under the fingers. A bulge or rapid contraction is evidence of contraction of the internal oblique muscle. The circle around the pelvis represents the "circle of integrity" produced by the co-contraction of transversus abdominis and the deep fibers of multifidus. (Reproduced with permission from © Diane G. Lee Physiotherapist Corp.)

can also gently cup the lower abdomen with the palm to provide feedback of where the contraction should be initiated. Observe the abdominal wall and trunk for signs of proper isolation without global muscle activation.

Correction technique – verbal and manual cues

Several verbal cues can help to facilitate an isolated contraction of transversus abdominis:

- "Breathe in, breathe out, then don't breathe as you slowly, gently draw your lower abdomen away from my fingers (or hand)."
- "Imagine that there is a slow tension coming up from the inner thighs into the front of your pelvic floor, then extend that tension up into my fingers in your lower abdomen."
- "Imagine that you are slowly and gently drawing these two bones [ASISs] together."
- "Imagine that you are slowly and gently drawing these two bones [ASISs] apart."
- "Imagine drawing your stomach away from your pubic bone." "Very lightly and slowly think of lifting up in your pelvic floor" (women can imagine lifting the vagina, while men can do a small lift of the testes).

Provide a sinking pressure into the abdomen as you give the verbal cues slowly and gently. Tactile pressure can also be given just above the pubic bone or with the hand cupping the abdomen; sink into the tissue slowly to encourage a slow, tonic contraction instead of a fast, phasic response. If there is excessive upper abdominal activity, the patient can continue to palpate at the ASIS points while the therapist provides gentle tactile pressure bilaterally into the upper medial thighs to take the focus away from the stomach. The patient is then encouraged to imagine the contraction starting lower.

Ideal and abnormal responses

A slow development of gentle tensioning under the fingers should be felt. It should be remembered that only a 10–15% contraction of this muscle is required. If the patient uses too much effort or performs a fast contraction, a bulge into the fingers will be felt, pushing the fingers away from the abdomen; this is the IO muscle. A similar IO bulge can often be felt with a cough or with lifting the head from the floor. There should be no movement of the pelvis or spine, and little movement in the upper abdomen. Rectus abdominis and the oblique abdominals should remain relaxed. If the ribcage is depressed and drawn in, this is a sign of EO activation. Perform a small "wiggle" of the ribcage by pushing it gently laterally; if there is a lot of resistance to your pressure this means the ribcage is being braced by overactive global muscles and an isolated TA contraction has not been achieved. The ribcage should still move easily in response to the lateral pressure in the presence of an isolated TA contraction.

The common abnormal responses are listed here and categorized according to patterns seen with real-time ultrasound imaging. The reader should note that real-time ultrasound is an adjunct to palpation and observation skills and is not an essential tool for teaching local muscle activation; however, it is often a useful tool for providing feedback to patients and objective assessment of dysfunction.

Ultrasound image – no TA recruitment, no substitution with IO

Imaging   On the real-time ultrasound image, the following is seen (Fig. 10.51):

- no widening (change in thickness) of the TA muscle layer
- no corseting of TA laterally or lateral slide of the medial fascia of TA
- no change in thickness in the IO muscle layer.

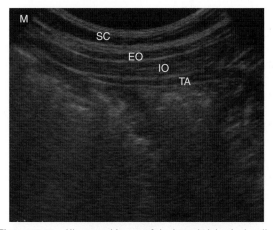

Figure 10.51   Ultrasound image of the lateral abdominal wall, transverse view. M, medial; SC, subcutaneous tissue; EO, external oblique; IO, internal oblique; TA, transversus abdominis. The ultrasound image appears the same as an image taken of the relaxed abdominal wall. This is consistent with an absent transversus abdominis contraction without internal oblique substitution. (Reproduced with permission from © Diane G. Lee Physiotherapist Corp.)

Palpation   On palpation, the following is felt:

- The lower abdomen remains soft and no tensioning or contraction is felt just medial to the ASIS, or
- A tensioning in the superficial fascia is palpated rather than a deep tension. This can occur due to a contraction of the EO muscle and the resultant tension in the EO fascia that occurs over the palpation point. The ultrasound image confirms that TA is not active. There may be no change in EO observed on the ultrasound image as the correlation between activity in the EO and change in the thickness of the muscle on the ultrasound screen is poor (Hodges et al 2003a). Activity in the EO can be palpated at the lower rib attachments of the muscle (Fig. 10.52). If there is no spinal movement then concurrent activity can be palpated in the erector spinae muscles. The rib wiggle test will be restricted.

Observation   On observation, the following is noted: if TA does not contract there will be no flattening or drawing in of the lower abdomen; however, there may be substitution patterns that are not observable from the ultrasound image. The possible scenarios include:

- EO contraction – movement of the abdominal wall is initiated from the upper abdomen and activity in the EO muscle fibers at their ribcage attachments will be observed. There may also be a horizontal skin crease in the abdomen just above the umbilicus, as well as an increase in the lateral diameter of the abdominal wall (widening at the waist). Lateral costal expansion will be reduced. If the erector spinae muscles remain relaxed there will be thoracolumbar flexion and narrowing of the infrasternal angle (Fig. 8.55b).

- Breath-holding – the upper abdomen will move superiorly and pull in; the ribcage will flare and may lift if there is a concurrent contraction of the erector spinae.

Correction technique   Several facilitation techniques can be used.

- Change patient position: if there is no activity in TA or any other abdominal muscle on cueing, choose a position that will provide more gravity pull on the abdomen such as sidelying (Fig. 10.53), four-point kneeling, or supported standing (Fig. 10.32). The increased proprioceptive input is often sufficient to produce the desired response. If the response is primarily in the EO (EO-dominant pattern), make sure that the patient is positioned in neutral spine. Sidelying or prone are good positions for allowing relaxation of the abdominal wall.

- For EO dominance: check for EO activity on expiration. Add the cue, "Breathe in, breathe out, *now really relax your stomach*, don't breathe, and gently think of lifting your lower abdomen away from your hand (or another image)." Use verbal cues that draw focus away from the abdomen; for example, thinking of the pelvic floor, tension coming up from

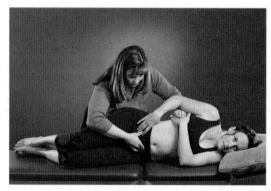

Figure 10.53   Facilitation of transversus abdominis isolation: sidelying position. In this example, the patient palpates for lateral costal expansion with the left hand and transversus abdominis contraction with the right hand; the therapist similarly palpates and provides manual facilitation. Note that patients often have more awareness of the lower abdomen lifting from the bottom side (in this case, the left side); for patients with an asymmetrical transversus abdominis contraction sidelying *on the side of poor activation* can facilitate more symmetrical recruitment. (Reproduced with permission from © Diane G. Lee Physiotherapist Corp.)

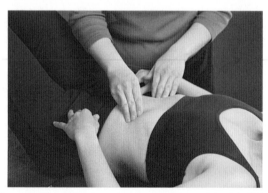

Figure 10.52   Palpation points for transversus abdominis (TA) and external oblique (EO). The patient is palpating just medial and inferior to the anterior superior iliac spine bones bilaterally to feel a contraction of the TA; the therapist palpates for substitution by the EO as the muscle comes off its attachment at the anterior surfaces of the lower ribs. (Reproduced with permission from © Diane G. Lee Physiotherapist Corp.)

the inner thighs, or a multifidus (deep fibers) contraction.

- For no abdominal muscle activity: try the verbal cues listed above, starting first with those that use palpation and focus on the lower abdomen to increase awareness of the area.

Ultrasound image – no TA, substitution with IO with or without EO and rectus abdominis

Imaging   On the real-time ultrasound image, the following is seen (Fig.10.54a, b)

- The IO layer increases in thickness with a fast, phasic response or with a slow, gradual increase. No increase in thickness of the TA layer is seen underneath, no lateral glide of the fascia is observed, and there is no corseting of the TA layer laterally.

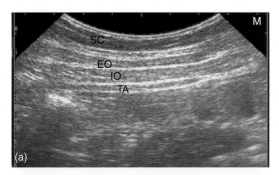

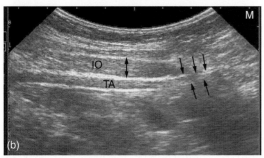

Figure 10.54   Ultrasound image of the lateral abdominal wall, transverse view. M, medial; SC, subcutaneous tissue; EO, external oblique; IO, internal oblique; TA, transversus abdominis. Dominant IO without precontraction of TA. (a) Relaxed abdominal wall. (b) Increased thickness in the IO layer is evident (double-head arrow) and the medial edge of the muscle bulges into the abdomen, with a resultant blurring of the fascial lines medially (small arrows). In this example a small TA contraction is occurring with the IO contraction, as evidenced by a change in thickness in the TA layer. However, there is no lateral corseting of TA and in real time the contraction did not occur before the IO contraction. (Reproduced with permission from © Diane G. Lee Physiotherapist Corp.)

Due to the lack of fascial tension a downward bulge (into the abdomen) at the medial edge of the IO will often be observed. This blurs the fascial lines medially. When the patient is asked to do the contraction slowly, the same pattern will be evident but occurs more slowly.

Palpation   On palpation, the following is felt:

- A fast or slow bulge (rather than a tensioning) can be felt medial to the ASIS.
- In order to determine if EO or rectus abdominis is also being recruited with the IO, palpate along the lower ribcage (below the eighth rib) and inferior to the sternum.

Observation   On observation, the following is noted:

- Bilateral contraction of only the IO will result in flaring (widening) of the infrasternal angle; in lean individuals the upper anterior fibers may be palpable and visible as an oblique band running superomedially from the anterior iliac crest to the ribs. If both the IO and EO are active, ribcage bracing and decreased lateral costal expansion will be observed along with lower abdominal bulging.
- Rectus abdominis activity will result in thoracolumbar flexion and/or a posterior pelvic tilt.
- Co-contraction of the erector spinae muscles will reduce the amount of thoracolumbar flexion observed but will result in trunk rigidity and a restricted "rib wiggle."
- If the dysfunctional substitution pattern is primarily unilateral, a lateral shift in the ribcage will occur with the contraction.

Correction technique   Several facilitation techniques can be used.

- Change patient position: choose a position that best facilitates relaxation of the trunk. This may be supine/crook lying (as long as the pelvis is not posteriorly tilted) or prone lying (Fig. 10.55). If the erector spinae are being recruited along with the superficial abdominal muscles a pillow can be placed under the stomach in prone to encourage relaxation.
- Start with verbal and tactile cues that draw focus away from the abdomen (activating the pelvic floor, tension coming up from the inner thighs, contracting multifidus (deep fibers)).
- Check for superficial abdominal activity on expiration. Add the cue, "Breathe in, breathe out, *now really relax your stomach*, don't breathe, and gently think of lifting in your pelvic floor."

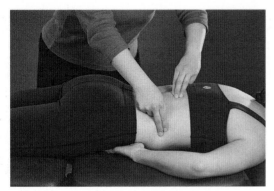

Figure 10.55 Facilitation of transversus abdominis (TA) isolation: prone lying position. To facilitate relaxation of the abdominal wall, ask the patient to "let the stomach relax on the bed" prior to attempting recruitment of the TA. The patient palpates for a TA contraction bilaterally while the therapist monitors the thoracic erector spinae and the lateral portions of the external oblique muscle for activity. (Reproduced with permission from © Diane G. Lee Physiotherapist Corp.)

Ultrasound image – TA contracting but not in isolation

When TA comes on first, followed by IO and the other abdominals (may occur quickly or more gradually), this indicates that proper timing of the muscles is occurring; however, the recruitment of the global system is happening too early and needs to be eliminated to get an isolated TA contraction.

Imaging On the real-time ultrasound image, the following is seen (Fig. 10.56a, b):

• The TA layer increases in thickness and moves laterally, drawing the medial fascial connection laterally. This is followed by an increase in thickness in the IO layer. There is less internal bulging and less fascial blurring of the medial portion of IO (as compared to an IO contraction without an underlying TA) due to the pretensioning of the underlying fascia by the TA contraction.

Palpation On palpation, the following is felt:

• A deep tensioning followed by a fast or slow bulge can be felt medial to the ASIS.

• In order to determine if EO or rectus abdominis is also being recruited with the IO, palpate along the lower ribcage (below the eighth rib, Fig. 10.52) and inferior to the sternum.

Observation On observation, the following is noted:

• The lower abdomen will gently flatten followed by signs of superficial abdominal muscle activity (described in sections above).

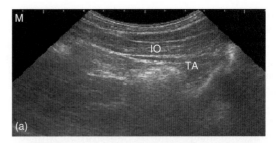

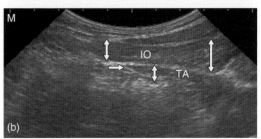

Figure 10.56 Ultrasound images of the lateral abdominal wall, transverse view. M, medial; IO, internal oblique; TA, transversus abdominis. (a) Relaxed abdominal wall. (b) TA contraction followed by IO contraction. When viewed in real time, an increase in thickness of the TA layer occurs first (small double-head arrow), with a lateral slide of the medial fascial attachments (horizontal arrow) and some corseting of TA laterally. This is quickly followed by a large increase in the thickness of the IO layer (large double-head arrows). Note that the medial fascial lines are still distinguishable, as compared to those in Figure 10.54b. (Reproduced with permission from © Diane G. Lee Physiotherapist Corp.)

Correction technique Several facilitation techniques can be used.

• Encourage a slower contraction; start with 50% of current speed, then 50% of the new speed, and so on.

• Encourage a lighter contraction; start with 50% of current effort, then 50% of the new effort, and so on. Remind patients that only 10–15% of maximal voluntary contraction is required and that they should be *imagining* a contraction rather than *doing* a contraction.

• If decreasing the speed and effort still results in global muscle activity, try changing the patient's position such that the global muscles are more relaxed.

• Direct the patient's attention to the ultrasound screen. Ask the patient to stop the contraction before movement in the global muscle layers (notably IO) occurs. Once this is mastered, have the patient perform the contraction without looking at the screen so that the new skill is internalized.

When the TA and IO (with or without EO and rectus abdominis) come on together, this indicates that there is incorrect timing and no separation of control of the local and global systems.

Imaging On the real-time ultrasound image, the following is seen:

• The TA layer increases in thickness and moves laterally, drawing the medial fascial connection laterally, but there is a concurrent increase in thickness in the IO layer. Often there is less lateral slide of the TA layer than usually observed with an isolated TA contraction and blurring of the medial fascia connections can occur depending on the amount of contraction in the TA (Fig. 10.54a, b). The lateral corseting occurs but there is concurrent inward movement of both the TA and IO layers.

Palpation On palpation, the following is felt:

• A fast or slow bulge can be felt medial to the ASIS (in this scenario palpation cannot identify if there is TA activity underneath or not as the bulge dominates the palpation result).
• In order to determine if EO or rectus abdominis is also being recruited with the IO, palpate along the lower ribcage (below the eighth rib, Fig. 10.52) and inferior to the sternum.

Observation On observation, the following is noted:

• The signs of superficial abdominal muscle activity will be evident and dependent on which global muscles are activated (see above).

Correction technique Several facilitation techniques can be tried.

• Consider using manual or other techniques to downtrain the global muscle activity (muscle energy, lateral costal breathing, treating thoracic joint restrictions, IMS, electromyogram biofeedback) prior to another attempt at TA isolation exercises.
• Change the patient position to one that maximizes relaxation of the abdominal wall.
• Encourage a slower contraction; start with 50% of current speed, then 50% of the new speed, and so on.
• Encourage a lighter contraction; start with 50% of current effort, then 50% of the new effort, and so on. Remind patients that only 10–15% of maximal voluntary contraction is required and that they should be *imagining* a contraction rather than *doing* a contraction.

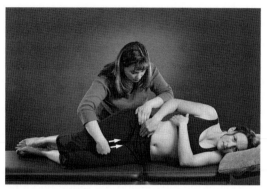

Figure 10.57 Facilitation of transversus abdominis isolation: sidelying. In this example, the patient palpates for lateral costal expansion with the left hand and transversus abdominis (TA) contraction with the right hand. The therapist palpates the right TA for evidence of an ideal contraction while the caudal hand provides gentle sinking pressure into the inner thighs bilaterally. While sliding the fingers up the thighs a short distance (arrows), give the cue, "Imagine tension coming up from my fingers in your inner thighs, moving up into the front of your pelvic floor." The image can be extended up to the lower abdomen if necessary. (Reproduced with permission from © Diane G. Lee Physiotherapist Corp.)

• Start with verbal and tactile cues that draw focus away from the abdomen (activating the pelvic floor, tension coming up from the inner thighs (Fig. 10.57), contracting multifidus).
• Check for superficial abdominal activity on expiration. Add the cue, "Breathe in, breathe out, *now really relax your stomach,* don't breathe, and gently think of lifting in your pelvic floor."

Ultrasound image – asymmetrical patterns

This is the most common clinical presentation and is often present with asymmetries in multifidus and/or pelvic floor function. Any of the above scenarios can occur asymmetrically, with one side producing an ideal response and the other side producing one of the abnormal responses, or with both sides showing abnormal but different responses. Correction of asymmetry will require a combination of the above facilitation techniques. The sidelying position (Figs 10.53 and 10.57) is useful for facilitating the TA on the side that the patient is lying. Successful correction of the asymmetry is often achieved by simply adding a small increase in patient focus and attention to the dysfunctional side when the isolation exercise is attempted. Images to address asymmetry in TA/multifidus will be addressed later under co-contraction strategies.

DEEP FIBERS OF MULTIFIDUS

Patient and therapist position

Choose the position where the patient can attain a neutral spine position and the global muscles are most relaxed, especially the erector spinae, the deep hip external rotators, and the posterior pelvic floor. Prone is a useful position for comparing right/left recruitment symmetry, but is not often the easiest position for patients first to practice isolation exercises. Sidelying is a useful position as it allows easy palpation of the muscle and relaxation into a neutral spine position. Positions such as supine and crook lying can also be beneficial for some patients.

Palpate multifidus just lateral to the spinous processes of the lumbar spine or sacrum bilaterally at the level of atrophy. To monitor the deep fibers, the muscle must be palpated close to the spine; in the lower lumbar and sacral segments the lateral muscle bulk consists of the more superficial fibers. Teach the patient how to find the dysfunctional segment ("feel for the soft part of the muscle") and how to sink into the muscle with the fingers.

Correction technique – verbal and manual cues

Several verbal cues can help to facilitate an isolated contraction of the deep fibers of multifidus.

- "Feel the muscle under my finger and think of a tension coming from inside your body to make this muscle bulge into my fingers."
- "Feel these two bones (palpate the PSISs) and imagine drawing them together."
- "Imagine that you are a Barbie doll, and that someone has pulled your leg off and left it lying at your pelvis, but disconnected. Imagine an energy from inside your spine that will draw the leg into your body and reconnect it." Or, "Imagine there is a string connected from the spine to the hip (in the groin); if you pull on this string from the muscle in your back you can connect the leg back into your body."

Images that create the idea of the spine being suspended are also effective for facilitating a contraction of the deep fibers of multifidus. Various descriptions can be used, but the common theme is that the spine is a central pole that needs to be suspended by tension wires from both sides. The tension in the wires needs to be equal on the right and left sides; if there is loss activity in one side of the

deep multifidus, it can be described as a loss of the connection in the wire, allowing rotation and collapse of the spine on that side. The image of energy coming up vertically along the wires to support the spine helps to create the sense of suspension. In each case, the deep multifidus is palpated bilaterally at the dysfunctional level; this is where the "guy wires" attach to. The inferior attachment of the wire can vary; the image ultimately chosen is the one that produces the best response in the deep multifidus. The timing of the tactile pressure from the therapist's hands creates the image and provides feedback as to how quickly the muscle should be contracted. The fingers should sink into the multifidus and provide a cranial pressure to encourage a lifted or suspended feeling. The inferior attachment of the wire can be just medial to the ASISs (Fig. 10.58a), superior to the pubic bone (Fig. 10.58b), or from the pelvic floor (Fig. 10.58c); the sequence of tactile feedback is from the anterior palpation point first, then up into the multifidus palpation point. Finally, cues to activate a TA or pelvic floor contraction can be used to activate a contraction in the deep multifidus.

Ideal and abnormal responses

A slow development of firmness in the muscle will be felt as a deep swelling and indentation of the pads of the palpating fingers. A fast contraction is indicative of the superficial multifidus and/or lumbar erector spinae activation; the fingers will be quickly pushed off the body. A fast generation of superficial tension can also be palpated if the thoracic erector spinae are contracting. The common tendon of the erector spinae muscle overlies the lumbar multifidus (Fig. 4.33) and activity in the muscle will change tension in the tendon, especially in individuals where this muscle is well-developed. It is important to teach the patient how easy it is to push the fingers into the muscle when it is relaxed ("feels like a mushy banana"), as compared to when the deep fibers of multifidus contract ("feel how it is firmer and harder to sink your fingers into the muscle"). There should be no pelvic or spinal motion observed, and no activity in the global abdominal muscles or in the hip musculature. A co-contraction of TA is acceptable and desired.

The common abnormal responses that occur are listed here and categorized according to patterns seen with real-time ultrasound imaging. The reader should note that real-time ultrasound is an adjunct

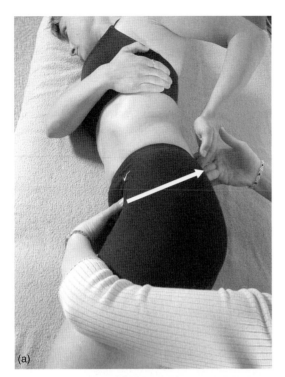

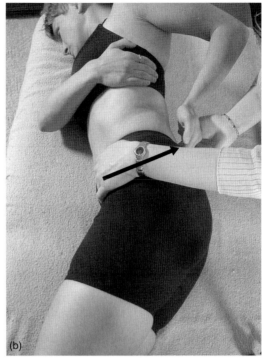

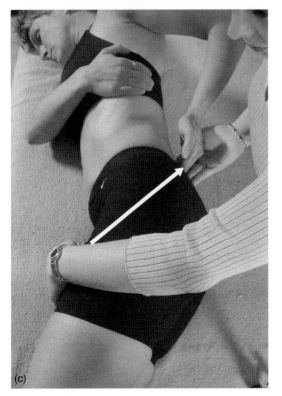

Figure 10.58   Describe the image to the patient: "Imagine that there is a tension wire or string that is going to suspend your spine. We are going to connect the wire from the front of your body, up and in through your body diagonally to my fingers in your spine. [The arrows in these illustrations represent the tension wire.] Breathe in, breathe out, now slowly connect a wire from this finger here [give pressure at anterior palpation point] to this finger here [give pressure into multifidus]." Options for anterior attachments include: (a) the therapist sinks the fingers and thumb just medial to the anterior superior iliac spine (ASIS) on each side, while the patient imagines two wires ascending diagonally and medially from the ASISs to the right and left side of the vertebra being palpated. (b) The therapist palpates just superior to the pubic bone and the patient imagines one wire ascending centrally and then splits to attach to the right and left sides of the spine at the palpated points. (c) The therapist uses pressure into the inner thighs bilaterally to cue a wire starting in the pelvic floor. (Reproduced with permission from © Diane G. Lee Physiotherapist Corp.)

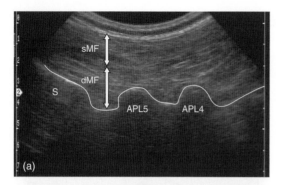

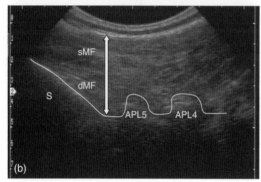

Figure 10.59   Ultrasound images of lumbosacral multifidus, longitudinal view. APL4, articular process L4; APL5, articular process L5; S, sacrum; dMF, deep multifidus; sMF, superficial multifidus. The arrows in both images indicate where muscle activity is seen when either the deep or superficial multifidus muscle contracts. (a) When no activity occurs in either the deep or superficial fibers of multifidus on a cue to recruit the muscle, the image does not change (there is no change in the thickness of the muscle layers) and resembles an image taken at rest. (b) Concurrent recruitment of the deep and superficial fibers of multifidus results in a change in thickness of the entire muscle from the lamina to the most superficial fibers. (Reproduced with permission from © Diane G. Lee Physiotherapist Corp.)

to palpation and observation skills and is not an essential tool for teaching local muscle activation; however, it is often a useful tool for providing feedback to patients and objective assessment of dysfunction.

Ultrasound image – no recruitment of the deep or superficial fibers of multifidus

Imaging   On the real-time ultrasound image, the following is seen (Fig. 10.59a):

- No change in the thickness of the muscle layers is seen on the ultrasound.

  Palpation   On palpation, the following is felt:

- The muscle remains soft and no tension is felt in the multifidus.

- Alternately, rapid tension in the superficial layers may be felt from the tensioning of the long tendons of the thoracic erector spinae muscles.
- Palpation of the abdomen may reveal a TA contraction or the TA may remain inactive.
- Activity is felt in any muscles being used in substitution (e.g., the oblique abdominals).

Observation   On observation, the following is noted:

- Breath-holding is commonly observed, as well as posterior tilting of the pelvis or segmental lumbar flexion as the patient attempts to push the muscle into the therapist's fingers. Abdominal bracing may also be evident.
- If the thoracic erector spinae muscles are active, the tone will be evident up into their origins in the thoracic spine, either symmetrically or asymmetrically, and spinal extension will occur unless there is co-contraction of the abdominals.

Correction technique   Several facilitation techniques can be tried.

- Try a variety of images until one is found that enables the patient to find the muscle. If lumbar flexion is occurring, use cues that emphasize a suspended or lifted feeling rather than "make the muscle swell."
- Check the posterior pelvic floor (ischiococcygeus) and posterior hip for hypertonicity (Fig. 10.33); if there is "butt gripping" it will inhibit activation of the multifidus. Change the patient position or use release techniques to decrease the tone prior to facilitating a multifidus contraction.
- If the thoracic erector spinae are active, choose a position that will maximize relaxation in these muscles, such as prone lying (Fig. 10.60).
- Check the breathing pattern and ensure there are no periods of breath-holding. Use the exhalation phase to encourage relaxation of the erector spinae muscles.

Ultrasound image – no recruitment of the deep fibers of multifidus, activity in the superficial layers

Imaging   On the real-time ultrasound image, the following is seen:

- No change in the width of the muscle layers is seen in the deep layers of multifidus. An increase in

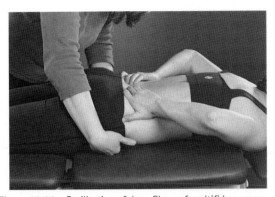

Figure 10.60 Facilitation of deep fibers of multifidus: prone. This position can reduce excessive activity in the thoracic erector spinae; placing a pillow under the stomach can increase support and further facilitate relaxation of the trunk. The patient palpates the multifidus bilaterally to monitor the contraction while the therapist checks for co-contraction of the transversus abdominis. The therapist's palpation points can be used to cue a "guy wire" image from the anterior abdomen. (Reproduced with permission from © Diane G. Lee Physiotherapist Corp.)

width of the superficial layers is observed, often a fast, phasic response.

Palpation On palpation, the following is felt:

- The fingers will be rapidly pushed out from the muscle, without any palpation of deep tension prior to the rapid contraction.
- Alternately, a fast contraction in the multifidus fibers lateral to the palpation point will be felt while the medial palpation point (deep fibers) stays soft and inactive.

Observation On observation, the following is noted:

- If the superficial multifidus is active without concurrent abdominal activity then an increase in the lumbar lordosis will be evident. No change in the lumbar curve will occur if there is concurrent abdominal bracing.

Correction technique Several facilitation techniques can be tried.

- Consider using manual or other techniques to decrease the tone and sensitivity in the superficial fibers prior to another attempt at isolation exercises for the deep layers.
- Try a variety of images until one is found that enables the patient to find the muscle. Avoid images that encourage an extension movement (e.g., "pretend you are arching your back but don't actually

move it") as these feed into the predisposition to recruit the superficial fibers.

- Check the breathing pattern and ensure there are no periods of breath-holding. Use the exhalation phase to encourage relaxation of the erector spinae and superficial multifidus.
- Change the patient's position to one where there is best relaxation of the superficial multifidus. A pillow under the abdomen is often effective.

Ultrasound image – concurrent phasic contraction of the deep and superficial fibers of multifidus

Imaging On the real-time ultrasound image, the following is seen (Fig. 10.59b):

- A change in thickness of the superficial and deep layers occurs simultaneously in a fast, phasic response.

Palpation On palpation, the following is felt:

- The fingers will be rapidly pushed out from the muscle, without any palpation of deep tension prior to the rapid contraction.

Observation On observation, the following is noted:

- If the multifidus is active without concurrent abdominal activity then an increase in the lumbar lordosis will be evident. No change in the lumbar curve will occur if there is concurrent abdominal bracing.

Correction technique Several facilitation techniques can be tried.

- Consider using manual or other techniques to decrease the tone and sensitivity in the superficial fibers prior to another attempt at isolation exercises for the deep layers.
- Encourage a much slower contraction, with much less effort. Often by repeatedly reducing speed and effort the pattern of activation can be altered such that the tension develops primarily in the deep layers of multifidus first. Use the ultrasound and manual cueing to teach the patient the point at which to stop the contraction (before the large bulge occurs).
- Try a variety of images until one is found that enables the patient to find the muscle. Avoid images that encourage an extension movement (e.g., "pretend you are arching your back but don't actually move it") as these feed into the predisposition to recruit the superficial fibers.

- Check the breathing pattern and ensure there are no periods of breath-holding. Use the exhalation phase to encourage relaxation of the erector spinae and superficial multifidus.

Ultrasound image – deep then superficial fibers of multifidus (correct timing but not isolated)

This is an acceptable recruitment pattern; however, the contraction of the superficial multifidus should be downtrained so that it is not excessive or phasic. The ultrasound image, palpation, and observation will be similar to that described above for the concurrent contraction of deep and superficial; however, the deep contraction can be observed on ultrasound and palpated prior to being overlaid with the superficial contraction. Cues for decreasing speed and effort are effective for reducing the activity in the superficial multifidus and thus bias the contraction to occur primarily in the deep layers.

Ultrasound image – asymmetrical activation

This is the most common clinical presentation and is often present with asymmetries in TA and/or pelvic floor function. The deep fibers of multifidus on one side will be poorly recruited, often in conjunction with excessive superficial multifidus activity on the ipsilateral or contralateral side. Correction of asymmetry will require a combination of the above facilitation techniques for all the local muscles. Using unilateral patient focus and attention is a key component. Images to address asymmetry in TA/multifidus will be addressed in the next section with co-contraction strategies.

CO-CONTRACTION AND ENDURANCE TRAINING FOR THE LOCAL SYSTEM

Once a successful strategy for creating an isolated contraction in the target local muscle has been identified, the patient is encouraged to work towards increasing the duration of the tonic contraction while maintaining normal breathing. It is important that the patient is taught how to recognize when the muscle stops working and/or when substitution patterns start (e.g., TA gradually fades and IO turns on). In this way, patients can monitor and progress their own program on a day-to-day basis, working towards 10 repetitions of 10-s holds, but varying the duration and number of contractions at each

practice session depending on how accurate the performance of the skill is at that time. Remind the patient that more practice sessions in a day, with smaller numbers of repetitions (e.g., 5-s holds, five repetitions, 10 times a day) is more effective at retraining the skill than one session of large numbers of repetitions (e.g., 5-s holds, 50 repetitions, once a day). As the skill is mastered in supported positions, more upright positions and activities are added to the program. The patient is instructed to perform the same contraction, but in positions such as sitting, supported standing, standing, and walking. The therapist must check the quality of the contraction in these new positions and ensure that activity in the global muscles is not excessive (use the checkpoints for global rigidity). More ideas on functional progressions are presented in the sections that follow.

If the patient presents with an asymmetric contraction, the verbal cueing and images can be altered such that more focus is directed towards the dysfunctional side. Careful palpation and observation by the therapist are crucial, as it is common to have one side with an ideal response in the muscle (isolated TA contraction), and a substitution response on the other side (IO contraction). In some cases, a bilateral contraction is cued first, and then the patient is instructed to think "a little bit more" about the side of the poor response ("pull the left tummy in a bit more," "think of drawing the left ASIS farther to the center," "create more tension in the guy wire to the right side of your low back"). In other cases, the best result is produced when only the dysfunctional side is cued ("just think of pulling in the left side of your tummy," "draw only the left ASIS to the center," "create a guy wire that only connects to the right side of your low back"). Although the patient is *thinking* of a unilateral contraction, a bilateral contraction is produced and palpated by the therapist. Usually this cueing needs to be progressed to a bilateral cueing as the global muscles on the dysfunctional side become less active and the isolated contraction more precise.

Ultimately the goal is a co-contraction of the local muscles – the pelvic floor, TA, and the deep fibers of multifidus – with normal breathing patterns (normal modulation of the diaphragm). Images can be combined or modified to produce co-contraction. The image of the guy wire for multifidus isolation often results in a co-contraction of TA and deep multifidus. Cues can be combined in many ways, for example, "Gently connect your two ASISs

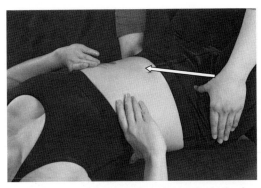

Figure 10.61   Cueing for correcting asymmetries in the deep local stabilizing system. The therapist provides deepening pressure at the palpation points as the verbal cue is given. In this example, the left thumb palpates the transversus abdominis and the right hand (under the trunk) palpates the deep multifidus. The arrow indicates the direction of the diagonal suspension wire. The patient palpates the ribcage bilaterally to self-cue a proper breathing pattern while the contraction is held. (Reproduced with permission from © Diane G. Lee Physiotherapist Corp.)

together [for TA], and imagine that they are connecting in the center at your pubic bone. Now connect a line from your pubic bone, through your body, and up into your spine on both sides where my fingers are [for multifidus]." In some cases palpation will reveal that cueing one muscle is sufficient to produce co-contraction in the others (the patient thinks of lifting in the pelvic floor and a co-contraction is felt in the TA and deep multifidus). For patterns of asymmetry, creating diagonal lines or guy wires can address a dysfunctional left TA and right multifidus simultaneously: "Think of connecting a wire from your right ASIS (or right pelvic floor) to the left low back where my finger is" (Fig. 10.61). When the ASLR indicates that asymmetrical compression is most beneficial, starting with asymmetrical images for asymmetrical co-contraction can often yield beneficial functional results (improved ASLR, improved stance phase of one-leg standing) more quickly than working on the muscles separately.

COORDINATING THE LOCAL AND GLOBAL SYSTEMS

Coordination of the local and global systems is essential for functional movement. Local system function can only control the segmental relationships of the joints and prevent excessive shearing.

It has very little ability to control the orientation of the ribcage in relation to the pelvis, or the limbs in relation to the trunk. It is essential to control spinal orientation, functional limb movement, and postural equilibrium of the global system. This section will cover exercises that promote optimal recruitment of the global muscles with a precontraction base of the local stabilizers. The goal is to maintain the co-contraction of the deep local system while sustaining positions and controlling movements that require global muscle activity. Care must be taken not to progress global exercises too quickly, and the ability voluntarily to isolate and tonically hold a segmental contraction should be reassessed often to ensure that control of the local system has not been lost. The specific exercise program used will vary depending on each patient's presentation, but a general protocol for progression is presented in Figures 10.62 and 10.63. This protocol is adapted from the guidelines developed by Richardson et al (1999).

Exercises can be designed to challenge control of flexion, extension, or rotation through the lumbar spine and pelvis depending on the direction that the limb is moved or the direction of the application of external forces (weights, resistive exercise bands, pulleys). Upright positions and movement of the limbs require activation of the global muscles and thus the global slings. For each progression focus should be first on *movement control*; in patients with lumbopelvic-hip dysfunction it is often most crucial to master dissociation of hip movement from trunk movement. Focus is on attaining proximal control first, and then adding the rest of the limb in functional patterns. As movement control is mastered, the exercises can be progressed to *resisted movements* to strengthen the muscles in functional patterns. It is important to identify the direction of loss of control and the area of loss of control (SIJs versus lumbar spine joints) so that the exercise program can be specific and not involve so many exercises that patient compliance is unlikely.

When the global muscles are activated in a coordinated, properly timed manner with a precontraction of the deep local stabilizers, the resultant movements will be performed with optimal alignment and fluidity of movement. Palpation of the poorly controlled segment will reveal maintained control of the neutral zone by the local stabilizers. Observation of the relative positions of the limbs in relation to the trunk and of the thorax in relation to the pelvis will reveal maintained alignment of all joints in the kinetic chain such that the entire body

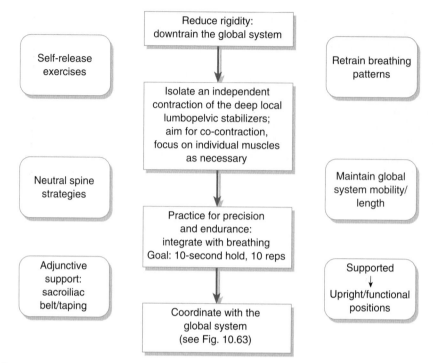

Figure 10.62   Program for stabilization of the lumbar spine and pelvis.

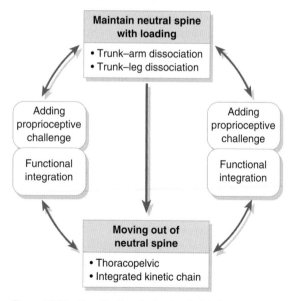

Figure 10.63   Coordinating the local and global systems.

is positioned to share and transmit forces equally. This overall body alignment is sustained by balanced length, strength, and timing in the global sling systems. Observation of the *quality* of muscle reactions during activities on unstable surfaces with

expected or unexpected challenges to balance will reveal control of postural equilibrium without long periods of excessive global muscle activation and trunk rigidity (Hodges 2003).

It is critical that for each new exercise the therapist palpates the segment(s) where failed load transfer was identified on assessment. This will reveal whether or not the local stabilizing system is continuing to function in the new movement and/or loading environment. Palpation points include:

● For the pelvic girdle, the innominate and the sacrum are palpated on the affected side to ensure that anterior rotation (or shearing) of the innominate does not occur with limb loading (Fig. 8.7).

● For the lumbar spine, the articular pillars or interspinous spaces are palpated to check for loss of control in the relevant direction (flexion, extension, rotation, or shearing).

● For the hip, the innominate and the greater trochanter of the femur are palpated to check for anterior displacement of the femoral head or loss of rotational control (change in hip position often reflects an altered stabilization strategy such that the hip muscles substitute for the lumbopelvic local stabilizers) (Fig. 8.6).

As exercises are added that include full limb movement, each joint in the kinetic chain should be observed/palpated for control of the optimal axis of movement and joint position. The position of the thorax in relation to the pelvis is monitored for alterations in the anteroposterior (sagittal), lateral (coronal), and rotational (transverse) planes. The femoral head should remain seated (centered in the acetabulum) without loss of control into internal/external rotation, abduction/adduction, flexion or extension. The knee should not excessively rotate or abduct/adduct (fall into a valgus or varus position); the foot should not excessively supinate or pronate. In closed kinetic chain exercises, the knee should stay aligned such that mid-patella is in line with the midpoint of the inguinal ligament and tracks over the second toe. By correcting deviations of alignment during the exercises with tactile cues, imagery, or proprioceptive input (e.g., via resistive exercise bands), the appropriate components of the global slings will be activated for total body movement control.

When adding the global muscles to the local stabilizers, the discerning clinician may ask, "How much is too much global activity?" It is evident that there needs to be enough global activity to control the imposed forces. However, excessive global activity is best avoided as it perpetuates too much compression through the joints and restricts mobility. Thus, the clinician needs to be able to identify when the added global muscle activity crosses over from "just enough" to "too much." Each patient will present with a specific pattern of global muscle hyperactivity; this pattern will have been identified during the assessment tests. By specifically palpating and observing these muscles during exercise progressions, the clinician will get an idea of how much activity is present; comparing for symmetry of activation between affected and non-affected sides is often revealing. Furthermore, the checkpoints for global rigidity as described above should be used often and even between repetitions of exercises; whenever rigidity is present there is "too much" global muscle activity. The patient can be taught how to monitor the specific muscles and pattern of substitution for the home exercise program.

GENERAL PRINCIPLES

- Connect first – teach the patient to perform a precontraction of the deep local stabilizers as the starting point for each exercise.

- Initially the patient may need to relax the local stabilizer co-contraction after each repetition of movement; however, the goal is to encourage a maintained local muscle co-contraction for several repetitions of movement, as long as substitution strategies are not observed. The number of repetitions possible with one local muscle activation will increase as control improves.
- Palpate and monitor the local muscle recruitment and control of the joint position during the exercises, especially when adding a new progression. Ensure that the muscles do not turn off and that there are no signs of loss of control into the direction of hypermobility.
- Focus on low load and control of movement.
- Aim for high repetitions. Start with only as many repetitions as the patient can perform with an effective local system co-contraction and control of the movement (sometimes as low as three to five repetitions), and progress to 15–20 repetitions where the exercise is easy and requires minimal concentration to control the movement.
- Use the manual cues and key points of control described above for attaining neutral spine and isolating the local stabilizers to provide tactile feedback and assist control at the levels where segmental hypermobility or multisegmental collapse occurs *during the exercise movements.*
- Avoid fast ballistic movements.
- Progress from stable to unstable surfaces to increase proprioceptive input and challenge.
- Check for excessive global muscle activity by monitoring the breathing pattern (should continue to see lateral costal and abdominal expansion) and by monitoring for bracing/rigidity (see checkpoints for global rigidity).
- Incorporate local muscle co-contraction into daily functional activities as early and as often as possible; break down functional tasks into component movements and use separate components as an exercise.
- Focus on co-contraction and control of position instead of single muscle strengthening.
- For SIJ dysfunction exercises that address rotational control need to be included in the program in order to restore full function.
- If high-load and high-speed activities are required for work or sport, add these at the end-stages of rehabilitation and ensure that low-load, slow-speed control is present for the same movement pattern first. High-speed/high-load activities should be only one part of the patient's exercise

program; low-load exercises should be continued concurrently to ensure continued function of the local system.

• There are many variations and options possible for each of the following categories. For each section, several progressions are presented, but the reader is encouraged to use the principles and guidelines in this chapter to guide the creation of other exercise progressions that may be necessary for a specific patient presentation.

MAINTAINING NEUTRAL SPINE WITH LOADING

The goal for all of the exercises in this section is to maintain co-contraction of the deep local stabilizers and control of the neutral spine position while adding the challenge of limb loading. The spinal curves should be monitored and the relationship between the lumbopelvic region and the thorax should be maintained throughout the exercises. The movements should be slow and controlled in both the concentric and eccentric phases of movement. Two types of exercises can be used: those that control dissociation of the arm from the trunk, and those that control dissociation of the leg from the trunk. Functional integration exercises are discussed later in the chapter.

Palpation of the poorly controlled joints and the local stabilizing muscle activation will reveal whether or not control of the neutral zone is maintained. Observation of the orientation of the pelvis, the orientation of the ribcage, and their relative alignment will reveal whether or not balanced and symmetrical activity in the global system is occurring. To correct loss of global muscle control, images of keeping connections of parts or of keeping tension along lines of force are used to cue correct alignment of parts of the kinetic chain. For thoracopelvic control during these exercises, the following cues can be used:

• If there is extension and right rotation of the thorax (Fig. 10.64), use the cue: "Keep the bottom of your ribcage on the right side connected to the left ASIS during the exercise" (this facilitates the anterior oblique sling).

• If there is flexion and rotation of the thorax to the right, use the cue: "Imagine that there is a line going from your left bottom rib at the back to your right hip (or PSIS); keep tension in that line throughout the exercise" (this facilitates the posterior oblique sling).

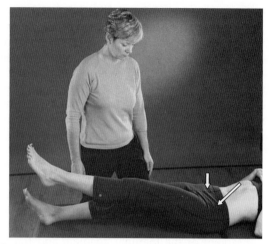

Figure 10.64   Images for correcting thoracopelvic alignment. In this example, the patient is unable to maintain a neutral spine position during leg loading. The thorax moves into extension and right rotation while the pelvis rotates to the left. The arrows indicate the direction and connections of the suspension wires created with imagery for thoracopelvic control. (Reproduced with permission from © Diane G. Lee Physiotherapist Corp.)

• If the pelvis is rotating left (Fig. 10.64), use the cue: "Imagine that there is a pin going through your right ASIS that is holding the right side of your pelvis down on the bed and keeping it still while you move your leg" (this facilitates contralateral anterior oblique sling and/or ipsilateral posterior oblique sling).

These cues are added after the initial co-contraction of the deep local stabilizing system occurs, and emphasized *during* movement of the arm or leg so that continued activation of the appropriate global sling occurs during increased limb loading.

Trunk and arm dissociation – supine or crook lying

Patient position   Crook lying in neutral spine on a flat surface. Arms are flexed to 90° so that the hands are vertically over the shoulder joints.

Exercise instruction   Cue the image that facilitates a co-contraction of the lumbopelvic local stabilizers. Palpate the TA and multifidus at the dysfunctional level(s), ensuring that recruitment occurs with your cue. Ask the patient to keep breathing and maintain the spinal position while performing various arm movements:

1. Triceps press (extension control) (Fig. 10.65): bend the elbows and bring the hands towards the

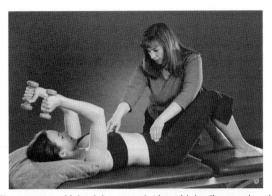

Figure 10.65 Maintaining neutral spine with loading: trunk and arm dissociation – crook lying triceps press (extension control). The therapist palpates for the recruitment and tonic contraction of the transversus abdominis while providing gentle pressure on the sternum to cue maintenance of the thoracic kyphosis and to prevent loss of neutral spine into thoracolumbar extension. (Reproduced with permission from © Diane G. Lee Physiotherapist Corp.)

head. The elbows are then straightened (triceps press movement). The shoulders should not flex or extend; movement occurs only at the elbow joints.

2. Overhead flexion (extension control): keep the arms straight while elevating the arms through flexion. The patient will require adequate length in the latissimus dorsi muscles to perform this progression with good control of the lumbar lordosis. The exercise can also be started with the arms at the sides instead of at 90° flexion.

3. One-arm fly (rotation control): keep the arm straight while lowering the arm through horizontal abduction one arm at a time. Palpate the dysfunctional area (lumbar spine, SIJs) to ensure no loss of control of the neutral position.

Progressions/other considerations   Progress to lying on a half-roll or other unsupported surface. Hand weights can be added to increase the challenge to the spine while concurrently strengthening the arm muscles. These exercises can be performed in sitting, sitting on a ball, and standing. The upright positions require more awareness and spinal control. If the triceps press and overhead flexion exercises are performed unilaterally with alternating arm movements, both extension and rotational control of the spine will be challenged.

Trunk and arm dissociation – sitting

Patient position   Sitting on a firm surface, feet flat on the floor, pelvis centered over the sitz bones,

in neutral spine position (optimal lumbopelvic pyramid). If an exercise band is being used as resistance, secure it such that when the patient moves the arm the band has a line of pull in the opposite direction to the movement.

Exercise instruction   Cue the image that facilitates a co-contraction of the lumbopelvic local stabilizers. Palpate the TA and multifidus at the dysfunctional level(s), ensuring that recruitment occurs with your cue. Ask the patient to keep breathing and maintain the spinal position while performing various arm movements:

1. Bilateral arm extension (flexion control): the hands are at shoulder level in front of the body, holding a resistive exercise band on slight tension. Both arms are pulled down to the sides as neutral spine is maintained (the tendency will be to flex the spine and posteriorly tilt the pelvis to pull the arms down). Use the rib wiggle and the hip internal and external rotation tests to ensure that there is no trunk bracing and no "butt gripping." The arms are returned smoothly to the starting position, controlling the movement against the pull of the resistive exercise band. This exercise can also be performed using pulleys. Unilateral movements will add a rotational challenge.

2. Diagonal arm extension: (flexion and rotation control): start with one arm in full flexion and adduction (across the body), holding a resistive exercise band attached above and lateral to the contralateral shoulder. The arm is pulled down into extension and across the body into abduction (to the ipsilateral hip). The tendency will be for the patient to flex and rotate the spine and pelvis to facilitate the arm movement. The therapist uses manual and verbal cues to prevent this substitution pattern.

3. Bilateral arm flexion with facilitation from a resistive exercise band (extension control): the patient starts with the elbows bent at the sides and palms facing. A light resistive exercise band is wrapped around the hands so that there is light tension present (Fig. 10.66). Instruct the patient to push gently into the band with the hands (5% abduction force), and then lift both arms into flexion as high as possible while controlling the spinal position. The arms are then lowered to the side. The light resistive exercise band is thought to increase proximal proprioceptive input and assist in learning movement control. The start position for this exercise is the same as that used in adding thoracopelvic rotation control (moving out of neutral spine, see below).

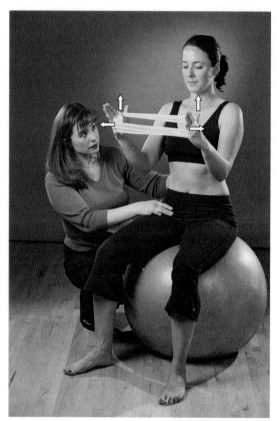

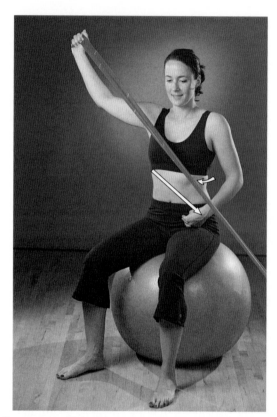

Figure 10.66   Maintaining neutral spine with loading: trunk and arm dissociation – sitting. Bilateral arm flexion (extension control). The therapist monitors the right transversus abdominis contraction and palpates multifidus bilaterally at the dysfunctional segment; a co-contraction of the local system should be performed first and then tonically maintained throughout the arm movements. The small arrows indicate the direction of the hands pressing into the resistive exercise band and the large arrows indicate the flexion movement of the arms. (Reproduced with permission from © Diane G. Lee Physiotherapist Corp.)

Figure 10.67   Maintaining neutral spine with loading: trunk and arm dissociation – sitting. Unilateral flexion diagonal (combined extension and rotation control). The patient monitors the left transversus abdominis contraction throughout the exercise. The right hand starts just lateral to the left hip and then pulls against the resistive exercise band diagonally into flexion and abduction to the end position, as shown. Note that there is a loss of the neutral position of the thorax over the pelvis into thoracolumbar extension and right rotation (short arrow). This should be corrected with a cue to connect the right ribcage to the left hand (diagonal arrow). (Reproduced with permission from © Diane G. Lee Physiotherapist Corp.)

Progressions/other considerations   Progress to sitting on a ball or sissel, sitting with the feet on a half-roll, or using other unsupported surfaces to increase proprioceptive challenge. These exercises can be performed in kneeling, supported standing, and standing. Diagonal arm patterns can be performed starting from either hip (Fig. 10.67) and either shoulder (four proprioceptive neuromuscular facilitation (PNF) patterns) and are good for functional integration and control of combined extension/rotation and flexion/rotation.

Trunk and arm dissociation – standing

The same arm movements described above and other variations can be performed in supported

standing, supported standing against a ball, or standing (Fig. 10.68). It is important to progress to these functional positions as early as possible. For the patient with lumbopelvic-hip dysfunction, arm movements in supported standing are a useful intermediate step before standing trunk–hip dissociation exercises such as a squat can be performed. Once the arm movements are mastered, the patient can be progressed to a squat (lower-extremity exercises). At the later stages of the rehabilitation exercise program, arm movements can be combined with modified leg positions to challenge the base of support further and integrate arm and leg movement with spinal control. For example, a split-squat

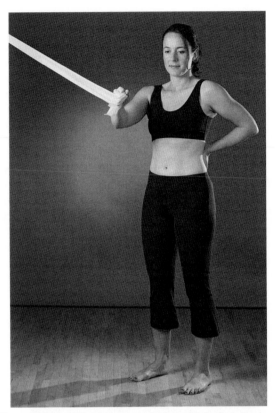

Figure 10.68   Maintaining neutral spine with loading: trunk and arm dissociation – standing. Unilateral extension diagonal (combined flexion and rotation control). The patient palpates the lumbosacral multifidus bilaterally at the dysfunctional segment to monitor precontraction and continued tonic activity during the performance of the arm movement. The right arm starts in abduction and elevation and pulls the resistive exercise band across the body to the left hip. (Reproduced with permission from © Diane G. Lee Physiotherapist Corp.)

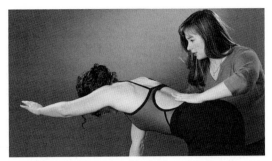

Figure 10.69   Maintaining neutral spine with loading: trunk and arm dissociation – four-point kneeling. The therapist's hand palpates the lumbopelvic spine to ensure that the lumbar lordosis is maintained during the arm lift and can also provide specific tactile feedback at the levels of poor control. (Reproduced with permission from © Diane G. Lee Physiotherapist Corp.)

stance or unilateral standing against a ball on the wall can be maintained while the arms move in diagonal patterns. Finally, the lower extremity and the arms move together (a dynamic lunge while the arm performs a diagonal pull) while continuing to maintain neutral spinal alignment.

Trunk and arm dissociation – four-point kneeling, four-point kneeling over a ball

If performed correctly, these positions are useful for training stability of the lumbopelvic region while maintaining an awareness of an open buttock (preventing "butt gripping").

Patient position   Kneeling prone over a ball with the thorax positioned so that the curve of the ball facilitates maintenance of the neutral thoracic kyphosis. The pelvis and lumbar spine should be unsupported and free to move into a neutral position over the hips. If there is a restriction of hip flexion range of motion, place the knees farther away from the ball so that they are not directly under the hips.

Exercise instruction   Cue the image that facilitates a co-contraction of the lumbopelvic local stabilizers. Palpate the TA and multifidus at the dysfunctional level(s), ensuring that recruitment occurs with your cue. Ask the patient to keep breathing, and maintain a still spine as the arm is lifted off the ball. This movement will challenge extension control of the spine.

Progressions/other considerations   Progress to performing the exercise without support from the ball (Fig. 10.69). Adding the challenge of a concurrent contralateral leg lift is a high-level exercise and requires significant control. Often the patient will be able to perform exercises in supported standing and standing positions before leg movements in four-point kneeling are possible. Decisions about how far to challenge control in any position will depend on the patient's functional demands and recreational goals (for example, if the patient performs activities that require prolonged forward-bent positions then progressions in four-point kneeling will likely be important).

Trunk and leg dissociation – crook lying

Various leg loading exercises and their progressions have been described by several authors (Hall & Brody 1999, Richardson et al 1999, Sahrmann 2001). Presented here are some specific examples and modified examples that we find useful in treating patients with lumbopelvic-hip dysfunction.

Patient position   Crook lying in neutral spine on a flat surface.

Exercise instruction   Cue the image that facilitates a co-contraction of the lumbopelvic local stabilizers ("connect" to the local system). Palpate the TA and multifidus at the dysfunctional level(s), ensuring that recruitment occurs with your cue. Ask the patient to keep breathing and maintain the neutral position of the lumbar spine and pelvis while performing various leg movements:

1. Heel slides (extension/rotation and flexion/rotation control): ensure that the feet can slide on the surface easily (have the patient wear socks). Ask the patient slowly to slide one heel away from the trunk (Fig. 10.70a), straightening the leg as far as possible without losing control of the neutral lumbopelvic position. Palpate the segment(s) of poor control to ensure that no rotation occurs in the lumbar spine or pelvis. This phase of the exercise challenges extension and rotation control; the return of the leg back to the flexed position challenges flexion and rotation control. The easiest position to start the slide from is the crook lying position; to increase the challenge, have the patient start the slide with the leg straight. The exercise can also be changed from a single-leg slide to alternating slides (from moving one leg at a time to moving both legs at the same time, one sliding down while the other slides up).

2. Bent knee fall-out (rotation control): from the crook lying position one knee is slowly taken to the side so that the hip abducts and externally rotates (Fig. 10.70b, arrow). The other leg stays stationary. Careful observation and palpation is necessary to ensure that the patient is not "butt gripping" and pushing the femoral head anterior. Palpate at the ASISs or in the lumbar spine interspinous spaces for rotation control. To progress the exercise, straighten the non-moving leg (Hall & Brody 1999).

3. Heel drops from 90° (extension control): to attain the starting position, the patient requires 90°

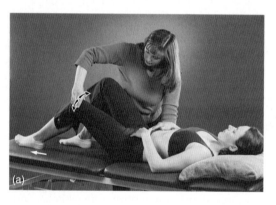

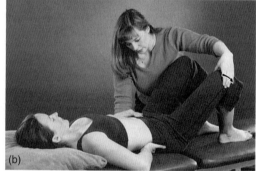

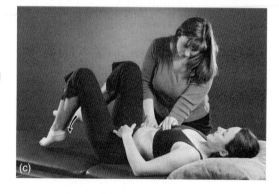

Figure 10.70   Maintaining neutral spine with loading: trunk and leg dissociation – crook lying exercises. (a) Heel slides in crook lying. The therapist palpates the lumbosacral multifidus bilaterally with the hand under the low back while the patient palpates the transversus abdominis (TA) bilaterally. The heel slides down the bed (white arrow) as far as the neutral spine position can be maintained and then returns to the start position. The therapist's hand on the knee guides the leg movement and periodically "wiggles" the knee laterally (hip internal and external rotation, small black arrows) to check for hip bracing. (b) Bent knee fall outs. The therapist palpates in the lumbar interspinous spaces to ensure that neutral is maintained (no rotation occurs); alternately the deep multifidus can be palpated. In this example the patient palpates the points to facilitate the image of a diagonal connection between the left TA and the right deep fibers of multifidus. (c) Heel drops from 90°. The therapist palpates the TA and multifidus on the right side; the patient palpates the left TA and the sternum. As the foot is lowered towards the table the tendency will be to lose the neutral spinal position and move into extension. The hand on the sternum helps to prevent thoracolumbar extension. (Reproduced with permission from © Diane G. Lee Physiotherapist Corp.)

of hip flexion (any articular or myofascial restrictions need to be addressed first). The patient lies with the hips flexed to 90° such that the knees are vertically over the hip joints. The lumbar lordosis should be checked for a neutral position. Cue a relaxation of the abdominal wall and breathing, and then instruct the patient to "connect" to the local stabilizers. The patient is then asked slowly to lower one foot, keeping the knee flexed, until the foot is placed on the floor (or until the spinal control is lost) (Fig. 10.70c). The foot is then lifted from the floor and returned to 90° hip flexion. Using the image "Keep the fold in the front of the hip deep and control the lowering of the knee from deep inside your groin" helps to prevent excessive activation of the tensor fascia latae and rectus femoris muscles. Progress the exercise by having the patient extend the knee as the foot is lowered (increase the lever arm). This exercise is a useful precursor to any exercise that involves lifting one foot off the ground in supine or sitting. It is also a key exercise to prescribe for those patients who have poor eccentric control in the hip flexion phase of the one-leg standing test.

4. Hip joint control progressions: these progressions are aimed at reducing tensor fascia latae, rectus femoris, and sartorius activity during hip flexion, and facilitate the underlying iliopsoas for control of the joint axis during movement. The therapist and patient should palpate around the greater trochanter and feel the activity in the lateral muscles during the exercise. The first level begins with the foot supported on a wall, with the hip flexed approximately 70–80°. The local system is precontracted, and then the patient is asked to "imagine an energy deep in your groin that is deepening your hip groove, and then fold the hip so that your knee comes towards your body" (Fig. 10.71a). Ankle plantarflexion (heel lift) can be used as an assist to

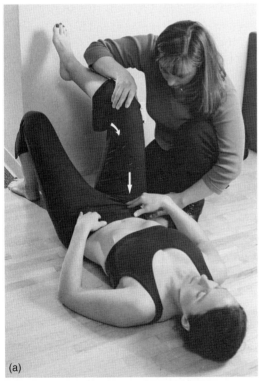

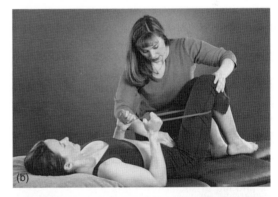

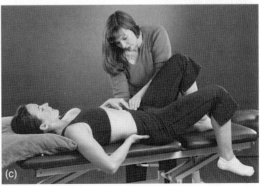

Figure 10.71 Maintaining neutral spine with loading: trunk and leg dissociation – hip control progressions. (a) Inner-range hip flexion off wall. The patient palpates in the anterior groin while the therapist palpates tensor fascia latae, rectus femoris, and sartorius laterally. The patient's left hand palpates transversus abdominis (TA). The idea of the femur sinking (vertical arrow) and the hip hinging will facilitate proper recruitment and patterning. (b) A resistive exercise band assist decreases the amount of load to control. In this example the therapist is palpating TA bilaterally to monitor the tonic activation during the exercise. (c) Moving into outer range. In this example the patient palpates a co-contraction of the left TA and right multifidus while the therapist monitors spinal position. As the leg moves into this outer-range position, the superficial hip flexors will turn on to some degree but this activity should not result in rigidity of the hip joint. (Reproduced with permission from © Diane G. Lee Physiotherapist Corp.)

get the foot off the wall. Alternately, if there is excessive tensor fascia latae, rectus femoris, or sartorius activity then use a resistive exercise band around the thigh to act as an assist to the hip flexion movement (Fig. 10.71b). At this inner range with the knee vertically over the hip there should be little need for a large contribution by the global hip muscles. The exercise is progressed by moving the patient farther and farther away from the wall. Finally, the exercise is performed over the edge of a table so that the foot can be lowered past the level of the table and the hip can move into full extension (Fig. 10.71c).

Progressions/other considerations Progress to lying on a half-roll or other unsupported surface. Initially the patient will only be able to move the leg through a small range of motion. As control improves, the leg can move through a larger range of motion. It is important to teach patients what it feels like when they lose control so that the exercise can be monitored and progressed at home. Be sure to use the rib wiggle, hip internal and external rotation, and to monitor lateral costal expansion breathing during the exercises to prevent excessive activation of the global muscles. Lifting the weight of the leg off the floor and lowering the leg into a fully extended position are high-level exercises, especially in those patients with muscular legs. In these cases, exercises in more upright positions such as sitting and supported standing can be added to the exercise program before the higher progressions of leg loading in supine are achieved.

Trunk and leg dissociation – prone

Patient position Prone lying, with the lumbar spine and pelvis in neutral position. Pillows or towels under the abdomen or thorax can be used to obtain the correct alignment.

Exercise instruction Instruct the patient to think of the image that facilitates the desired local muscle co-contraction, palpating the TA and multifidus to provide feedback and check recruitment. Ask the patient to bend one knee to 90° flexion, lifting the foot and then lowering it to the table (Fig. 10.72). Repeat on the other side.

Other considerations This movement can also be used as a test for effective load transfer. Before cueing a local system contraction, ask the patient to bend the knee (without thinking of controlling the pelvis or spine). Palpate the innominate and the sacrum as the movement is performed. If the innominate anteriorly rotates relative to the sacrum, especially in the early stages of the movement as the

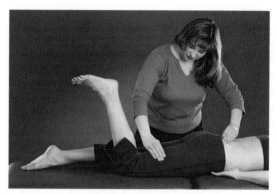

Figure 10.72 Maintaining neutral spine with loading: trunk and leg dissociation – prone knee bend. In this example the therapist is palpating the sacral multifidus bilaterally to ensure that a precontraction and continued tonic activity of the deep fibers is maintained while the patient lifts the right foot from the table and bends the knee. The therapist also monitors medial and lateral hamstring activity for equal recruitment. The patient cues and monitors the transversus abdominis anteriorly. (Reproduced with permission from © Diane G. Lee Physiotherapist Corp.)

weight of the leg is moved and before tension occurs in the rectus femoris muscle, this is considered a positive test for failed load transfer of the SIJ. Palpation of the medial and lateral hamstrings often reveals asymmetrical activation. Manual stabilization of the SIJ (nutate the sacrum) often makes the movement easier to initiate and changes the balance in the recruitment of the medial/lateral hamstrings. If this test is positive, the SIJ must be monitored during the performance of the exercise to ensure that the local muscle co-contraction controls the neutral zone; the patient can monitor the innominate anteriorly with a hand under the ASIS to feel for any anterior rotation. For this specific patient, exercises such as resisted hamstring curls without conscious local control of the SIJ usually increase and perpetuate symptoms. These patients often complain of vague medial or lateral hamstring aching or insertional hamstring pain unrelated to a traumatic incident. A specific hamstrings muscle test may reveal "weakness"; however, on retesting the hamstrings strength with the SIJ manually stabilized (nutated), the strength will be normal. This illustrates the importance of monitoring for proximal control as the lower limb is added in exercise progressions.

Trunk and leg dissociation – sitting

In this position exercises can focus on either movement of the trunk on the hips or movement of the legs under the trunk.

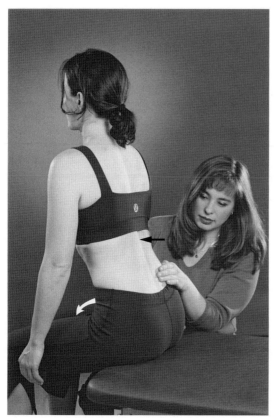

Figure 10.73 Maintaining neutral spine with loading: trunk and leg dissociation – sitting lean-forward. The therapist palpates the lumbar lordosis posteriorly and the right hip crease (not visible). Neutral spine position should be maintained as the patient anteriorly tilts the pelvis forward over the femurs (white arrow); in this example the patient has moved into extension in the lower thorax as the exercise is attempted (black arrow). (Reproduced with permission from © Diane G. Lee Physiotherapist Corp.)

Sitting lean-forward – patient position Sitting on the edge of a plinth, chair, or ball. If there is a restriction of hip flexion, the surface should be high enough to allow the pelvis to flex over the femoral heads. The feet are supported on the floor.

Exercise instruction Cue a neutral spine position (optimal lumbopelvic pyramid) and palpate the anterior hip crease (unilaterally or bilaterally). Have the patient "connect" to the local system, and then instruct the patient to hinge at the hips to bring the trunk forward over the hips while keeping the spine neutral (Fig. 10.73). Only allow movement through a range of motion where there is no loss of neutral spine. Start with small amounts of movement and progress to larger ranges. This exercise can be progressed to standing (Sahrmann's "waiter's bow" (2001)). Hamilton & Richardson (1998) studied the

ability to control spinal position during the sitting lean-forward movement in subjects with and without low back pain. They found that low back pain patients showed a consistently earlier loss of control of the neutral position, and that the displacement of the curvature between T12 and S2 in low back pain subjects was almost twice the displacement in non-low back pain subjects.

Sitting knee extension or hip flexion – patient position Sitting in neutral spine (optimal lumbopelvic pyramid), feet supported on the floor; to progress the exercises have the patient sit on a ball or other unstable surface.

Exercise instruction "Connect to the deep local stabilizers, then slowly let the foot slide on the floor as you straighten one knee. Keep the curve in your low back and your spine still as you move the leg." Or, ask the patient to palpate the anterior hip in the groin and lift the heel (ankle plantarflexion), feeling the anterior hip fold, keeping the "outside muscles" (tensor fascia latae) relaxed, and keeping the weight equal on the buttocks as the hip flexes. Alternate with the other foot. This exercise can be progressed to lifting the toe off the ground, which is a much higher load, especially in patients with long or muscular legs. If training hip flexion/extension control is an important component for the patient, this exercise should be used in conjunction with progressions in the supine position above.

Trunk and leg dissociation – four-point kneeling

If performed correctly, these positions are useful for training stability of the lumbopelvic-hip region while maintaining an awareness of an open buttock (preventing "butt gripping"). The "hip rock" exercise (Fig. 10.24) and the "hip rock'n'roll" exercise (Fig. 10.25) for maintaining hip mobility can be combined with a co-contraction of the deep stabilizers to incorporate mobility training with lumbopelvic stability training. Exercises involving lifting one leg from this position require significantly higher levels of stability and should be added later in the rehabilitation program. Examples include one-leg lifts, alternating arm/leg lifts, and leg press into extension against a resistive exercise band (Fig. 10.74). The lumbopelvic position must be carefully monitored to ensure no tilting or rotation.

Trunk and leg dissociation – supported standing

Patient position Standing in neutral spine against a wall. The feet are approximately 15 cm (6 in.) away

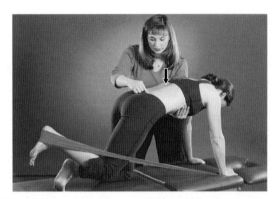

Figure 10.74 Maintaining neutral spine with loading: trunk and leg dissociation – four-point kneeling. Resistive exercise band leg press. The patient first finds a neutral spine position. A resistive exercise band is wrapped around the heel and arch of the working foot; the other end is held secure with the ipsilateral hand. With a precontraction of the local stabilizers, hip extension and knee extension are performed by pressing back into the resistive exercise band. Here, the therapist cues the maintenance of the thoracic curve and ensures a continued contraction of the lumbosacral multifidus throughout the exercise. The patient has lost some of the upper lumbar lordosis (arrow) due to overrecuitment of the oblique abdominals. (Reproduced with permission from © Diane G. Lee Physiotherapist Corp.)

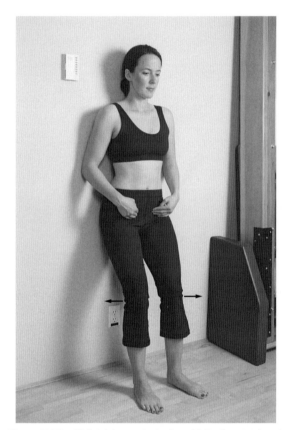

Figure 10.75 Maintaining neutral spine with loading: trunk and leg dissociation – supported standing. The chicken: the patient starts by finding neutral spine in supported standing. In this example the patient is palpating and self-cueing the transversus abdominis component bilaterally. The arrows indicate movement of the knees for the chicken exercise. (Reproduced with permission from © Diane G. Lee Physiotherapist Corp.)

from the wall. The hips should be in approximately 20° flexion, so that the pelvis and spine are inclined forward on the hips and the upper thorax and head are away from the wall. The hips should be in neutral rotation, the knees flexed under the hips, the second toe of each foot in line with the middle of the patella, and equal body weight distributed over each foot. In correcting technique and position in the standing position, it is important to use all of the checkpoints for global rigidity from the ribcage to the toes.

Exercise instruction Advise the patient that movement is to occur only in the legs; the spine stays still and suspended by the "guy wires." Have the patient "connect" to the local system, and then continue breathing while moving the knees in and out (hip internal and external rotation). For the chicken exercise the right and left knees are moved away from each other and then together (Fig. 10.75). If the patient is "butt gripping" there will be a restriction of the movement. Alternately, the patient may have more difficulty controlling one hip than the other (shudders of movement, uneven speed of movement). The focus should be on smooth, even movement of the legs under a stable lumbopelvis and spine. The feet are allowed to roll in and out as needed, but not excessively. The exercise is progressed to the skier, where

both knees are moved in the same direction simultaneously. This produces more rotational challenge to the lumbopelvic position. The patient should feel equal pressure on both sides of the buttock during both of these exercises, indicating that there is no rotation of the pelvis occurring. Both the chicken and the skier can be performed in varying amounts of knee and hip flexion (deeper squat position).

Trunk and leg dissociation – standing flexion control

Patient position Standing in neutral spine, feet shoulder-width apart. In the initial stages of this exercise the weight of the upper body and trunk can be supported by resting the hands on the back of a chair or counter.

Exercise instruction Advise the patient that movement is to occur only at the hips; the spine stays still and suspended by the "guy wires." Have the patient "connect" to the local system, then imagine bending forward "like a Barbie doll," hinging at the hips as the buttocks move backwards and the trunk moves forwards (waiter's bow – Sahrmann 2001). Only allow forward inclination of the trunk as far as the lumbar lordosis can be maintained. The trunk then returns to the upright position. Useful palpation points for the patient are in the lumbar lordosis, or around the greater trochanters to feel the hips "folding" and moving backwards. Ensure that there is symmetrical flexion of the hips.

Trunk and leg dissociation – standing rotation control

Patient position Standing in neutral spine, with the legs in stance position. The back leg is supported on the ball of the foot (heel lifted). Weight is focused on the front leg. Ensure that the knee faces anterior with the middle of the patella in line with the hip joint and the second toe.

Exercise instruction Cue recruitment of the lumbopelvic local muscles. Instruct the patient to keep the leg still and the knee forward while rotating the pelvis and trunk as one unit over the leg (spin the pelvis over the femoral head). Cue the initiation of the rotation movement to come from just inside the ASIS (the movement comes from the pelvis).

Progressions/other considerations Do not allow any lateral or posterior pelvic tilting as the pelvis rotates. Monitor the knee and give tactile cues to keep the knee facing forward, and the hip centered (no "butt gripping"). Monitor the segments of poor control, either at the SIJ (sacrum and innominate) or in the lumbar spine. Progress the exercise to weight-bearing only on the front leg (Fig. 10.76). Alternately, lateral control of the pelvis on the innominate can be trained by having the patient perform a controlled drop of the pelvis on the front hip, then return the pelvis to neutral lateral tilt by using the gluteus medius. This movement should be carefully monitored to ensure that the opposite quadratus lumborum is not performing the movement.

MOVING OUT OF NEUTRAL SPINE

Control of movements out of neutral spine is essential for stability during many functional activities.

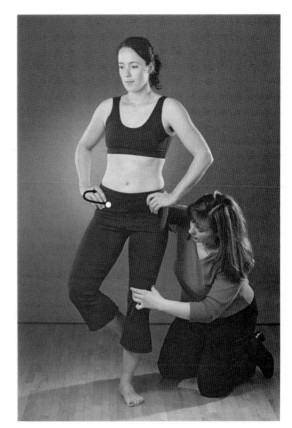

Figure 10.76 Maintaining neutral spine with loading: trunk and leg dissociation – standing rotation control, unilateral weight-bearing. The therapist monitors the maintenance of the position of the weight-bearing leg; the femur and rest of the lower extremity should remain still as the pelvis rotates to the right (arrow) and to the left. In this example, for right rotation of the pelvis the patient thinks of a point medial to the right anterior superior iliac spine and imagines drawing the pelvis back from that point (white circle). (Reproduced with permission from © Diane G. Lee Physiotherapist Corp.)

The therapist must carefully monitor the intervertebral, intrapelvic, and hip (innominate/femur) relationships during these movements to ensure that there is equal movement and loading occurring at each segment and from each component in the kinetic chain of movement. For functional load transfer, the hypermobile segment(s) must be controlled during changes in *thoracopelvic* orientation and as a component part of an *integrated functional kinetic chain* movement.

Changes in the thoracopelvic orientation will result in movement in the lumbar spine: flexion, extension, lateral bending, rotation, or combinations of these movements. The ability to control thoracopelvic movement is an essential requirement of many functional activities, from those as basic as walking to more complex sport maneuvers. Exercises can be designed such that the thorax moves on the pelvis or the pelvis moves under the thorax. These exercises focus on training the ability to dissociate movement of the thorax from the pelvis and vice versa. Some examples are provided here, and then the concept is applied to retraining the pelvic component of a functional movement (the golf swing). Ultimately, restoring optimal movement specific to a patient's activities requires breaking down complex functional, work, or sport movements into component parts. Once a base of isolation/recruitment and co-contraction endurance has been established for the lumbopelvic local stabilizers and integration of the global system has progressed to the point where functional positions can be attained, training of component parts of work- or sport-specific movements can begin. The first step for this category of movement retraining involves teaching control of the thoracopelvic movement component.

Thoracopelvic control – rowing back

Patient position   The patient starts sitting with the knees bent on a plinth or the floor. A small ball can be placed between the upper inner thighs to facilitate a "connection" to the anterior pelvic floor and maintenance of neutral hip alignment during the exercise. The ball is not to be squeezed, but merely held in place by the thighs sinking into the sides of the ball. Correct for neutral spine position (optimal lumbopelvic pyramid), then cue a recruitment of the lumbopelvic local stabilizers.

Exercise instruction   Ask the patient to maintain the position of the thorax and shoulders and gently roll slightly back on the pelvis (posteriorly tilt) (Fig. 10.77). Only a small movement is required. The patient is then asked slowly to rotate the thorax to the right and then to the left, imagining that the ribcage is a lid on a jar that is turning while the jar (pelvis) stays still. The therapist provides manual feedback to ensure that the distance between the ribcage and iliac crests does not change and that no lateral shift or collapse of the thorax occurs during the rotation. The pelvis should not rotate as a unit or undergo any intrapelvic torsions. This exercise trains flexion and rotation control; alternately, cueing pure rotation only (no pelvic tilt) will train rotation in neutral spine.

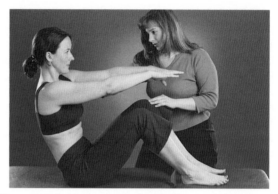

Figure 10.77   Moving out of neutral spine: thoracopelvic control. Rowing back. The pelvis is slightly rolled back prior to rotating the arms and thorax to the right and left. The pelvis remains facing forward throughout the exercise (no rotation in the transverse plane). (Reproduced with permission from © Diane G. Lee Physiotherapist Corp.)

Thoracopelvic control – bridge and rotate

Patient position   The patient starts in crook lying. Check for lateral costal expansion during breathing.

Exercise instruction   At the end of a breath out, cue a co-contraction of the deep local stabilizers, then instruct the patient to roll the pelvis back into a posterior pelvic tilt by pushing through the feet and lifting the hips off the floor. Cue a continued lumbar spine flexion as the hips are lifted. The mid-thorax remains on the floor. At the top of the "bridge" position, the patient is asked to release the hips and pelvis into a neutral pelvic tilt position ("let the buttocks drop and the hip creases fold"), creating a neutral lumbar lordosis. Once this is mastered, rotation of the pelvis under the thorax is added ("rotate the jar under the lid") (Fig. 10.78). Cue folding of the hip as the pelvis is slowly rotated to one side; to return to neutral, have the patient think of drawing the pelvis up from just inside the ASIS. Repeat the rotation to the opposite side. Movement must be controlled through both phases of the rotation. Return to the starting position by flexing the thorax ("let the chest go heavy"), then flexing the lumbar spine ("bring your low back down to the bed"), and finally releasing into a neutral lumbar lordosis ("let the pelvis tilt forward and the buttocks go wide").

Modifications/considerations   In patients with a poor connection to their anterior oblique sling (oblique abdominals and contralateral adductors), a ball between the upper inner thighs can be used to facilitate control during the exercise. If the ribcage extends unilaterally during the movements (loss of

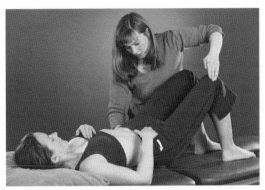

Figure 10.78   Moving out of neutral spine: thoracopelvic control. Bridge and rotate. From neutral spine in a bridge position, the patient is rotating the pelvis to the right (arrow) while maintaining the thoracic position. The therapist cues control of the right femur in neutral alignment and palpates the lumbar multifidus. The pelvis returns to neutral by pulling the left anterior superior iliac spine back. (Reproduced with permission from © Diane G. Lee Physiotherapist Corp.)

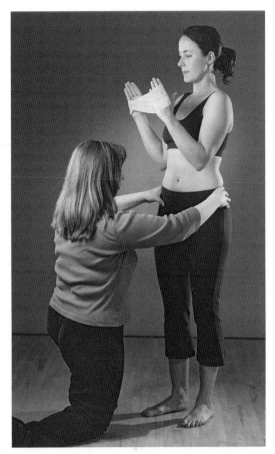

Figure 10.79   Moving out of neutral spine: thoracopelvic control. Standing trunk rotation. The therapist palpates the transversus abdominis bilaterally while also providing feedback to keep the pelvis still and facing forward during the thoracic rotation. (Reproduced with permission from © Diane G. Lee Physiotherapist Corp.)

neutral thoracic spine position), then the EO component of the anterior oblique sling needs to be cued on that side ("think of keeping a line of tension between your left ribcage and the right ASIS throughout the exercise"). Alternately, for patients with a poor connection to their lateral sling (especially the gluteus medius portion), a resistive exercise band can be tied around the thighs to facilitate better control during the exercise.

Thoracopelvic control – lateral bending

Patient position   The patient sits on a ball in neutral spine, with the weight centered over the sitz bones and the spine suspended by co-contraction of the local stabilizers.

Exercise instruction   The patient is asked to keep the thorax still and suspended in space, while the pelvis is rocked laterally side to side, inducing lateral bending of the lumbar spine. Ensure that lateral costal expansion continues with breathing, and that the movement is smooth in both the concentric and eccentric phases in both directions.

Thoracopelvic control – standing trunk rotation

Patient position   The patient stands in neutral spine with the feet hip-width apart. A light-resistance exercise band is wrapped around the hands with the palms facing each other and shoulder-width apart. The hands start relaxed in front of the patient. Cue a connection to the local stabilizers, then ask the patient gently to abduct the shoulders to push against the resistive exercise band (5% effort), then raise the arms with the elbows bent until the hands are at approximately eye level. The spine should remain neutral during this movement.

Exercise instruction   The patient is then asked to rotate the thorax to the right (Fig. 10.79) and to the left while breathing and maintaining the distance between the ribcage and pelvis. The use of the resistive exercise band and arm elevation is thought to increase proximal proprioception and prevent collapse of the ribcage or overactivation of the latissimus dorsi during the trunk rotation.

Thoracopelvic control – standing pelvic rotation

Patients with lumbopelvic dysfunction often have difficulty dissociating pelvic rotation from the thorax. This affects performance of many functional and sport activities. This exercise can be applied to a variety of sport maneuvers; the starting position may vary but the principles are the same. For golfers, this exercise retrains the use of the pelvis for rotation during both phases of the swing by first isolating the movement and then integrating it into proper timing of the swing.

Patient position The patient starts standing in a neutral spine position. Cue a connection to the lumbopelvic local stabilizers, then have the patient assume the position of the start of a golf swing (the approach to the ball, holding an imaginary golf club). The therapist checks for equal flexion of the hips and maintenance of the neutral lumbopelvic curve.

Exercise instruction Maintaining the local stabilizer co-contraction and breathing normally, the patient is then asked to rotate the pelvis under the thorax in the direction of the backswing, initiating the movement from just inside the ASIS on the same side (Fig. 10.80). The movement will be small, and no movement in the thorax should be noted. The patient is then asked to rotate the pelvis in the opposite direction fully, again, initiating from just inside the ASIS on the same side as the rotation (into the swing and follow-through direction). The patient then returns to the neutral starting position. This pelvic movement is practiced at slow speeds to begin with and then the other components of the golf swing are added. For the backswing portion, the sequence would proceed as follows: pelvis rotation, then thorax rotation but no arm back swing → pelvis rotation, thorax rotation, then arm back swing → all three movements together at slow pace → all three movements at faster speeds. The other parts of the swing are similarly broken down, practiced, and reintegrated.

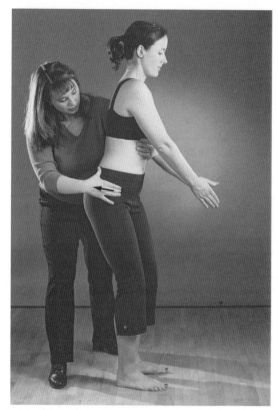

Figure 10.80 Moving out of neutral spine: thoracopelvic control. Standing pelvic rotation. The therapist supports the ribcage to inhibit movement of the thorax as the cue is given to "draw the right hip bone [anterior superior iliac spine] back" to spin the pelvis under the thorax (arrow). The right hip undergoes flexion and relative internal rotation during this movement. To return to neutral and move into left rotation, a similar image is used from just medial to the left anterior superior iliac spine. (Reproduced with permission from © Diane G. Lee Physiotherapist Corp.)

Integrated functional kinetic chain

At this stage in the rehabilitation exercise program the patient should be performing several of the functional integration exercises (see below) that involve maintaining the neutral spine position and moving the trunk over the hips or moving the arms in relation to the trunk. As the patient learns to perform exercises moving out of neutral spine successfully (above), exercises that incorporate an increasing number of joints in a movement chain are added. The previous golf simulation exercise is an example of this progression for one specific activity. Other exercises are described below, but the reader should recognize that by following the principles presented in this chapter, many more exercises can be created that are specific to each patient's work, sport, and recreational goals.

FUNCTIONAL INTEGRATION

Many functional activities require the ability to maintain neutral spine while moving the trunk on the hips (squatting to sit down), moving the arms on the trunk (driving), or both of these movements simultaneously (lifting). In addition, activities of daily life, work, and sport require the ability to control movements of the spine in and out of neutral while the arms and legs are moving. Certain activities may require prolonged positions such as sitting at a desk or kneeling while leaning forward to work with the hands. These different functional conditions illustrate that both dynamic and static control of the spine need to be trained, in both the neutral and non-neutral position of the spine.

In order to facilitate the automatic and tonic function of the local stabilizing muscles, it is important to include functional integration exercises in the rehabilitation program as early as possible. Every few treatment sessions, a functional activity that is challenging or uncomfortable for the patient should be identified and targeted for training. Two approaches can be used: first, educate and provide cues to change the way the patient performs a specific functional activity, so that whenever the activity is performed, the patient "checks in" and spends a moment thinking about the position of the spine, breathing, and the contraction of the local system, and second, design an exercise that breaks the activity down into components and practice the base components first, then add complexity as the patient's ability and movement control improve. Depending on the patient's level of control, choose an appropriate activity to modify. For example, for a patient who is at the level of practicing neutral spine and exercises in the sitting position, education of driving position can be initiated. The patient is instructed how to sit equally on both sitz bones, relax the buttocks, and lightly contract the deep local stabilizing muscles while driving. This is performed whenever possible: before starting the car, at stop lights, or whenever the patient thinks about it. This same patient may not be ready for integration of new stabilization strategies into lifting or more complex movements in standing. These can be introduced later in the rehabilitation process as new levels of control are gained. The key is that functional integration activities are introduced at each stage of the stabilization program.

Training of static positions follows the guidelines and uses the techniques described above in the section Postural re-education, neutral spine and releasing the "butt gripper" to apply neutral spine awareness to patient-specific functional tasks. The key is to educate the patient on ways to avoid rigidity when maintaining prolonged postures. Normal function in static postures involves small reactive movements in response to limb movements (arm movements while sitting at a desk), to shifts in the center of gravity due to trunk movements (e.g., turning or shifting the trunk) and to postural effects of respiration (Hodges 2003). A spine made rigid

with excessive bracing in the global system is unable to use these small dampening movements to maintain stability and postural equilibrium. Patients can use the checkpoints for global rigidity periodically while in prolonged positions to ensure maintenance of mobile stability.

The exercises that follow are examples of training control of neutral spine during dynamic activities involving the lower-extremity kinetic chain. They are progressed to movements that require spinal control while moving in and out of neutral spine. During the exercise performance, areas of poor control or give will become apparent, either at a segmental level or at a global orientation level. Loss of segmental control will require specific cueing and attention to the local system precontraction and endurance; these techniques have been described extensively above. A loss of global orientation (thorax on pelvis, pelvis on hip, hip on knee, knee on foot) will require specific cueing and attention to muscles of the global slings that are being insufficiently activated. This is performed by using imagery and manual cues to facilitate proper alignment during the exercise movement. Some of these have been described previously in relation to the thoracopelvic alignment (see section Coordinating the local and global systems: Maintaining neutral spine with loading). When adding the lower extremity, the imagery is extended to include all joints in the movement. For example, a common pattern is a decrease in activation in the adductors and/or vastus medialis obliquus, evidenced by a palpable decrease in tone and often observable atrophy. This creates a deficiency in the anterior oblique sling and the continuation of the connections of this sling into the lower leg and foot (tibialis posterior and the medial arch). Excessive internal rotation of the tibia and pronation of the foot can be observed. Rather than prescribing a specific exercise for each muscle in this medial sling (adductors, vastus medialis obliquus, tibialis posterior, foot intrinsics), an image of a suspension wire coming up from the medial arch, to the medial knee, and into the groin is used (Fig. 10.81). In the early stages a small ball is placed between the upper inner thighs and the patient is instructed gently to "connect" to the ball, lightly squeezing it and increasing facilitation to the adductors. Manual palpation is used as the image is created for the patient, and a new position and alignment will be observed. The patient can then think about tension and support along the tension wire during any standing exercise. In some cases,

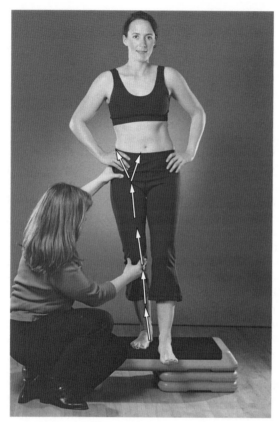

Figure 10.81 Functional integration: imagery for facilitating optimal alignment during a step-down. In this case, to cue the medial sling and its connections into the lower leg and foot, ask the patient to "imagine a suspension wire coming from under the inside of your arch, tracing up to the inside of the knee and inner thigh, and into the groin" (arrow). From the groin, the suspension wire can continue medially up to the lumbar multifidus, or laterally to the posterior gluteus medius, depending on where the patient is losing control. (Reproduced with permission from © Diane G. Lee Physiotherapist Corp.)

especially where there has been peripheral injuries (e.g., a sprained ankle), additional strengthening exercises will be necessary. In cases where proximal control is the primary problem, restoring lumbo-pelvic control and then integrating the new motor pattern into functional patterns with cueing of proper alignment is often sufficient.

Squats

Patient position   Standing in neutral spine against the wall. The feet are approximately 15 cm (6 in.) away from the wall. The hips should be in approximately 20° flexion, so that the pelvis and spine are inclined forward on the hips and the upper thorax and head are away from the wall. The hips should be in neutral rotation, the knees under the hips, the second toe of each foot in line with the middle of the patella, with equal body weight distributed over each foot. In correcting technique and position in the standing position, it is important to use all of the checkpoints for global rigidity from the ribcage to the toes.

Exercise instruction   Advise the patient that movement is to occur only in the legs; the spine stays still and suspended by the "guy wires." The patient is asked to squat "as if sitting in a chair," flexing at the hips, knees, and ankles, while maintaining the neutral spine position and sliding the buttocks equally down the wall. The therapist can palpate in the lumbar spine, or at the sacrum and innominate to ensure that there is no loss of control during the movement. For patients with failed load transfer of the SIJ the innominate will be felt to rotate anteriorly relative to the sacrum on the side of failed load transfer. During the return to starting position, watch for and correct any "butt gripping" as the hips extend.

Progressions/other considerations

• The wall provides feedback for maintaining the pelvis in the same frontal plane; if any rotation occurs, the pressure on one buttock will change. The eventual goal is to have the patient perform this squatting exercise in a free-standing position.

• The depth of the squat movement is varied depending on the control of the movement but is not usually progressed to lower than 90° knee flexion (unless sport or work demands require it).

• The wall squat is progressed to a sling squat: the patient squats down, then lifts both heels to stand on the balls of the feet (Fig. 10.82), then straightens the knees and hips to come up to standing but remaining on the toes, then lowers the heels to return to the exercise starting position. This pattern can be performed in reverse to challenge eccentric control. Using a ball between the thighs and cueing the medial leg sling image is helpful for optimal exercise performance.

• Other progressions include performing the squat and the sling squat against a ball. The ball should be placed such that it supports the lumbar lordosis and does not restrict the movement of the thorax into a neutral kyphosis. As the squat occurs the lumbar lordosis should be maintained and the hips should move posteriorly under the ball.

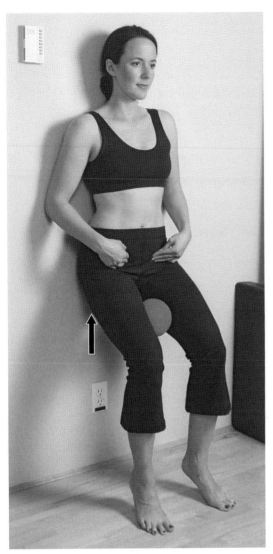

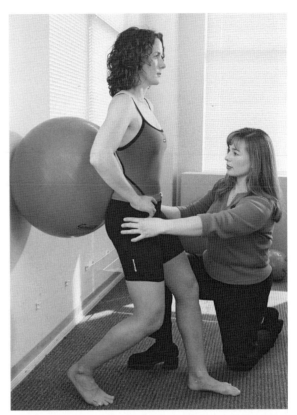

Figure 10.83 Functional integration: split squat. The base of support is reduced by placing one foot forward and one foot back with the heel lifted (as compared to a basic squat). The body weight should be distributed equally over both legs as the hips and knees flex. In this example the therapist provides tactile feedback at the anterior hip creases to facilitate folding (flexion) of the hips equally and maintenance of pelvic position during the movement. (Reproduced with permission from © Diane G. Lee Physiotherapist Corp.)

Figure 10.82 Functional integration: sling squat, progression of wall squat. The starting position is neutral spine in supported standing against a wall. In this example the patient is palpating transversus abdominis bilaterally for a symmetrical contraction. The ball in the medial thighs is then gently squeezed without any hip internal or external rotation; this pressure is sustained throughout the exercise. (Reproduced with permission from © Diane G. Lee Physiotherapist Corp.)

• Squats with the ball can then be progressed to split squats (Fig. 10.83). Again, this exercise should be practiced both free-standing and against the ball.

• Using a resistive exercise band tied around the lower thigh during the initial introduction of these exercises will provide facilitation to the posterior fibers of the gluteus medius muscle. The patient is asked to maintain pressure against the band at the knee with a 5% effort during the exercise. There should be no visible external rotation movement of the hip or change in alignment of the knee and foot; however, an increase in the activity of the posterior fibers of gluteus medius will be palpated. The exercise is progressed by *removing* the band and having the patient maintain the control and activity in the gluteus medius.

• The patient's arm position depends on where tactile feedback is required for correct exercise performance. Initially the multifidus and TA may need to be palpated. Alternately, palpation at the hip can facilitate folding anteriorly and maintenance of the axis for hip movement during the exercise. As the movement pattern becomes more automatic, use less tactile feedback and have the patient swing

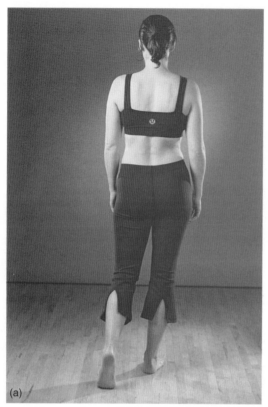 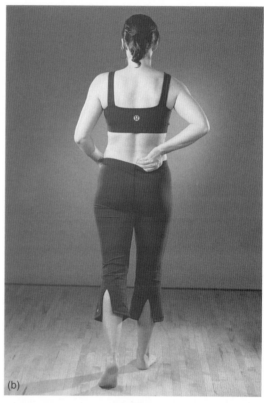

(a)　(b)

Figure 10.84 Functional integration: step forward, step back. (a) Poor performance of weight shift component. The patient is losing control of the right sacroiliac joint and hip as weight is taken on the right leg. Note the Trendelenburg on the right side. (b) Correct technique. Prior to shifting weight on to the front leg, the patient palpates and "connects" to the right deep multifidus with an image, then continues to keep the muscle active as weight is taken on to the right leg. The cue to "keep the pelvis vertically over the hip" is also helpful to control the hip and correct the Trendelenburg. (Reproduced with permission from © Diane G. Lee Physiotherapist Corp.)

the arms while moving the legs. During squatting motions, the arms are lifted bilaterally in front of the body. In split squats the arms move in a contralateral pattern to the legs (if the left leg is forward, as the left knee bends, the left arm extends behind the body and right arm flexes forward).

Step forward, step back

The goal of these exercises is to simulate components of the gait cycle in a progressive manner. Initially, the exercise is performed in stride standing as a weight shift from front to back (Fig. 10.84a, b). The patient palpates the key muscles to focus on (multifidus, posterior fibers gluteus medius, TA, etc.). The exercise is repeated with the opposite leg forward. The exercise is progressed from bilateral weight-bearing to unilateral weight-bearing as follows. The same weight shift exercise is performed, but the back foot is lifted from the ground at the end of the weight shift forward, held for a few seconds, and then a step back is performed and the front foot is lifted from the ground at the end of the weight shift backwards. The next progression involves performing a swing phase with one leg; from bilateral stride stance the weight is shifted forward on to the front leg, the back foot is lifted, and the hip flexes to bring the leg forward into a new step. The same leg is then swung back and a backward step is taken. Arm swings are added as less tactile feedback is required. The size of the steps is gradually increased to a functional stride length. In the first stages of this exercise, the goal is to maintain a neutral spine as weight is transferred forward and back, but as the exercise progresses to become more like normal gait, the spinal position will move in and out of neutral position (but not excessively so).

Lunges and variations

Patient position   Standing in neutral spine. The patient palpates the muscles that need extra cueing and attention for correct performance; this may be the TA and/or multifidus, or the posterior gluteus medius, or the anterior hip (to cue relaxation and folding). The therapist initially palpates the area of dysfunctional load transfer (sacrum and innominate, lumbar spine, around the greater trochanter, etc.), and then uses different palpation points as needed to correct the exercise technique.

Exercise instruction   Cue a co-contraction of the lumbopelvic local stabilizers. The patient steps forward with one foot, landing heel first, and allowing the heel of the back foot to come off the ground so that weight-bearing is performed through the ball of the back foot. Ask the patient to bend both knees so that the body drops down between the legs, while keeping the weight equally distributed between both legs. The front knee should be vertically in line with the ankle joint as the knee bends. Cue folding of both hips and maintenance of the neutral lumbopelvic curve as the hips bend. To return to the starting position, the hips and knees are straightened as the patient pushes backwards off the heel of the front foot and brings the legs back together into a neutral standing posture.

Progressions/other considerations   The depth of the lunge can be varied depending on the patient's control. Watch for any lateral tilting or excessive rotation of the pelvis. During the step forward, observe the stationary leg (the back leg). Poor load transfer at the SIJ or decreased gluteus medius activation in the back leg is often a cause for compensatory hip strategies in the other leg such as hip hiking and pelvic rotation because of the unstable base for movement. Using a resistive exercise band tied around the lower thigh during the initial introduction of these exercises will provide facilitation to the posterior fibers of the gluteus medius muscle (Fig. 10.85). The patient's arm position depends on where tactile feedback is required for correct exercise performance. As the movement pattern becomes more automatic, use less tactile feedback and have the patient swing the arms while moving the legs. During forward and diagonal lunges use the arms in a contralateral swing pattern; during side lunges both arms can move together in front of the body as for squats (see above).

Progressions include a lunge with one knee lift progressing to walking lunges. The basic lunge is

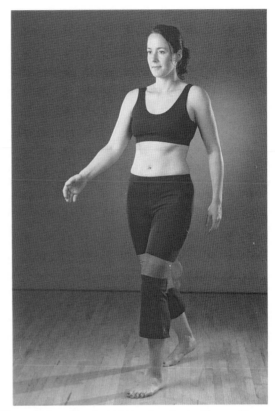

Figure 10.85   Functional integration: forward lunge with resistive exercise band facilitation. In normal standing, the band is secured around the patient's thighs; the patient then performs a variety of functional exercises, for example a forward lunge. Progression of the exercise is achieved by removing the band (reducing proprioceptive input). (Reproduced with permission from © Diane G. Lee Physiotherapist Corp.)

performed to the point where the body drops between the two legs. Now, instead of pushing back off the front leg to return the legs together, the body moves forward on to the front leg while lifting the back knee and hip forward into flexion (unilateral weight-bearing on the front leg). This end position resembles the one-leg standing test and is held for a few seconds to challenge control of balance. To return to the start position, a step backwards is performed by the non-weight-bearing leg. The exercise is then performed on the other side. A further progression is to remove the final step backwards and link alternating lunge knee lifts together so that the patient moves forward with each lunge. These are now walking lunges. Using brief holds where the patient stops with the knee lifted in between several walking lunges adds proprioceptive challenge to the exercise.

• Backward lunges: one leg moves into extension to land on the ball of the foot so that the squatting motion is performed in the same position as the forward squat, but the initiation of the exercise requires different muscle patterning. It is useful to target eccentric gluteus maximus control in one-leg standing.

• Side or diagonal lunges: the stepping leg moves in a side step, and a squat is performed so that the body weight is equal between the legs. Alternately, the stepping leg moves in a forward and diagonal line or a backwards and diagonal line. Correct the body position when the foot lands to teach the patient how to land with the weight already equally distributed between both feet; this retraining helps to correct and facilitate better awareness of body center, which is often altered in patients with lumbopelvic-hip dysfunction. The body centre awareness exercise can be performed at different speeds to increase automatic reactions.

• Lunge against a resistive exercise band: a piece of resistive exercise band is secured behind the patient at shoulder level. The patient stands in neutral spine, holding the band with one hand at the ipsilateral shoulder (elbow is bent). With a precontraction of the local stabilizing system, the patient performs a dynamic lunge against the unilateral resistance of the band (Fig. 10.86). The lunge can be performed on the leg ipsilateral or contralateral to the arm holding the band. In both cases a rotational force is imparted to the trunk. The patient is instructed to keep the spine in neutral throughout the performance of the movement.

• Cross-tubing lunges: these exercises are adapted from Alex McKechnie and Rick Celebrini's Hard Core Strength exercise protocol. These clinicians have incorporated the use of light-weight resistive exercise bands in a cross pattern (Fig. 10.87a) to facilitate proper motor patterns and exercise performance in end-stage rehabilitation training programs. Two long pieces of bands are used for the arm connections. Each piece is tied together at the ends, forming one large circle. A loop is formed in one end and the patient steps into the loop so that it can be slid up the leg and secured around the thigh. The other end of the circle is placed around the contralateral hand. The same pattern is repeated on the other leg with the second piece of exercise band; this completes the upper-body cross-tubing set-up. Another smaller circular piece of exercise band is used around the ankles. For these lunge variation exercises, the start position is a supported

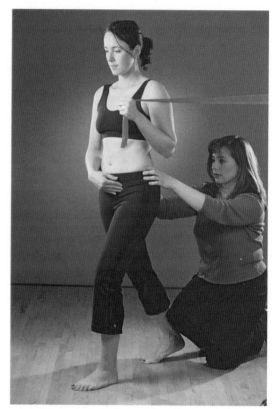

Figure 10.86 Functional integration: forward lunge against a resistive exercise band. As the lunge is performed the patient is cued to maintain the neutral spinal position and not allow rotation towards the band. This trains isometric control through the anterior oblique slings (against rotation and extension). In this example the therapist is palpating the left innominate and sacrum to ensure control of the left sacroiliac joint during the movement. (Reproduced with permission from © Diane G. Lee Physiotherapist Corp.)

standing position against a ball on the wall with the knees bent. The lumbar spine lordosis is supported by the ball and the thoracic kyphosis is maintained. The pelvis should be in neutral position with the hips folded symmetrically; do not allow any posterior tilt, flexion of the lumbar spine, or "butt gripping." The hands are together in front of the mid-thorax (Fig. 10.87a). Cue a co-contraction of the deep local stabilizing muscles, and then ask the patient to perform a side squat to one side, transferring the weight so that it remains equally distributed between both legs. As the leg moves laterally, the arms are moved up and out in a diagonal flexion pattern (Fig. 10.87b). Depending on the patient's control and balance, the height the arms are raised can be increased to above the shoulders (hands

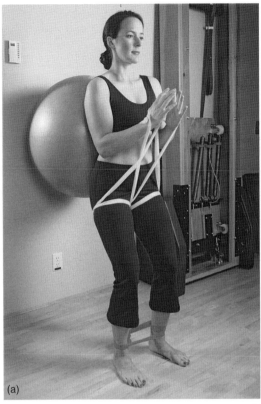 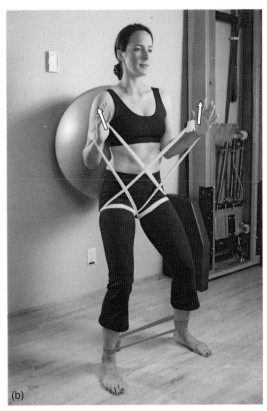

(a)   (b)

Figure 10.87   Functional integration: cross-tubing lunges. (a) Light-weight yellow resistive exercise band is used for the upper-body cross-tubing set-up; red resistive exercise band for the ankle tubing (from McKechnie & Celebrini). The start position is a neutral spinal curve in supported standing with the lordosis supported against the ball. (b) A precontraction of the deep local stabilizers is performed and the right leg steps to the side to perform a squat. The arrows indicate the direction of arm movement; as the patient gets better control, the arms can be lifted higher. (Reproduced with permission from © Diane G. Lee Physiotherapist Corp.)

level with the top of the head) and the depth of the squat movement can be varied. A progression of the side step is a diagonal lunge, where one leg moves back into extension and abduction in a diagonal pattern to land on the ball of the foot. Concurrently, the ipsilateral arm moves into an extension diagonal (down, back and out, following the leg) and the contralateral arm lifts into a flexion/abduction diagonal (as before).

 • Lunge with contralateral trunk rotation: this exercise integrates incongruent rotation between the thorax and the pelvis during movement of the full kinetic chain. The patient performs a lunge with the lower extremity while simultaneously rotating the trunk against a resistive exercise band. For lunges with the right leg, the band is secured above and anterior to the right shoulder. The left arm holds the band in elevation across the body (Fig. 10.88a). The patient is instructed to step forward and lunge with the right foot, then straighten the

right leg and lift the left hip and knee into flexion. As the right leg is straightened the left arm draws the band down across the body in the direction of the left hip (extension and abduction diagonal) and the thorax is rotated to the left (Fig. 10.88b).

One-leg squats

Patient position   Standing in neutral spine. The patient palpates the muscles that need extra cueing and attention for correct performance. The therapist initially palpates the area of dysfunctional load transfer (sacrum and innominate, lumbar spine, around greater trochanter, etc.), and then uses different palpation points as needed to correct the exercise technique. More cueing and attention will be needed for the weight-bearing leg.

 Exercise instruction   Cue a co-contraction of the lumbopelvic local stabilizers. The patient lifts one foot, bending the knee and hip to clear the foot off

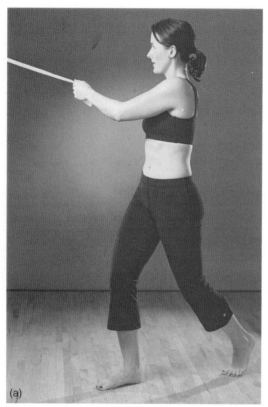 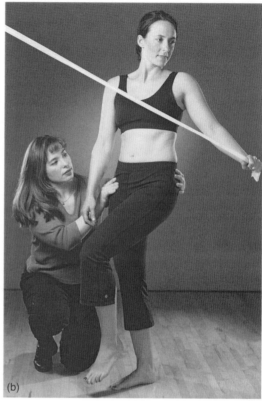

Figure 10.88 Functional integration: lunge with contralateral trunk rotation. (a) The patient performs a co-contraction of the deep local stabilizers, steps forward with the right leg, and performs a lunge. (b) The final phase of the exercise involves right pelvis rotation and left thoracic rotation, thus challenging control of contralateral thoracopelvic motion. The therapist is monitoring pelvic control. (Reproduced with permission from © Diane G. Lee Physiotherapist Corp.)

the ground. The pelvis should remain level and in neutral rotation. A squat is performed on the other leg. The hip should fold and the pelvis move anteriorly over the femur. Cue, "Imagine you are dropping down to sit in a chair and your hip is moving back to the chair." The knee should track in line with the second toe and the femur should not excessively internally or externally rotate. Watch for toe gripping and trunk bracing. The exercise repetition is completed by straightening the leg; further squat repetitions can be repeated on the same leg or the legs can be alternated.

Progressions/other considerations The depth of the squat can be varied depending on the patient's control. Watch for any lateral tilting or rotation of the pelvis. The position of the non-weight-bearing leg can be varied so that the foot is in front of the body, in line with the body, or behind the body. If the patient cannot control full unilateral weight-bearing, the non-weight-bearing toe can be placed on the floor slightly behind the other foot in a

featherweight-bearing role. The patient's arm position depends on where tactile feedback is required for correct exercise performance. As the movement pattern becomes more automatic, use less tactile feedback and have the patient swing the arms in a contralateral swing pattern with the squat.

Step up

Patient position Standing in neutral spine in front of a step. The patient palpates the muscles that need extra cueing and attention for correct performance. The therapist initially palpates the area of dysfunctional load transfer (sacrum and innominate, lumbar spine, around greater trochanter, etc.) during subsequent exercise repetitions; different palpation points are used as needed to correct the exercise technique.

Exercise instruction Cue a co-contraction of the lumbopelvic local stabilizers. The patient steps forward on to the step with one foot, landing heel first,

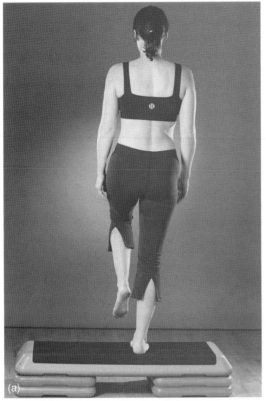
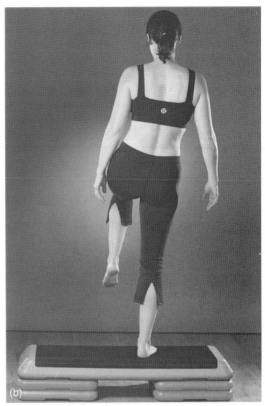

Figure 10.89   Functional integration: step-up. (a) Good exercise technique. The pelvis is level and there is minimal lateral shift of the trunk. (b) Poor control. The trunk is excessively shifted to the right, the left hip is hiked, and the right buttock is "gripping" (note the divot posterior to the greater trochanter). (Reproduced with permission from © Diane G. Lee Physiotherapist Corp.)

and then transfers the body-weight forward to perform the full step-up. The other leg lifts from the ground and is then brought forward into hip and knee flexion to simulate stepping up on to another step (Fig. 10.89a). The exercise is completed reaching the non-weight-bearing leg backwards into extension and stepping back down off the step. The exercise is repeated on the other leg.

Progressions/other considerations   Watch for substitution strategies on both legs (e.g., Trendelenburg or hip hiking), on the back leg as the patient lifts the foot to place it on the step and on the front leg as weight is transferred on to the step into unilateral weight-bearing (Fig. 10.89b). Watch for any lateral tilting or excessive rotation of the pelvis. "Butt gripping" will result in an inability to dissociate hip movement (e.g., flexion as the leg moves forward) from pelvic movement. If this occurs unilaterally, a posterior tilt, lateral tilt, and/or rotation of the pelvis will occur when an attempt to flex the hip is made. Check alignment and monitor the checkpoints for global rigidity throughout the kinetic

chain. Weak links in the global slings will result in altered alignment in the lower extremity during the movement. Use manual palpation and imagery to correct any deviations. Encourage arm swing as during a normal gait pattern; initially the hands may need to be placed on the iliac crests or palpate specific muscles to ensure optimal exercise performance. Progressions include stepping up on a diagonal (to a corner on the step) and adding thoracopelvic rotation (as in the lunge with contralateral trunk rotation, see above).

Step down

Patient position   Standing in neutral spine on a step. The patient palpates the muscles that need extra cueing and attention for correct performance; having both hands on the iliac crests provides good feedback for maintaining pelvic position. The therapist initially palpates the area of dysfunctional load transfer (sacrum and innominate, lumbar spine, around greater trochanter, etc.), then uses different palpation points as needed to correct exercise technique. To correct alignment it is helpful to kneel or stand on the same side as the leg that will be unilaterally weight-bearing.

Exercise instruction Cue a co-contraction of the lumbopelvic local stabilizers and then cue any sling imagery that is needed to maintain thoracopelvic and lower-extremity alignment. The patient lifts one foot off the step, and then bends the weight-bearing hip, knee, and ankle to lower the foot to the ground (Fig. 10.81). The center of gravity is slowly moved forward as the foot is lowered. The ball of the foot should contact the ground first, then the rest of the foot. As weight is transferred on to the front leg, the knee and hip are allowed to flex as part of the shock-absorbing mechanism and in simulation of continuing to proceed down stairs. The repetition can be completed by bringing the feet together on the floor, then stepping back up on to the step. The exercise is then repeated on the other leg.

Progressions/other considerations Start with a small step, as low as a phone book. Progress by increasing the height of the step. The exercise can be broken up into stages and performed as progressions: at first just the hip and knee flexion component are practiced without the shift in the center of gravity, then the shift is added with a small lowering of the foot, then the foot is lowered completely to the ground but only the toe touches, then finally the full weight transfer is allowed. Watch for any lateral tilting or excessive rotation of the pelvis. Palpate the femur for internal or external rotation, observe for medial knee tracking, medial arch collapse, and toe gripping. Using a resistive exercise band tied around the lower thigh will provide facilitation to the posterior fibers of the gluteus medius muscle and help correct excessive internal rotation of the femur.

Low to high pulleys

This exercise integrates congruent rotation through multiple joints in a functional kinetic chain. The movement can be performed from low to high (flexion to extension) or from high to low (extension to flexion). The feet need to be able to pivot to allow movement through the whole chain; start with the feet facing the pulleys and then finish the movement with the feet pointing 180° from the start position. Aim to maintain the normal sagittal curves of the spine throughout (flexion and extension should occur at the hips and knees). The arms start low at the pulleys by flexing at the hips and knees, and then rotation occurs through the legs, pelvis, and thorax as the arms are taken in a diagonal extension and elevation pattern, the front hip and knee extends and weight is transferred to the other leg. There should be no segmental shifting or anteroposterior loss of curves in the spine. The goal is a smooth controlled transition and integration of the rotation and extension at all joints along the chain. Use only light resistance as the focus is on control.

Many work and sport activities require control along with power and speed. The exercises presented in this chapter can be modified and performed at varying speeds, and many can be adapted to add jumps and coordinated with plyometric exercise protocols to address these functional goals. However, there is evidence that performing ballistic forms of exercise increases activity preferentially in the superficial global muscles and may be inhibitory to the deep local stabilizing system (Richardson et al 1999). Thus, care should be taken whenever ballistic exercises are used. Slow-speed and low-load exercises for motor recruitment and control should be continued throughout the exercise program and the therapist should check the ability to isolate and maintain a tonic contraction in the local system muscles on a regular basis.

ADDING PROPRIOCEPTIVE CHALLENGE

Using uneven surfaces and equipment that challenge proprioception and balance is an important component in the rehabilitative exercise program. When combined with a conscious co-contraction of the local stabilizers and cues to prevent long periods of global rigidity, adding proprioceptive challenge facilitates the retraining of the automatic recruitment of the local system and trains the ability to maintain postural equilibrium. In general, the patient should be able to maintain co-contraction of the deep local stabilizers, providing neutral zone control, and maintain low-load activity in various postural global muscles depending on the direction of change of the center of gravity. Thus, the previously described checkpoints for global rigidity can be used. However, brief periods of high levels of activity in the global muscles are to be expected when there are large deviations in the center of gravity such that muscles are activated to prevent a fall. Many different variables can be used and combined to create proprioceptive challenges. Some of these include: removing visual input (close the eyes), changing the base of support (single- or double-leg stance, uneven surfaces), moving other body parts while on an altered base of support (head, arms, one leg), performing arm activities concurrently with an altered base of support (bouncing a ball, throwing/catching a medicine ball, resistive exercise band diagonals), and holding static positions in between dynamic activities (perform hops on one foot and then hold a one-leg stance position between varying numbers of repetitions). The following exercises provide some ideas for adding proprioceptive challenge in functional positions, but many more adaptations and options can be used by combining different variables in light of the patient's goals.

Rocker board squats

Patient position The patient stands on a rocker board in neutral spine with the knees and hips in some flexion. The board can be positioned so that the unstable direction is in an anteroposterior direction or in a mediolateral direction. The patient holds on to a support to find a still balance point and pre-connect to the local stabilizing muscles, and then releases the support.

Exercise instruction Maintaining control of the neutral spine position, the patient is asked to perform a squat, keeping the board in the horizontal position (Fig. 10.90). Generally patients with poor flexion/extension control will have more difficulty with the anteroposterior control and patients with poor rotational control will have more difficulty with the mediolateral control. Both directions should be checked; often starting with the position of better control builds confidence and reinforces good motor control strategies to apply in the more challenging position.

Lunge on a sissel

Patient position A static lunge (split squat) position is assumed with the front foot placed on a sissel or other unstable surface. Instruct the patient to co-contract the lumbopelvic stabilizers and use small-range hip internal and external rotation to check for "butt gripping," especially in the front leg.

Exercise instruction Have the patient perform a lunge, dropping the body between the legs and keeping equal weight between the front and back legs (Fig. 10.91). A resistive exercise band around the thighs can be used for extra facilitation of control and gluteus medius activation.

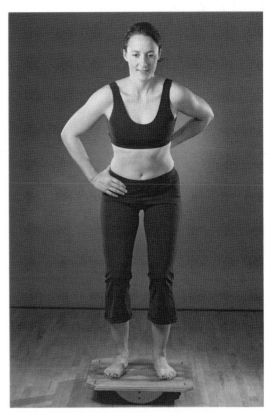

Figure 10.90 Adding proprioceptive challenge: rocker board squats. Here the patient is monitoring the left deep multifidus and right transversus abdominis as these are the portions of the "circle of integrity" that she recruits poorly. (Reproduced with permission from © Diane G. Lee Physiotherapist Corp.)

Kneeling on the ball

The patient holds on to a stable object with the hands while positioning the legs on a ball in a kneeling position. The hands then let go and the patient works on maintaining neutral spine while kneeling on the ball. This exercise provides a large degree of challenge to the trunk control system, and is highly beneficial if performed without "butt gripping" and trunk rigidity. The therapist needs to provide close supervision and support in the early stages, and the patient should be reminded of checkpoints for global rigidity.

ADDRESSING SPECIFIC GLOBAL MUSCLE "WEAKNESS"

Often by using functional movements, cueing proper alignment, and using imagery to "connect"

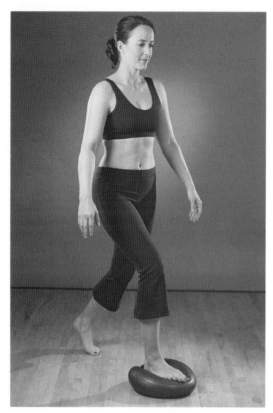

Figure 10.91 Adding proprioceptive challenge: lunge on sissel. In this example the patient has developed an internal sense of the images required to achieve recruitment of the lumbopelvic local stabilizers to the point where manual facilitation is no longer required. The arms are allowed to swing in a normal functional contralateral pattern as the lunge is performed. (Reproduced with permission from © Diane G. Lee Physiotherapist Corp.)

the patient to inactive muscles in the sling, under-recruited global muscles will be properly recruited and strengthened. On some occasions, however, specific focus is required for some of the global muscles. The following exercises are for muscles of the lumbopelvic-hip region that may require specific attention. The goal is to prescribe an exercise that targets isolation and awareness of the dysfunctional muscle. Of course, this is not true isolation, as first, the deep local stabilizers need to be cued and activated underneath these global muscles, and second, movement synergists need to be active to perform the exercises. However, certain exercises can facilitate activity *predominantly* in certain key agonists. Once recruitment is successful, movements to strengthen the muscle are performed with protocols for strength (increased resistance, 8–12 repetitions, two to three sets). Again, identification of substitution patterns will enable

the therapist to modify patient position and movement to ensure that the target muscle is the prime mover. These exercises are early-stage isolation and strengthening exercises. They should be progressed to functional integration exercises as soon as the movements can be controlled, providing that activity is monitored and maintained in the dysfunctional muscle during the functional exercise.

GLUTEUS MEDIUS – POSTERIOR FIBERS

Clamshell

Patient position   Sidelying with the target limb facing up. The spine is passively positioned into neutral spine, and the top hip is rolled slightly forward. The patient is reminded to relax the hip and let the sitz bones go wide. The therapist palpates posteriorly in the posterior fibers of gluteus medius and anterolaterally in the tensor fascia latae muscle on the uppermost hip.

Exercise instruction   Cue a contraction of the deep local stabilizers, checking particularly for a contraction in the deep fibers of multifidus. Ask the patient gently to lift the top knee from the bottom knee, opening the knees like a clamshell (Fig. 10.92). Watch for activity in the deep hip external rotators (the femoral head will move anteriorly and a groove behind the greater trochanter will appear or deepen). Palpate for activity in the tensor fascia latae. If activity is noted in either of these muscles, try the following cues: "Imagine there is a string connecting the top of your hip [palpate in the posterior gluteus medius] to your knee: try to lift the knee by shortening the string." "Draw the leg (along the femur) into your body to lift the leg rather than just thinking of lifting the knee."

Correct response   A swelling in the deep multifidus is felt prior to the leg lift. A contraction in the posterior fibers of gluteus medius is palpated and no activity in the tensor fascia latae is present. The femoral head stays centered in the acetabulum. If the exercise cannot be performed without tensor fascia latae dominance, an alternate exercise should be used for gluteus medius (see below).

Progressions/other considerations   The clamshell is an excellent progression for patients with marked atrophy of the deep fibers of multifidus. The patient is taught to palpate for a maintained deep tension in the multifidus as the leg is lifted and to keep the leg lifted for up to 10s as long as the multifidus contraction is held. The exercise is progressed by lifting

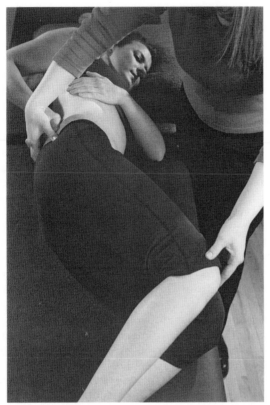

Figure 10.92   Addressing specific global muscle "weakness": clamshell. The patient is monitoring lateral costal expansion and palpating multifidus. The therapist palpates multifidus and the right posterior fibers of gluteus medius while cueing the knee lift. (Reproduced with permission from © Diane G. Lee Physiotherapist Corp.)

the foot after lifting the knee, or by adding resistance with exercise bands around the knees.

Isometric wall press

Patient position   Sidelying with the back to the wall, the head and shoulders farther away from the wall than the hips. The pelvis is rolled slightly forward and the uppermost hip is placed in external rotation and extended so that the heel rests against the wall. Check that the lumbar spine is not excessively lordosed (as close to neutral position as possible). The therapist palpates the posterior fibers of gluteus medius and the tensor fascia latae muscle on the uppermost hip.

Exercise instruction   Cue a co-contraction of the deep local stabilizers, and then ask the patient gently to push the heel into the wall (isometric extension). The exercise is progressed by sliding the heel

up the wall so that the hip abducts, while the extension push into the wall is maintained. Watch that the trunk does not shift or twist during any part of the exercise.

Correct response   A contraction in the posterior fibers of the gluteus medius is palpated and no activity in the tensor fascia latae is present.

Progressions/considerations   If the patient cannot maintain trunk control or excessive global activity is noted, the exercise can be performed in the standing position against a wall. The key components are external rotation and extension of the hip. Poles can be used to help support the weight of the trunk. This exercise is then progressed by using resistive exercise bands or pulleys for resistance instead of the wall; this option requires more trunk control and balance.

Lunge with isometric external rotation

Patient position   In standing, a resistive exercise band is tied around the patient's lower thighs. The patient then moves into a static lunge position (also known as a split squat position). The body weight is distributed equally between the front and back legs. The back foot is plantarflexed such that the weight is supported on the ball of the foot. Check that the hip, knee, and foot are in correct alignment for both the front and back legs (described previously).

Exercise instruction   Cue a co-contraction of the deep local stabilizers, and then ask the patient to think of gently pushing both knees into the band without moving the knees (Fig. 10.85). This first stage of the exercise should result in a palpable increase in the activity of the posterior fibers of gluteus medius bilaterally. The patient is shown how to feel the muscle, and instructed to keep the activity in the muscle (and the pressure against the band) constant as the body is lowered farther into a lunge (both knees and hips flex), then returned to the starting position.

Correct response   Activity in the posterior fibers of gluteus medius is maintained throughout the lunge movement, and activity in the tensor fascia latae is not excessive to the point of restricting the hip flexion component of the exercise.

Progressions/considerations   This exercise works both to increase gluteus medius activity and to integrate the muscle into functional movement. It is important to monitor the lower-extremity alignment and all checkpoints for global rigidity during the exercise and teach the patient how to self-monitor technique. For patients who are "butt grippers," use tactile and verbal cues to facilitate flexion of the hip during the lunge portion. Flexion should occur bilaterally ("think of folding the hip in the front and sticking the buttock backwards"). The principles used in this exercise can be applied to other functional integration exercises that have been described (step forward, step up or step down, etc.).

Prone hip extension and abduction

Patient position Prone lying in neutral spine. A resistive exercise band can be tied around the lower thighs; in some cases this makes the exercise harder for the patient (due to increased resistance to abduction) and in other cases it makes the exercise easier for the patient (due to increased proprioceptive feedback).

Exercise instruction Cue a co-contraction of the deep local stabilizers, and then ask the patient to lift the leg off the floor (hip extension) as far as possible without losing the lumbopelvic position. Then, the lift of the leg is maintained while the leg is abducted ("take your leg out to the side"). Provide feedback to ensure that the lumbopelvic posture does not change and that the leg does not drop as abduction is performed.

Progressions/other considerations This exercise requires significant lumbopelvic stability in order to control the spine while the weight of the leg is lifted. It is a useful progression of the previous gluteus medius exercises and usually prescribed when increased strength is required for functional integration exercises in one-leg weight-bearing positions. By this stage of the stabilization program the patient should have sufficient lumbopelvic control to be able to perform the exercise correctly.

GLUTEUS MAXIMUS

Seated gluteus maximus squeeze and sit to stand

Patient position Sitting on a firm surface with the feet planted on the floor, in an optimal lumbopelvic pyramid and neutral spine. If there is any restriction of hip flexion (common in "butt grippers") a raised surface should be used so that the hips do not restrict a neutral tilt of the pelvis on the femurs. As the patient progresses a lower surface is used.

Exercise instruction Cue a co-contraction of the deep local stabilizers, and then ask the patient to squeeze the buttocks *while maintaining the neutral spine position and the wide pyramid base*. Do not allow the pelvis to rock backwards. This is essential; if the patient performs a posterior pelvic tilt with the activation of the gluteus maximus, symptoms can be exacerbated. Furthermore, the muscle is not activated in a functional position. Palpate the muscle for equal activation and use tactile feedback to increase recruitment.

Progressions/other considerations If the patient has difficulty with the sitting recruitment, the prone position can be used. Again, neutral spine must be monitored. The sitting exercise is progressed from an isometric recruitment exercise to a functional concentric/eccentric contraction by asking the patient *slowly* to perform a sit-to-stand movement. The feet are moved back under the sitting surface, the trunk inclines forward at the hips, and the patient thinks of using the buttocks to push off from the seat and rise to standing. The return to sitting should also be slow and controlled, with both hips flexing equally and smoothly during the movement. It is particularly important to monitor the last phase as the patient comes close to sitting; this outer range often reveals eccentric weakness (watch for a fast drop into the seat). Do not allow the use of momentum or speed during the lift from the seat. Start with a high surface and progress to a lower surface. A ball can also be used instead of a stable surface. If the patient has weakness of both the gluteus medius and gluteus maximus, use a resistive exercise band around the lower thighs for extra facilitation.

Bridging

The bridge position in the Moving out of neutral spine: Thoracopelvic control – bridge and rotate exercise, above, can be used to increase the loading of an isometric gluteus maximus contraction in a neutral spine position. The exercise can be progressed by lifting one foot off the ground and weight-bearing on one leg at a time. The neutral spine and hip position must be carefully monitored to prevent "butt gripping" and posterior pelvic tilting.

Prone hip extension – knee flexed

To increase loading in concentric and eccentric contractions, the test position described in Chapter 8 (Fig. 8.65c) can be modified so that the patient performs the bent-knee hip extension movement over the end of a bed. This allows increased range of motion. Again, as for the prone gluteus medius exercise, this progression requires significant lumbopelvic stability. It is not always a necessary progression if successful activation of the muscle is occurring during functional integration exercises and their progressions. However, in cases where marked atrophy is present, the prone hip extension exercise may be indicated.

ADDUCTORS AND VASTUS MEDIALIS OBLIQUUS

It is common to observe poor activation unilaterally or bilaterally in the adductors and/or vastus medialis obliquus during functional tests, evidenced by a palpable decrease in tone and often observable atrophy. This creates a deficiency in the anterior oblique sling and the continuation of the connections of this sling into the lower leg and foot (tibialis posterior and the medial arch). Usually this poor recruitment pattern can be facilitated during functional integration exercises by simply placing a small compressible ball between the upper inner thighs and asking the patient to "connect" to the ball with the thighs, lightly squeezing it without any internal or external rotation at the hips. Activity will be palpated in the adductors and vastus medialis obliquus and should be maintained during exercise movements. In some cases additional strengthening is required.

Patient position   Sidelying with the top hip and knee flexed so that the knee or foot can be placed in front of the bottom leg. The bottom leg is flexed at the knee so that the exercise targets the short adductors of the thigh (Comerford M – Kinetic Control, unpublished course notes).

Exercise instruction   Cue a co-contraction of the deep local stabilizers, and then ask the patient to lift the bottom thigh while maintaining the position of the spine and pelvis (no tilting or rotation). Allow only the range of motion where the lumbopelvic position can be controlled.

Progressions/other considerations   A lift with the leg straight will activate the long adductors. Both movements can be tested and the position prescribed based on the weaker component. Alternate exercise options include standing adduction with pulleys (or adduction against resistive exercise band). The standing position requires sufficient lumbopelvic stability and hip control in the unaffected leg (weight-bearing leg). In patients with chronic low back or pelvic pain it is common for load transfer performance to be affected bilaterally, consequently exercises in one-leg standing are less optimal.

ILIOPSOAS

Exercises that facilitate hip control and activation of the iliopsoas (and downtrain the dominance of the tensor fascia latae) have been described above in Maintaining neutral spine with loading: Trunk and leg dissociation – Crook lying. See Figure 10.71a–c. The crook lying progressions can be used in sitting and standing to challenge strength and control of iliopsoas further.

HAMSTRINGS

The medial and lateral hamstring muscles have different fascial and ligamentous connections to the pelvis, and asymmetry in activation and strength is often present in patients with lumbopelvic-hip dysfunction. This affects torsional forces through the knee joint. Palpation of the medial (semitendinosus/semimembranosus) and lateral hamstrings (biceps femoris) during the prone knee-bend exercise (see Maintaining neutral spine with loading: Trunk and leg dissociation – prone, Fig. 10.72) will reveal the asymmetry. Resisting knee flexion in this position combined with medial or lateral rotation of the tibia will provide a measure of strength. However, if the SIJ is poorly controlled, this dysfunction needs to be addressed first. Only then can hamstring retraining begin. Several options are available for strengthening the hamstrings: closed-chain exercises such as squats, split squats, and lunges provide the best environment to train symmetrical medial/lateral recruitment. To uptrain the less recruited hamstring muscle(s), use tactile cues ("find this muscle") and verbal cues ("Imagine there is a wire from the outside of your knee [touch patient's fibula] to the outside of your hip: keep tension in the wire throughout the exercise.") to increase activity in the muscle during movement. If open-chain hamstring curls are used, the muscles must be palpated to ensure equal activity, and the tibia must stay neutral (the foot should not turn in or out) during the exercise.

ADDRESSING SPECIFIC GLOBAL MUSCLE "TIGHTNESS"

As previously discussed, lumbopelvic-hip dysfunction often results in hypertonicity and/or shortening of the global muscles, with resultant limitations of movement through specific global slings. Careful assessment (Ch. 8) will reveal whether there is true muscle shortening or a neurological sensitivity/hypertonicity in the muscles, and subsequently direct the type of manual intervention required. In both cases, supplementary home exercises should be prescribed with the goal of increasing the extensibility of a shortened muscle and/or maintaining the mobility gained in a hypertonic muscle. This section covers home exercises for the lumbopelvic-hip muscles that are often short/hypertonic. The reader is reminded that many of the muscle length test positions (Ch. 8) can be modified into home exercises. The exercise parameters prescribed will vary depending on the goal of the exercise; to maintain and increase length in a short muscle, a prolonged hold of at least 20–30 s (up to a minute), repeated two to three times, is necessary. This can be combined with slow, rhythmic movements through range with 10 s holds to teach the patient new movement patterns with full muscle lengthening. Several images have been described thus far with the techniques to release the "butt gripper," to restore neutral spine, and to restore optimal breathing patterns; these can be used in conjunction with these exercises to optimize results.

LATISSIMUS DORSI

The patient starts in four-point kneeling with the hands together. The spine is allowed to flex as the patient sits back on the feet and walks the hands forward, farther away from the body. The thoracic and lumbar spines should remain flexed as the arms are extended overhead, and the hands kept close together. To bias one side more than the other, the hands can be walked to the right or left, inducing lateral bending of the spine. This exercise will also lengthen components of the quadratus lumborum muscle.

ERECTOR SPINAE

If the patient has more restriction in the erector spinae than in the latissimus dorsi, the above stretch will be an effective technique for the erector spinae. An alternate exercise is the "ball hang" (Fig. 10.93). The patient kneels prone over a large ball, then pushes from the feet and rolls forward on the ball so that the spine is parallel to the floor. The weight of the legs provides a gentle flexion force to

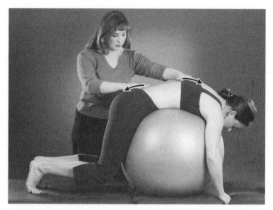

Figure 10.93 Addressing specific global muscle "tightness": erector spinae. The therapist can provide a gentle traction force with both hands and encourage "lengthening or opening" of the back as the legs hang from the ball. (Reproduced with permission from © Diane G. Lee Physiotherapist Corp.)

the spine while the arms rest on the floor and provide some lateral stability. Posterolateral costal expansion breathing is encouraged and a conscious "melting" of the muscles is cued during each exhale.

OBLIQUE ABDOMINALS

Asymmetries in the oblique abdominals will result in altered thoracopelvic alignment; correction of the neutral spine position and maintenance of this position using imagery during the progression of stabilization exercises is an effective way to activate the weak or poorly recruited oblique abdominal muscles while providing an active stretch of the opposing oblique muscles (Fig. 10.64). Lateral costal breathing is another useful technique that requires lengthening in the oblique muscles (Fig. 10.36). Lying prone with the trunk raised into extension and supported on the elbows opens the anterior ribcage and can be combined with breathing techniques to stretch the external oblique abdominals and rectus abdominis bilaterally. Supine trunk rotation stretches can also be prescribed (crook lying, knees rock gently to one side and then the other) but must be carefully monitored. If there is a rotational hypermobility of the lumbar spine or hypermobility of the SIJ, a co-contraction of the local stabilizers should be cued prior to rotating the hips so that the hypermobilities are controlled. The thorax should also be observed for compensatory movements (unilateral flexion, extension, lateral

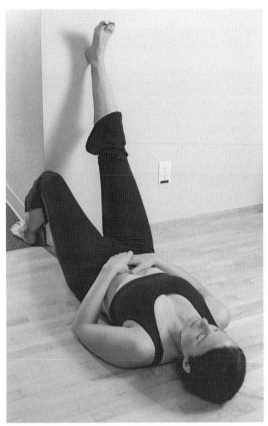

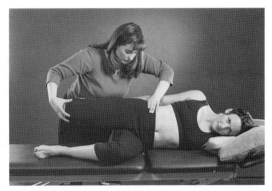

Figure 10.95 Addressing specific global muscle "tightness": rectus femoris and tensor fascia latae. The therapist ensures that the pelvis remains still as the right hip is moved into extension. (Reproduced with permission from © Diane G. Lee Physiotherapist Corp.)

(see Maintaining neutral spine with loading: Trunk and leg dissociation – sitting) is an effective active stretch of the hamstrings, with the added benefit of reciprocal inhibition due to the activity in the quadriceps muscle. If the foot is kept in neutral rotation, both the medial and lateral hamstrings will be required to lengthen equally.

RECTUS FEMORIS AND TENSOR FASCIA LATAE

Several variations of this exercise can be performed. The key component is control of the pelvic position as the hip and leg are moved into extension. For both muscles, a posterior pelvic tilt is cued to stabilize the pelvis and resist the pull of the rectus femoris and tensor fascia latae muscles. To stretch the rectus femoris, the patient is sidelying with the bottom hip and knee flexed to 90°. The patient bends the top knee to grasp the ankle. A posterior pelvic tilt is performed, then the patient pulls the leg into hip extension and knee flexion until a gentle stretch along the front of the thigh is felt. The therapist monitors the pelvis for any signs of anterior tilt (Fig. 10.95). To bias the stretch into the tensor fascia latae muscle, the knee flexion is slightly released, the hip is externally rotated (while the pelvis remains neutral – no rolling back) and the leg is adducted *while maintaining the hip extension component*. If the hip is allowed to flex or the pelvis rolls back the stretch will be removed from the tensor fascia latae. A stretch should be felt in the muscle belly at the ilium or may be felt along the fascial connections of the iliotibial band. The tensor fascia

Figure 10.94 Addressing specific global muscle "tightness": hamstrings wall stretch. (Reproduced with permission from © Diane G. Lee Physiotherapist Corp.)

shift, or rotation) that take the restricted muscles off stretch and thus render the exercise ineffective.

HAMSTRINGS

This exercise is a modification of the test described in Chapter 8 (Fig. 8.70c–e). The patient lies on the floor with the hip flexed, knee bent, and the foot supported on a wall or doorframe. The other leg lies through the door, with the knee slightly bent or straight. The stretch is performed by slowly sliding the foot up the wall, straightening the knee until a stretch is felt in the posterior thigh. Alternately, the patient places the straight leg against the wall. The amount of stretch is varied by how close the body moves towards the wall (Fig. 10.94). The medial or lateral hamstring is biased by rotating the tibia/fibula and foot into external rotation (for the medial hamstrings) and internal rotation (for the lateral hamstring). The seated knee extension exercise latae can also be stretched in a kneeling position, with one foot on the ground and the other knee on the ground behind and in line with the heel of the foot. The kneeling leg is positioned in hip adduction and external rotation. The pelvis is posteriorly tilted and then the body sways forward on to the front foot to move the hip into extension. Again, it is important for an effective tensor fascia latae stretch that the pelvic tilt and hip extension components are maintained as the body moves forward.

POSTERIOR BUTTOCK – PIRIFORMIS/DEEP EXTERNAL ROTATORS OF THE HIP

The four-point kneeling rock exercise has been described previously (Fig. 10.24) and can be performed as a motor patterning exercise (to teach trunk–hip dissociation) and held at the end-position of hip flexion to stretch the muscles of the posterior buttock. A further stretch is obtained by positioning the hips into some internal rotation at the start of the exercise ("slightly turn the knees in"). Alternately, slightly different fibers of the muscles will be targeted with the pretzel stretch. The patient lies supine with the knees bent. To stretch the right posterior hip muscles, the right ankle is crossed over the left knee, placing the right hip into external rotation and flexion. The patient then grasps the left posterior thigh. Ask the patient to "let the right buttock go wide and let the hip sink" as the left knee is pulled up towards the chest with the hands. This movement is stopped when a gentle stretch is felt in the posterior buttock. There should be no sensation of pinching or impingement in the groin of either hip. By gently adducting and abducting the left thigh, the patient can vary the abduction and adduction of the right hip and find the position where the most restriction is perceived.

Summary

A primary requirement of the lumbopelvic-hip region is to transfer load and this depends on:

1. optimal function of the bones, joints, and ligaments (form closure)
2. optimal function of the muscles and fascia (force closure)
3. appropriate neural function (motor control, emotional state).

The effective management of lumbopelvic-hip pain and dysfunction requires thorough analysis (Ch. 8) and treatment of form closure, force closure, motor control, and an understanding of the impact of the emotional state on motor control and posture. Ultimately, the goal is to teach the patient a healthier way to live and move such that sustained compression and/or tensile forces on any one structure are avoided. The key is to restore confident stability with mobility. The therapist uses manual skills (mobilization, manipulation, and touch), education, and exercise to facilitate this process.

If you are interested in learning more about this model and the international researchers and clinicians who embrace it, please join us at the Interdisciplinary World Congress on Low Back and Pelvic Pain (www.worldcongresslbp.com). For courses and other education products relevant to this text check www.dianelee.ca and www.ljptconsulting.ca.

References

Abergel R P 1984 Biostimulation of procollagen production by low energy lasers in human skin fibroblast cultures. Journal of Investigative Dermatology 82:395

Abitbol M M 1995 Energy storage in the vertebral column. In: Vleeming A, Mooney V, Dorman T, Snijders C (eds) Second interdisciplinary world congress on low back pain: the integrated function of the lumbar spine and sacroiliac joint, Part 1. San Diego, California, p 257

Abitbol M M 1997 Quadrupedalism, bipedalism, and human pregnancy. In: Vleeming A, Mooney V, Dorman T, Snijders C, Stoeckart R (eds) Movement, stability and low back pain. Churchill Livingstone, Edinburgh, p 395

Adams J C 1973 Outline of orthopaedics, 7th edn. Churchill Livingstone, Edinburgh

Adams M, Dolan P 1995 Recent advances in lumbar spinal mechanics and their clinical significance. Clinical Biomechanics 10(1):3

Adams M A, Dolan P 1997 The combined function of spine, pelvis, and legs when lifting with a straight back. In: Vleeming A, Mooney V, Dorman T, Snijders C, Stoeckart R (eds) Movement, stability and low back pain. Churchill Livingstone, Edinburgh, p 195

Albee F H 1909 A study of the anatomy and the clinical importance of the sacroiliac joint. Journal of the American Medical Association 53:1273

Allen R E, Hosker G L, Smith A R B, Warrell D W 1990 Pelvic floor damage and childbirth: a neurophysiological study. British Journal of Obstetrics and Gynaecology 97:770

Arendt-Nielsen L, Graven-Nielsen T, Svarrer H, Svensson P 1996 The influence of low back pain on muscle activity and coordination during gait: a clinical and experimental study. Pain 64(2):231

Ashton-Miller J A, Howard D, DeLancey J O L 2001 The functional anatomy of the female pelvic floor and stress continence control system. Scandinavian Journal of Urology and Nephrololgy Supplement 207

Astrom J 1975 Pre-operative effect of fenestration upon intraosseous pressures in patients with osteoarthrosis of the hip. Acta Orthopaedica Scandinavica 46:963

Barker P J, Briggs C A 1999 Attachments of the posterior layer of the lumbar fascia. Spine 24(17):1757

Basmajian J V, Deluca C J 1985 Muscles alive: their functions revealed by electromyography. Williams & Wilkins, Baltimore

Bassett C A L 1968 Biologic significance of piezoelectricity. Calcified Tissue Research 1:252

Bellamy N, Park W, Rooney P J 1983 What do we know about the sacroiliac joint? Seminars in Arthritis and Rheumatism 12:282

Bergmark A 1989 Stability of the lumbar spine. A study in mechanical engineering. Acta Orthopedica Scandinavica 230(60):20

Bernstein I, Juul N, Gronvall S, Bonde B, Klarskov P 1991 Pelvic floor muscle thickness measured by perineal ultrasonography. Scandinavian Journal of Nephrology Supplement 137:131

Blaney F, Sawyer T 1997 Sonographic measurement of diaphragmatic motion after upper abdominal surgery: a comparison of three breathing manoeuvres. Physiotherapy Theory and Practice 13:207

Blaney F, Seaman English C, Sawyer T 1999 Sonographic measurement of diaphragmatic displacement during tidal breathing manoeuvres – a reliability study. Australian Journal of Physiotherapy 45:41

Bo K, Borgen J S 2001 Prevalence of stress and urge urinary incontinence in elite athletes and controls. Medical Science Sports Exercise 33(11):1797

Bo K, Hagen R H, Dvarstein B, Jorgensen J, Larsen S 1990 Pelvic floor muscle exercise for the treatment of female stress urinary incontinence: III Effects of two different degrees of pelvic floor muscle exercises. Neurourology and Urodynamics 9:489

Bo K, Stein R 1994 Needle EMG registration of striated urethral wall and pelvic floor muscle activity patterns during cough, Valsalva, abdominal, hip adductor, and gluteal muscles contractions in nulliparous healthy females. Neurourology and Urodynamics 13:35

Bo K, Lilleas F, Talseth T, Hedland H 2001 Dynamic MRI of the pelvic floor muscles in an upright sitting position. Neurourology and Urodynamics 20:167

Bogduk N L T 1983 The innervation of the lumbar spine. Spine 8:286

Bogduk N L T 1997 Clinical anatomy of the lumbar spine and sacrum, 3rd edn. Churchill Livingstone, New York

Bowen V, Cassidy J D 1981 Macroscopic and microscopic anatomy of the sacroiliac joint from embryonic life until the eighth decade. Spine 6:620

Bradlay K C 1985 The posterior primary rami of segmental nerves. In: Glasgow E F, Twomey L T, Scull E R, Kleynhans A M (eds) Aspects of manipulative therapy, 2nd edn. Churchill Livingstone, Melbourne, p 59

Brooke R 1924 The sacro-iliac joint. Journal of Anatomy 58:299

Brooke R 1930 The pelvic joints during and after parturition and pregnancy. The Practitioner, London, p 307

Brukner P, Khan K 2002 Clinical sports medicine, 2nd edn. McGraw-Hill, Sydney, Australia

Bullock-Saxton J E, Janda V, Bullock M I 1993 Reflex activation of gluteal muscles in walking: an approach to restoration of muscle function for patients with low back pain. Spine 18(6):704

Bullock-Saxton J E, Janda V, Bullock M I 1994 The influence of ankle sprain injury on muscle activation during hip extension. International Journal of Sports Medicine 15(6):330

Bump R C, Hurt G W, Fantl J A, Wyman J F 1991 Assessment of Kegal pelvic muscle exercise performance after brief verbal instruction. American Journal of Obstetrics and Gynecology 165:322

Bunce S M, Moore A P, Hough A D 2002 M-mode ultrasound: a reliable measure of transversus abdominis thickness? Clinical Biomechanics 17:315

Butler D S 2000 The sensitive nervous system. NOI Group Publications, Adelaide, Australia

Butler D S, Moseley G L 2003 Explain pain. NOI Group Publications, Adelaide, Australia

Buyruk H M, Stam H J, Snijders C J, Vleeming A, Laméris J S, Holland W P J 1995a The use of colour Doppler imaging for the assessment of sacroiliac joint stiffness: a study on embalmed human pelvises. European Journal of Radiology 21:112

Buyruk H M, Snijders C J, Vleeming A, Laméris J S, Holland W P J, Stam H J 1995b The measurements of sacroiliac joint stiffness with colour Doppler imaging: a study on healthy subjects. European Journal of Radiology 21:117

Buyruk H M, Stam H J, Snijders C J, Vleeming A, Laméris J S, Holland W P J 1997 Measurement of sacroiliac joint stiffness with color Doppler imaging and the importance of asymmetric stiffness in sacroiliac pathology. In: Vleeming A, Mooney V, Dorman T, Snijders C, Stoeckart R (eds) Movement, stability and low back pain. Churchill Livingstone, Edinburgh, p 297

Buyruk H M, Stam H J, Snijders C J, Laméris J S, Holland W P J, Stijnen W P 1999 Measurement of sacro-iliac joint stiffness in peripartum pelvic pain patients with Doppler imaging of vibrations (DIV). European Journal of Obstetrics and Gynecological Reproduction Biology 83(2):159

Carmichael J P 1987 Inter- and intra-examiner reliability of palpation for sacroiliac joint dysfunction. Journal of Manipulative Physical Therapy 10(4):164

Chaitow L, Bradley D, Gilbert C 2002 Multidisciplinary approaches to breathing pattern disorders. Churchill Livingstone, Edinburgh

Chamberlain W E 1930 The symphysis pubis in the Roentgen examination of the sacroiliac joint. American Journal of Roentgenology 24:621

Christensen L L, Djurhuus J C, Constantinou C E 1995 Imaging of pelvic floor contractions using MRI. Neurourology and Urodynamics 14:209

Colachis S C, Worden R E, Bechtol C O, Strohm B R 1963 Movement of the sacroiliac joint in the adult male: a preliminary report. Archives of Physical Medicine and Rehabilitation 44:490

Comerford M J, Mottram S L 2001 Movement and stability dysfunction – contemporary developments. Manual Therapy 6(1):15

Constantinou C E, Govan D E 1982 Spatial distribution and timing of transmitted and reflexly generated urethral pressures in healthy women. Journal of Urology 127:964

Cooperman J M, Riddle D L, Rothstein J M 1990 Reliability and validity of judgments of the integrity of the anterior cruciate ligament of the knee using the Lachman's test. Physical Therapy 70(4):225

Cresswell A 1993 Responses of intra-abdominal pressure and abdominal muscle activity during dynamic loading in man. European Journal of Applied Physiology 66:315

Crock H V 1980 An atlas of the arterial supply of the head and neck of the femur in man. Clinical Orthopaedics and Related Research 152:17

Cyriax J 1954 Textbook of orthopaedic medicine. Cassell, London

Damen L, Buyruk H M, Guler-Uysal F, Snijders C J, Lotgering F K, Stam H J 2001 Pelvic pain during pregnancy is associated with asymmetric laxity of the sacroiliac joints. Acta Obstetrica Gynecologica Scandinavica 80:1019

Damen L, Stijnen T, Roebroeck M E, Snijders C J, Stam J H 2002a Reliability of sacroiliac joint laxity measurement with Doppler imaging of vibrations. Ultrasound in Medicine and Biology 28:407

Damen L, Buyruk H M, Guler-Uysal F, Lotgering F K, Snijders C J, Stam H J 2002b Prognostic value of asymmetric laxity of the sacroiliac joints in pregnancy-related pelvic pain. Spine 27(24):2820

Damen L, Spoor C W, Snijders C J, Stam H J 2002c Does a pelvic belt influence sacroiliac joint laxity? Clinical Biomechanics 17(7):495

Damen L, Mens J M A, Snijders C J, Stam J H 2002d The mechanical effects of a pelvic belt in patients with pregnancy-related pelvic pain. PhD thesis, Erasmus University, Rotterdam, The Netherlands

Dangaria T, Naesh O 1998 Changes in cross-sectional area of psoas major muscle in unilateral sciatic caused by disc herniation. Spine 23(8):928

Danneels L A, Vanderstraeten G G, Cambier D C, Witvrouw E E, De Cuyper H J 2000 CT imaging of trunk muscles in chronic low back pain patients and healthy control subjects. European Spine 9(4):266

Danneels L A, Vanderstraeten G, Cambier D, Witvrouw E, Raes H, de Cuyper H 2001 A randomized clinical trial of three rehabilitation programs for the lumbar multifidus in patients with chronic low back pain. In: Proceedings from the 4th interdisciplinary world congress on low back and pelvic pain. Montreal, Canada

De Diemerbroeck I 1689 The anatomy of human bodies. Translated by W Salmon Brewster, London

DeLancey J O L 1994 Structural support of the urethra as it relates to stress urinary incontinence: the hammock hypothesis. American Journal of Obstetrics and Gynecology 170(6):1713

DeRosa C 2001 Functional anatomy of the lumbar spine and sacroiliac joint. In: Proceedings from the 4th Montreal proceedings of the interdisciplinary world congress on low back and pelvic pain. Montreal, Canada

DeTroyer A D 1989 The mechanism of the inspiratory expansion of the rib cage. Journal of Laboratory Clinical Medicine 114(2):97

Dietz H P, Wilson P D, Clarke B 2001 The use of perineal ultrasound to quantify levator activity and teach pelvic floor muscle exercises. International Urogynecological Journal of Pelvic Floor Dysfunction 12(3):166

Dietz H P, Steensma A B, Vancaillie T G 2003 Levator function in nulliparous women. International Urogynecological Journal 14:24

DonTigny R L 1985 Function and pathomechanics of the sacroiliac joint: a review. Physical Therapy 65:35

DonTigny R L 1990 Anterior dysfunction of the sacroiliac joint as a major factor in the etiology of idiopathic low back pain syndrome. Physical Therapy 70:250

DonTigny R L 1997 Mechanics and treatment of the sacroiliac joint. In: Vleeming A, Mooney V, Dorman T, Snijders C, Stoeckart R (eds) Movement, stability and low back pain. Churchill Livingstone, Edinburgh, p 461

Dorman T 1994 Failure of self bracing at the sacroiliac joint: the slipping clutch syndrome. Journal of Orthopaedic Medicine 16:49

Dorman T 1997 Pelvic mechanics and prolotherapy. In: Vleeming A, Mooney V, Dorman T, Snijders C, Stoeckart R (eds) Movement, stability and low back pain. Churchill Livingstone, Edinburgh, p 501

Dreyfuss P, Dreyer S, Griffin J, Hoffman J, Walsh N 1994 Positive sacroiliac screening tests in asymptomatic adults. Spine 19:1138

Dreyfuss P, Michaelsen M, Pauza D, McLarty J, Bogduk N 1996 The value of history and physical examination in diagnosing sacroiliac joint pain. Spine 21:2594

Egund N, Olsson T H, Schmid H 1978 Movements in the sacro-iliac joints demonstrated with Roentgen stereophotogrammetry. Acta Radiologica 19:833

Encyclopedia Britannica 1981 15th edn, vol 7. William Benter, Chicago

Faflia C P, Prassopoulos P K, Daskalogiannaki M E, Gourtsoyiannis N C 1998 Variation in the appearance of the normal sacroiliac joint on pelvic CT. Clinical Radiology 53(10):742

Fantl J A, Newman D K, Colling J et al 1996 Managing acute and chronic urinary incontinence, clinical practice guideline, no. 2. Rockville MD, US Department of Health and Human Services

Farfan H F 1973 Mechanical disorders of the low back. Lea & Febiger, Philadelphia

Farfan H F 1978 The biomechanical advantage of lordosis and hip extension for upright activity. Spine 3:336

Farrell J, Drye C, Koury M 1994 Therapeutic exercises for back pain. In: Twomey L T, Taylor J R (eds) Physical therapy of the low back, 2nd edn. Churchill Livingstone, New York

Fortin J D, Dwyer A, West S, Pier J 1994a Sacroiliac joint pain referral patterns upon application of a new injection/arthrography technique. I: Asymptomatic volunteers. Spine 19(13):1475

Fortin J D, Dwyer A, Aprill C, Ponthieux B, Pier J 1994b Sacroiliac joint pain referral patterns. II: Clinical evaluation. Spine 19(13):1483

Fortin J D, Pier J, Falco F 1997 Sacroiliac joint injection: pain referral mapping and arthrographic findings. In: Vleeming A, Mooney V, Dorman T, Snijders C, Stoeckart R (eds) Movement, stability and low back pain. Churchill Livingstone, Edinburgh, p 271

Fortin J D, Kissling R O, O'Connor B L, Vilensky J A 1999 Sacroiliac joint innervation and pain. American Journal of Orthopedics December: 687

Franklin E 1996 Dynamic alignment through imagery. Human Kinetics, Illinois

Fryette H H 1954 Principles of osteopathic technique. American Academy of Osteopathy, Colorado

Gamble J G, Simmons S C, Freedman M 1986 The symphysis pubis. Anatomic and pathologic considerations. Clinical Orthopedics (203):261

Gandevia S C 1992 Some central and peripheral factors affecting human motorneuronal output in neuromuscular fatigue. Sports Medicine 13(2):93

Gandevia S C 1999 Mind, muscles and motoneurones. Journal of Science and Medicine in Sport 2(3):167

Gibbons S, Comerford M, Emerson P 2002 Rehabilitation of the stability function of psoas major. Orthopaedic Division Review Jan/Feb:9

Gilmore K L 1986 Biomechanics of the lumbar motion segment. In: Grieve G P (ed) Modern manual therapy of the vertebral column. Churchill Livingstone, Edinburgh, p 103

Goldthwait J E, Osgood R B 1905 A consideration of the pelvic articulations from an anatomical, pathological and clinical standpoint. Boston Medical and Surgical Journal 152:593

Goodall J 1979 Life and death at Gombe. National Geographic 155(5):592

Gottschalk F, Kourosh S, Leveau B 1989 The functional anatomy of tensor fasciae latae and gluteus medius and minimus. Journal of Anatomy 166:179

Gracovetsky S 1990 Musculoskeletal function of the spine. In: Winters J M, Woo S L Y (eds) Multiple muscle systems: biomechanics and movement organization. Springer Verlag, New York

Gracovetsky S 1997 Linking the spinal engine with the legs: a theory of human gait. In: Vleeming A, Mooney V, Dorman T, Snijders C, Stoeckart R (eds) Movement, stability and low back pain. Churchill Livingstone, Edinburgh, p 243

Gracovetsky S, Farfan H F 1986 The optimum spine. Spine 11:543

Gracovetsky S, Farfan H F, Lamy C 1981 The mechanism of the lumbar spine. Spine 6:249

Gracovetsky S, Farfan H, Helluer C 1985 The abdominal mechanism. Spine 10:317

Greenman P E 1990 Clinical aspects of sacroiliac function in walking. Journal of Manual Medicine 5:125

Greenman P E 1997 Clinical aspects of the sacroiliac joint in walking. In: Vleeming A, Mooney V, Dorman T, Snijders C, Stoeckart R (eds) Movement, stability and low back pain. Churchill Livingstone, Edinburgh, p 235

Grieve G P 1981 Common vertebral joint problems. Churchill Livingstone, Edinburgh

Grieve G P 1986 Modern manual therapy of the vertebral column. Churchill Livingstone, Edinburgh

Grob K R, Neuhuber W L, Kissling R O 1995 Innervation of the sacroiliac joint of the human. Zeitschrift für Rheumatologie 54:117

Gunn C C 1996 The Gunn approach to the treatment of chronic pain. Intramuscular stimulation for myofascial pain of radicolopathic origin. Churchill Livingstone, New York

Hagen R 1974 Pelvic girdle relaxation from an orthopaedic point of view. Acta Orthopaedica Scandinavica 45:550

Hall C M, Brody L T 1999 Therapeutic exercise – moving toward function. Lippincott/Williams & Wilkins, Philadelphia

Hamilton C, Richardson C 1998 Active control of the neutral lumbopelvic posture; a comparison between back pain and non back pain subjects. In: Third interdisciplinary world congress on low back and pelvic pain. European Conference Organizers, Rotterdam, p 295

Hanson P, Sonesson B 1994 The anatomy of the iliolumbar ligament. Archives of Physical Medicine and Rehabilitation 75:1245

Hartman L 1997 Handbook of osteopathic technique, 3rd edn. Chapman & Hall, London

Herrington L 2000 The inter-tester reliability of a clinical measurement used to determine the medial/lateral orientation of the patella. Manual Therapy 7(3):163

Herzog W, Read L, Conway P J W, Shaw L D, McEwen M C 1989 Reliability of motion palpation procedures to detect sacroiliac joint fixations. Journal of Manipulative and Physical Therapy 12(2):86

Hesch J 1997 Evaluation and treatment of the most common patterns of sacroiliac joint dysfunction. In: Vleeming A, Mooney V, Dorman T, Snijders C, Stoeckart R (eds) Movement, stability and low back pain. Churchill Livingstone, Edinburgh, p 535

Hesch J, Aisenbrey J, Guarino J 1992 Manual therapy evaluation of the pelvic joints using palpatory and articular spring tests. In: Vleeming A, Mooney V, Snijders C J, Dorman T (eds) First interdisciplinary world congress on low back pain and its relation to the sacroiliac joint. San Diego, California, p 435

Hewitt J D, Glisson R R, Guilak F, Parker Vail T 2002 The mechanical properties of the human hip capsule ligaments. Journal of Arthroplasty 17(1):82

Hides J A, Cooper D H, Stokes M J 1992 Diagnostic ultrasound imaging for measurement of the lumbar multifidus muscle in normal young adults. Physiotherapy Theory and Practice 8:19

Hides J A, Stokes M J, Saide M, Jull G A, Cooper D H 1994 Evidence of lumbar multifidus muscles wasting ipsilateral to symptoms in patients with acute/subacute low back pain. Spine 19(2):165

Hides J A, Richardson C A, Jull G A 1995a Magnetic resonance imaging and ultrasonography of the lumbar multifidus muscle; comparison of two different modalities. Spine 20(1):54

Hides J A, Richardson C A, Jull G A, Davies S 1995b Ultrasound imaging in rehabilitation. Australian Journal of Physiotherapy 41(3):187

Hides J A, Richardson C A, Jull G A 1996 Multifidus recovery is not automatic following resolution of acute first episode low back pain. Spine 21(23):2763

Hides J A, Jull G A, Richardson C A 2001 Long-term effects of specific stabilizing exercises for first-episode low back pain. Spine 26(11):E243

Hodges P W 1997 Feedforward contraction of transversus abdominis is not influenced by the direction of arm movement. Experimental Brain Research 114:362

Hodges P W 2000 The role of the motor system in spinal pain: implications for rehabilitation of the athlete following lower back pain. Journal of Science and Medicine in Sport 3:242

Hodges P W 2001 Changes in motor planning of feed-forward postural responses of the trunk muscles in low back pain. Experimental Brain Research 141:261

Hodges P W 2003 Neuromechanical control of the spine. PhD thesis. Karolinska Institutet, Stockholm, Sweden

Hodges P W, Gandevia S C 2000a Changes in intra-abdominal pressure during postural and respiratory activation of the human diaphragm. Journal of Applied Physiology 89:967

Hodges P W, Gandevia S C 2000b Activation of the human diaphragm during a repetitive postural task. Journal of Physiology 522(1):165

Hodges P W, Moseley G L 2003 Pain and motor control of the lumbopelvic region: effect and possible mechanisms. Journal of Electromyography and Kinesiology 13:361

Hodges P W, Richardson C A 1996 Inefficient muscular stabilization of the lumbar spine associated with low back pain. A motor control evaluation of transversus abdominis. Spine 21(22):2640

Hodges P W, Richardson C A 1997 Contraction of the abdominal muscles associated with movement of the lower limb. Physical Therapy 77:132

Hodges P W, Gandevia S C, Richardson C A 1997a Contractions of specific abdominal muscles in postural tasks are affected by respiratory maneuvers. Journal of Applied Physiology 83(3):753

Hodges P W, Butler J E, McKenzie D K, Gandevia S C 1997b Contraction of the human diaphragm during rapid postural adjustments. Journal of Physiology 505(2):539

Hodges P W, Cresswell A G, Thorstensson A 1999 Preparatory trunk motion accompanies rapid upper limb movement. Experimental Brain Research 124:69

Hodges P W, Cresswell A G, Daggfeldt K, Thorstensson A 2001a In vivo measurement of the effect of intra-abdominal pressure on the human spine. Journal of Biomechanics 34:347

Hodges P W, Cresswell A G, Thorstensson A 2001b Perturbed upper limb movements cause short-latency postural responses in trunk muscles. Experimental Brain Research 138:243

Hodges P W, Heinjnen I, Gandevia S C 2001c Postural activity of the diaphragm is reduced in humans when respiratory demand increases. Journal of Physiology 537(3):999

Hodges P W, Pengel L H M, Herbert R D, Gandevia S C 2003a Measurement of muscle contraction with ultrasound imaging. Muscle Nerve 27:682.

Hodges P W, Kaigle Holm A, Holm S et al 2003b Intervertebral stiffness of the spine is increased by evoked contraction of transversus abdominis and the diaphragm: in vivo porcine studies. Spine (submitted)

Holstege G, Bandler R, Saper C B 1996 The emotional motor system. Elsevier Science, Amsterdam

Howard D, Miller J M, DeLancey J O L, Aston-Miller J A 2000 Differential effects of cough, Valsalva, and continence status on vesical neck movement. Obstetrics and Gynecology 95(4):535

Hungerford B A 2002 Patterns of intra-pelvic motion and muscle recruitment for pelvic instability. PhD thesis. University of Sydney, Australia

Hungerford B, Gilleard W, Lee D 2001 Alteration of sacroiliac joint motion patterns in subjects with pelvic motion asymmetry. In: Proceedings from the fourth world interdisciplinary congress on low back and pelvic pain. Montreal, Canada

Inman V T, Ralston H J, Todd F 1981 Human walking. Williams & Wilkins, Baltimore

Jacob H A C, Kissling R O 1995 The mobility of the sacroiliac joints in healthy volunteers between 20 and 50 years of age. Clinical Biomechanics 10(7):352

Janda V 1978 Muscles, central nervous motor regulation and back problems. In: Korr I (ed) The neurobiologic mechanisms in manipulative therapy. Plenum Press, London, p 27

Janda V 1986 Muscle weakness and inhibition (pseudoparesis) in back pain syndromes. In: Grieve G P (ed) Modern manual therapy of the vertebral column. Churchill Livingstone, Edinburgh, p 197

Jarcho J 1929 Value of Walcher position in contracted pelvis with special reference to its effect on true conjugate diameter. Surgery, Gynecology and Obstetrics 49:854

Jull G A, Richardson C A 2000 Motor control problems in patients with spinal pain: a new direction for therapeutic exercise. Journal of Manipulative and Physiological Therapeutics 23(2):115

Jull G A, Bogduk N, Marsland A 1988 The accuracy of manual diagnosis for cervical zygapophyseal joint pain syndromes. Medical Journal of Australia 148:233

Kaigle A M, Wessberg P, Hansson T H 1998 Muscular and kinematic behavior of the lumbar spine during flexion-extension. Journal of Spinal Disorders 11(2):163

Kampen W U, Tillmann B 1998 Age-related changes in the articular cartilage of human sacroiliac joint. Anatomy and Embryology (Berlin) 198(6):505

Kapandji I A 1970 The physiology of the joints II: the lower limb, 2nd edn. Churchill Livingstone, Edinburgh

Kapandji I A 1974 The physiology of the joints III: the trunk and vertebral column, 2nd edn. Churchill Livingstone, Edinburgh

Kappel D A, Zilber S, Ketchum L D 1973 In vivo electro-physiology of tendons and applied current during tendon healing. In: Llaurado J G, Battocletti J H (eds) Biologic and clinical effects of low-frequency magnetic and electric fields. C C Thomas, Illinois, p 252

Keagy R D, Brumlik J 1966 Direct electromyography of the psoas major muscle in man. Journal of Bone and Joint Surgery 48A:1377

Kendall F P, Kendall McCreary E, Provance P G 1993 Muscles testing and function, 4th edn. Williams & Wilkins, Baltimore

Kirkaldy-Willis W H (ed) 1983 Managing low back pain. Churchill Livingstone, New York

Kirkaldy-Willis W H, Wedge J H, Yong-Hing K, Reilly J 1978 Pathology and pathogenesis of lumbar spondylosis and stenosis. Spine 3:319

Kissling R O, Jacob H A C 1997 The mobility of sacroiliac joints in healthy subjects. In: Vleeming A, Mooney V, Dorman T, Snijders C, Stoeckart R (eds) Movement, stability and low back pain. Churchill Livingstone, Edinburgh, p 177

Kristiansson P 1997 S-Relaxin and pelvic pain in pregnant women. In: Vleeming A, Mooney V, Dorman T, Snijders C, Stoeckart R (eds) Movement, stability and low back pain. Churchill Livingstone, Edinburgh, p 421

Laslett M 1997 Pain provocation sacroiliac joint tests: reliability and prevalence. In: Vleeming A, Mooney V, Dorman T, Snijders C, Stoeckart R (eds) Movement, stability and low back pain. Churchill Livingstone, Edinburgh, p 287

Laslett M, Williams W 1994 The reliability of selected pain provocation tests for sacroiliac joint pathology. Spine 19(11):1243

Lavignolle B, Vital J M, Senegas J et al 1983 An approach to the functional anatomy of the sacroiliac joints in vivo. Anatomica Clinica 5:169

Lawson T L, Foley W D, Carrera G F, Berland L L 1982 The sacroiliac joints: anatomic, plain roentgenographic, and computed tomographic analysis. Journal of Computer Assisted Tomography 6(2):307

Lee D G 1992 Intra-articular versus extra-articular dysfunction of the sacroiliac joint – a method of differentiation. IFOMT Proceedings, 5th international conference. Vail, Colorado, p 69

Lee D G 1997a Instability of the sacroiliac joint and the consequences for gait. In: Vleeming A, Mooney V, Dorman T, Snijders C, Stoeckart R (eds) Movement, stability and low back pain. Churchill Livingstone, Edinburgh, p 231

Lee D G 1997b Treatment of pelvic instability. In: Vleeming A, Mooney V, Dorman T, Snijders C, Stoeckart R (eds) Movement, stability and low back pain. Churchill Livingstone, Edinburgh, p 445

Lee D G 1999 The pelvic girdle, 2nd edn. Churchill Livingstone, Edinburgh

Lee D G 2001a Imagery for core stabilization. Diane G. Lee Physiotherapist Corporation, Surrey, Canada. Available online at: www.dianelee.ca

Lee D G 2001b An integrated model of "joint" function and its clinical application. In: Proceedings from the 4th interdisciplinary world congress on low back and pelvic pain. Montreal, Canada, p 137

Lee D G 2002 The compressor. Available online at: www.optp.com

Lee D G 2003 The thorax – an integrated approach. Diane G. Lee Physiotherapist Corporation, Surrey, Canada. Available online at: www.dianelee.ca

Lee L J 2003 Restoring force closure/motor control of the thorax. In: The thorax – an integrated approach. Diane G Lee Physiotherapist Corporation, Surrey, Canada. Available online at: www.dianelee.ca

Lee D G, Vleeming A 1998 Impaired load transfer through the pelvic girdle – a new model of altered neutral zone function. In: Proceedings from the 3rd interdisciplinary world congress on low back and pelvic pain. Vienna, Austria

Lee D G, Vleeming A 2003 The management of pelvic joint pain and dysfunction. In: Jull G (ed) Grieve's modern manual therapy of the vertebral column, 3rd edn. Elsevier Science, Edinburgh (in press)

Lee D G, Walsh M C 1996 A workbook of manual therapy techniques for the vertebral column and pelvic girdle, 2nd edn. Nascent, Vancouver

Levin S M 1997 A different approach to the mechanics of the human pelvis: tensegrity. In: Vleeming A, Mooney V, Dorman T, Snijders C, Stoeckart R (eds) Movement, stability and low back pain. Churchill Livingstone, Edinburgh, p 157

Lovett R W 1903 A contribution to the study of the mechanics of the spine. American Journal of Anatomy 2:457

Lucas D, Bresler B 1961 Stability of the ligamentous spine. In: Technical report no. 40. Biomechanics Laboratory, University of California, San Francisco

Luk K D K, Ho H C, Leong J C Y 1986 The iliolumbar ligament: a study of its anatomy, development and clinical significance. Journal of Bone and Joint Surgery 68B:197

Lynch F W 1920 The pelvic articulations during pregnancy, labor, and the puerperium. Surgery, Gynecology and Obstetrics 30:575

MacConaill M A, Basmajian J V 1977 Muscles and movements; a basis for human kinesiology, 2nd edn. Krieger, New York

MacDonald G R, Hunt T E 1951 Sacro-iliac joint observations on the gross and histological changes in the various age groups. Canadian Medical Association Journal 66:157

MacNab I 1977 Backache. Williams & Wilkins, Baltimore

Maigne J Y 1997 Lateral dynamic X-rays in the sitting position and coccygeal discography in common coccydynia. In: Vleeming A, Mooney V, Dorman T, Snijders C, Stoeckart R (eds) Movement, stability and low back pain. Churchill Livingstone, Edinburgh, p 385

Maigne J Y, Aivaliklis A, Pfefer F 1996 Results of sacroiliac joint double block and value of sacroiliac

pain provocation tests in 54 patients with low back pain. Spine 21:1889

Mattila M, Hurme M, Alaranta H et al 1986 The multifidus muscle in patients with lumbar disc herniation. Spine 11(7):732

McArdle W D, Katch F I, Katch V L 1991 Exercise physiology. Energy, nutrition, and human performance, 3rd edn. Lea & Febiger, Malvern, PA

McGill S 2002 Low back disorders – evidence-based prevention and rehabilitation. Human Kinetics, Canada

McGill S, Norman R W 1987 Effects of an anatomically detailed erector spinae model on L4/L5 disc compression and shear. Journal of Biomechanics 20(6):591

McKenzie D K, Gandevia S C, Gorman R B, Southon F C G 1994 Dynamic changes in the zone of apposition and diaphragm length during maximal respiratory efforts. Thorax 49:634

McNeill A R 1995 Elasticity in mammalian backs. In: Vleeming A, Mooney V, Dorman T, Snijders C (eds) Second interdisciplinary world congress on low back pain: the integrated function of the lumbar spine and sacroiliac joint, Part 1. European Conference Organizers, Rotterdam, p 7

McNeill A R 1997 Elasticity in human and animal backs. In: Vleeming A, Mooney V, Dorman T, Snijders C, Stoeckart R (eds) Movement, stability and low back pain. Churchill Livingstone, Edinburgh, p 227

Meisenbach R O 1911 Sacro-iliac relaxation; with analysis of eighty-four cases. Surgery, Gynecology and Obstetrics 12:411

Melzak R, Wall P D 1965 Pain mechanisms: a new theory. Science 150:971

Mens J M A, Vleeming A, Snijders C J, Stam H J 1997 Active straight leg raising test: a clinical approach to the load transfer function of the pelvic girdle. In: Vleeming A, Mooney V, Dorman T, Snijders C, Stoeckart R (eds) Movement, stability and low back pain. Churchill Livingstone, Edinburgh, p 425

Mens J M A, Vleeming A, Snijders C J, Stam H J, Ginai A Z 1999 The active straight leg raising test and mobility of the pelvic joints. European Spine 8:468

Mens J M A, Vleeming A, Snijders C J, Koes B J, Stam H J 2001 Reliability and validity of the active straight leg raise test in posterior pelvic pain since pregnancy. Spine 26(10):1167

Mens J M, Vleeming A, Snijders C J, Koes B W, Stam H J 2002 Validity of the active straight leg raise test for measuring disease severity in patients with posterior pelvic pain after pregnancy. Spine 27(2):196

Mester E 1971 Effects of laser rays on wound healing. American Journal of Surgery 122:532

Meyer G H 1878 Der Mechanismus der Symphysis sacroiliaca. Archiv für Anatomie und Physiologie 1:1

Miller J A A, Schultz A B, Andersson G B J 1987 Load-displacement behavior of sacro-iliac joints. Journal of Orthopedic Research 5:92

Mitchell F L, Mitchell P K G 2001 The muscle energy manual – evaluation and treatment of the pelvis and sacrum, 2nd edn. MET Press, East Lansing, Michigan

Mixter W J, Barr J S 1934 Rupture of intervertebral disc with involvement of the spinal cord. New England Journal of Medicine 211:210

Mooney V 1997 Sacroiliac joint dysfunction. In: Vleeming A, Mooney V, Dorman T, Snijders C, Stoeckart R (eds) Movement, stability and low back pain. Churchill Livingstone, Edinburgh, p 37

Moseley G L 2002 Combined physiotherapy and education is efficacious for chronic low back pain. Australian Journal of Physiotherapy 48:297

Moseley G L 2003 Unraveling the barriers to reconceptualization of the problem in chronic pain: the actual and perceived ability of patients and health professionals to understand the neurophysiology. Journal of Pain 4(4):184

Moseley G L, Hodges P W, Gandevia S C 2002 Deep and superficial fibers of the lumbar multifidus muscle are differentially active during voluntary arm movements. Spine 27(2):E29

Moseley G L, Hodges P W, Gandevia S C 2003 External perturbation of the trunk in standing humans differentially activates components of the medial back muscles. Journal of Physiology 547(2):581

Murphy M 1992 The future of the body: explorations into the further evolution of human nature. Tarcher Putnam, New York

Nelson H, Jurmain R 1985 Introduction to physical anthropology, 3rd edn. West Publishing, St Paul

Nygaard I E, Thompson F L, Svengalis S L, Albright J P 1994 Urinary incontinence in elite nulliparous athletes. Obstetrics and Gynecology 84(2):183

O'Sullivan P 2000 Lumbar segmental "instability": clinical presentation and specific stabilizing exercise management. Manual Therapy 5(1):2

O'Sullivan P, Twomey L, Allison G 1997. Evaluation of specific stabilising exercise in the treatment of chronic low back pain with radiological diagnosis of spondylolysis and spondylolisthesis. Spine 15(24):2959

O'Sullivan P B, Grahamslaw K M, Kendell M M, Lapenski S C, Moller N E, Richards K V 2001 The effect of different standing and sitting postures on trunk muscle activity in a pain free population. In: 4th interdisciplinary world congress on low back and pelvic pain. Montreal, Canada, p 180

O'Sullivan P B, Beales D, Beetham J A et al 2002 Altered motor control strategies in subjects with sacroiliac joint pain during the active straight leg raise test. Spine 27(1):E1

O'Sullivan P, Bryniolfsson G, Cawthorne A, Karakasidou P, Pederson P, Waters N 2003 Investigation of a clinical test and transabdominal ultrasound during pelvic floor muscle contraction in subjects with and without lumbosacral pain. In: 14th international WCPT congress proceedings. Barcelona, Spain, CD ROM abstracts

Ostgaard H C 1997 Lumbar back and posterior pelvic pain in pregnancy. In: Vleeming A, Mooney V, Dorman T, Snijders C, Stoeckart R (eds) Movement, stability and low back pain. Churchill Livingstone, Edinburgh, p 411

Ostgaard H C, Zetherstrom G, Roos-Hansson E 1994 The posterior pelvic pain provocation test in pregnant women. European Spine Journal 3:258

Panjabi M M 1992a The stabilizing system of the spine. Part I: function, dysfunction, adaptation, and enhancement. Journal of Spinal Disorders 5(4):383

Panjabi M M 1992b The stabilizing system of the spine. Part II. Neutral zone and instability hypothesis. Journal of Spinal Disorders 5(4):390

Panjabi M M, Abumi K, Duranceau J, Oxland T 1989 Spinal stability and intersegmental muscle forces – a biomechanical model. Spine 14(2):194

Paydar D, Thiel H, Gemmell H 1994 Intra- and interexaminer reliability of certain pelvic palpatory procedures and the sitting flexion test for sacroiliac joint mobility and dysfunction. Journal of Neuromusculoskeletal Medicine 2(2):65

Peacock E E 1984 Wound repair, 3rd edn. W B Saunders, London

Pearcy M, Tibrewal S B 1984 Axial rotation and lateral bending in the normal lumbar spine measured by three-dimensional radiography. Spine 9:582

Peschers U M, Vodusek D B, Fanger G et al 2001a Pelvic muscle activity in nulliparous volunteers. Neurourology and Urodynamics 20:269

Peschers U M, Ganger G, Schaer G N et al 2001b Bladder neck mobility in continent nulliparous women. British Journal of Obstetrics and Gynaecology 108:320

Pitkin H C, Pheasant H C 1936 Sacroarthrogenetic telalagia II. A study of sacral mobility. Journal of Bone and Joint Surgery 18:365

Potter N A, Rothstein J 1985 Intertester reliability for selected clinical tests of the sacroiliac joint. Physical Therapy 65(11):1671

Pranathi Reddy A, DeLancey J O L, Zwica L M, Ashton-Miller J A 2001 On screen vector-based ultrasound assessment of vesical neck movement. American Journal of Obstetrics and Gynecology 185:65

Radebold A, Cholewicki J, Panjabi M M, Patel T C 2000 Muscle response pattern to sudden trunk loading in healthy individuals and in patients with chronic low back pain. Spine 25(8):947

Radebold A, Cholewicki J, Polzhofer G K, Greene H S 2001 Impaired postural control of the lumbar spine is associated with delayed muscle response times in patients with chronic idiopathic low back pain. Spine 26(7):724

Reid D C 1992 Sports injury assessment and rehabilitation. Churchill Livingstone, New York

Reilly J, Yong-Hing K, MacKay R W, Kirkaldy-Wallis W H 1978 Pathological anatomy of the lumbar spine. In: Helfet A J, Gruebel-Lee D M (eds) Disorders of the lumbar spine. J B Lippincott, Philadelphia

Resnick D, Niwayama G, Goergen T G 1975 Degenerative disease of the sacroiliac joint. Journal of Investigative Radiology 10:608

Richardson C A, Jull G A 1995 Muscle control – pain control. What exercises would you prescribe? Manual Therapy 1:2

Richardson C A, Jull G A, Hodges P W, Hides J A 1999 Therapeutic exercise for spinal segmental stabilization in low back pain – scientific basis and clinical approach. Churchill Livingstone, Edinburgh

Richardson C A, Snijders C J, Hides J A, Damen L, Pas M S, Storm J 2002 The relationship between the transversely oriented abdominal muscles, sacroiliac joint mechanics and low back pain. Spine 27(4):399

Rizk N N 1980 A new description of the anterior abdominal wall in man and mammals. Journal of Anatomy 131:373

Rodman P S, McHenry M 1980 Bioenergetics and the origin of hominid bipedalism. American Journal of Physical Anthropology 52:103

Rohen J W, Yokochi C 1983 Color atlas of anatomy, a photographic study of the human body. F K Schattauer, Stuttgart/Igaku-Shoin, Tokyo

Romer A S 1959 A shorter version of the vertebrate body. W B Saunders, Philadelphia

Rothman R H, Simeone F A 1975 Spine, vol IV. W B Saunders, London

Rowinski M J 1985 Afferent neurobiology of the joint. In: Gould J A, Davies J D (eds) Orthopaedic and sports physical therapy. C V Mosby, St. Louis, p 50

Sahrmann S 2001 Diagnosis and treatment of movement impaired syndromes. Mosby, St Louis

Sapolsky R M, Spencer E M 1997 Insulin growth factor 1 is suppressed in socially subordinate male baboons. American Journal of Physiology 273(4 Pt 2):1346

Sapolsky R M, Alberts R C, Altmann J 1997 Hypercortisolism associated with social subordinance isolation among wild baboons. Archives of General Psychiatry 54(12):1137

Sapsford R, Bullock-Saxton J, Markwell S 1998 Women's health: a textbook for physiotherapists. W B Saunders, London

Sapsford R R, Hodges P W, Richardson C A, Cooper D H, Markwell S J, Jull G A 2001 Co-activation of the abdominal and pelvic floor muscles during voluntary exercises. Neurourology and Urodynamics 20:31

Sashin D 1930 A critical analysis of the anatomy and the pathologic changes of the sacro-iliac joints. Journal of Bone and Joint Surgery 12:891

Schamberger W 2002 The malalignment syndrome. Implications for medicine and sport. Churchill Livingstone, Edinburgh

Schunke G B 1938 The anatomy and development of the sacro-iliac joint in man. Anatomical Record 72:313

Schwarzer A C, Aprill C N, Bogduk N 1995 The sacroiliac joint in chronic low back pain. Spine 20:31

Shibata Y, Shirai Y, Miyamoto M 2002 The aging process in the sacroiliac joint: helical computed tomography analysis. Journal of Orthopedic Science 7(1):12

Siffert R S, Feldman D J 1980 The growing hip. Acta Orthopaedica Belgica 46:443

Singleton M C, LeVeau B F 1975 The hip joint: structure, stability, and stress. Physical Therapy 55:957

Smidt G L 1995 Sacroiliac kinematics for reciprocal straddle positions. In: Vleeming A, Mooney V, Dorman T, Snijders C (eds) Second interdisciplinary world congress on low back pain: the integrated function of the lumbar spine and sacroiliac joint, part 2. San Diego, California, p 695

Snijders C J, Vleeming A, Stoeckart R 1993a Transfer of lumbosacral load to iliac bones and legs. 1: Biomechanics of self-bracing of the sacroiliac joints and its significance for treatment and exercise. Clinical Biomechanics 8:285

Snijders C J, Vleeming A, Stoeckart R 1993b Transfer of lumbosacral load to iliac bones and legs. 2: Loading of the sacroiliac joints when lifting in a stooped posture. Clinical Biomechanics 8:295

Snijders C J, Vleeming A, Stoeckart R, Mens J M A, Kleinrensink G J 1997 Biomechanics of the interface between spine and pelvis in different postures. In: Vleeming A, Mooney V, Dorman T, Snijders C, Stoeckart R (eds) Movement, stability and low back pain. Churchill Livingstone, Edinburgh, p 103

Solonen K A 1957 The sacro-iliac joint in the light of anatomical roentgenological and clinical studies. Acta Orthopaedica Scandinavica Supplement 26

Stark S D 1997 The stark reality of stretching. Peanut Butter, Vancouver

Stein P L, Rowe B M 1982 Physical anthropology, 3rd edn. McGraw-Hill, New York

Stokes I A F 1986 Three-dimensional biplanar radiography of the lumbar spine. In: Grieve G P (ed) Modern manual therapy of the vertebral column. Churchill Livingstone, Edinburgh, p 576

Strayer L M 1971 Embryology of the human hip joint. Clinical Orthopaedics 74:221

Strender L, Sjoblom A, Sundell K, Ludwig R, Taube A 1997 Interexaminer reliability in physical examination of patients with low back pain. Spine 22(7):814

Sturesson B 1997 Movement of the sacroiliac joint: a fresh look. In: Vleeming A, Mooney V, Dorman T, Snijders C, Stoeckart R (eds) Movement, stability and low back pain. Churchill Livingstone, Edinburgh, p 171

Sturesson B, Selvik G, Uden A 1989 Movements of the sacroiliac joints: a Roentgen stereophotogrammetric analysis. Spine 14(2):162

Sturesson B, Uden A, Vleeming A 2000 A radiosteriometric analysis of movements of the sacroiliac joints during the standing hip flexion test. Spine 25(3):364

Sunderland S 1978 Traumatized nerves, roots and ganglia: musculo-skeletal factors and neuropathological consequenes. In: Korr I (ed) The neurobiologic mechanisms in manipulative therapy. Plenum Press, London, p 137

Swindler D R, Wood C D 1982 An atlas of primate gross anatomy: baboon, chimpanzee, and man. Robert E Krieger, Florida

Taylor J R, Twomey L T 1986 Age changes in lumbar zygapophyseal joints: observations on structure and function. Spine 11(7):739

Taylor J T, Twomey L T 1992 Structure and function of lumbar zygapophyseal (facet) joints: a review. Journal of Orthopaedic Medicine 14(3):71

Taylor J T, Twomey L T, Corker M 1990 Bone and soft tissue injuries in post-mortem lumbar spines. Paraplegia 28:119

Thind P, Lose G, Jorgensen L, Colstrup H 1991 Urethral pressure increment preceding and following bladder pressure elevation during stress episode in healthy and stress incontinent women. Neurourology and Urodynamics 10:177

Travell J G, Rinzler S H 1952 The myofascial genesis of pain. Postgraduate Medicine 11:425

Trotter M 1937 Accessory sacro-iliac articulations. American Journal of Physical Anthropology 22:247

Tuttle R H (ed) 1975 Primate functional morphology. Mouton, The Hague

Twomey L T, Taylor J R 1985 A quantitative study of the role of the posterior vertebral elements in sagittal movements of the lumbar vertebral column. In: Glasgow E F, Twomey L T, Scull E R, Kleynhans A M (eds) Aspects of manipulative therapy, 2nd edn. Churchill Livingstone, Melbourne, p 34

Twomey L T, Taylor J R 1986 The effects of aging on the lumbar intervertebral discs. In: Grieve G P (ed) Modern manual therapy of the vertebral column. Churchill Livingstone, Edinburgh, p 129

Twomey L T, Taylor J R, Taylor M M 1989 Unsuspected damage to lumbar zygapophyseal (facet) joints after motor-vehicle accidents. Medical Journal of Australia 151:210

Uhlig Y, Weber B R, Grob D, Muntener M 1995 Fiber composition and fiber transformations in neck muscles of patients with dysfunction of the cervical spine. Journal of Orthopaedic Research 13:240

Uhtoff H K 1993 Prenatal development of the iliolumbar ligament. Journal of Bone and Joint Surgery (Britain) 75:93

Urquhart D, Hodges P, Story I 2001 Regional variation in transversus abdominis recruitment. In: 4th interdisciplinary world congress on low back and pelvic pain. Montreal, Canada, p 358

Van Wingerden J P, Vleeming A, Snijders C J, Stoeckart R 1993 A functional-anatomical approach to the spine-pelvis mechanism: interaction between the biceps femoris muscle and the sacrotuberous ligament. European Spine Journal 2:140

Van Wingerden J P, Vleeming A, Buyruk H M, Raissadat K 2001 Muscular contribution to force closure; sacroiliac joint stabilization in vivo. In: Proceedings from the 4th interdisciplinary world congress on low back and pelvic pain. Montreal, Canada, pp 153–159

Van Wingerden J P, Vleeming A, Buyruk H M, Raissadat K Stabilization of the sacroiliac joint in vivo: verification of muscular contribution to force closure of the pelvis. European Spine Journal (submitted)

Vicenzino G, Twomey L 1993 Sideflexion induced lumbar spine conjunct rotation and its influencing factors. Australian Physiotherapy 39(4):299

Vlaeyen J W S, Kole-Snijders A M J, Heuts P H T G, van Eek H 1997 Behavioral analysis, fear of movement/(re)injury and behavioral rehabilitation in chronic low back pain. In: Vleeming A, Mooney V, Dorman T, Snijders C, Stoeckart R (eds) Movement, stability and low back pain. Churchill Livingstone, Edinburgh, p 435

Vleeming A, Stoeckart R, Snijders C J 1989a The sacrotuberous ligament:a conceptual approach to its dynamic role in stabilizing the sacroiliac joint. Clinical Biomechanics 4:201

Vleeming A, van Wingerden J P, Snijders C J, Stoeckart R, Stijnen T 1989b Load application to the sacrotuberous ligament: influences on sacroiliac joint mechanics. Clinical Biomechanics 4:204

Vleeming A, Stoeckart R, Volkers A C W, Snijders C J 1990a Relation between form and function in the sacroiliac joint. 1: Clinical anatomical aspects. Spine 15(2):130

Vleeming A, Volkers A C W, Snijders C J, Stoeckart R 1990b Relation between form and function in the sacroiliac joint. 2: Biomechanical aspects. Spine 15(2):133

Vleeming A, van Wingerden J P, Dijkstra P F, Stoeckart R, Snijders C J, Stijnen T 1992a Mobility in the SI-joints in old people: a kinematic and radiologic study. Clinical Biomechanics 7:170

Vleeming A, Mooney V, Snijders C, Dorman T (eds) 1992b First interdisciplinary world congress on low back pain and its relation to the sacroiliac joint. San Diego, California

Vleeming A, Buyruk H, Stoechart R, Karamursel S, Snijders C J 1992c An integrated therapy for peripartum pelvic instability: a study of the biomechanical effects of pelvic belts. American Journal of Obstetrics and Gynecology 166(4):1243

Vleeming A, Pool-Goudzwaard A L, Stoeckart R, van Wingerden J P, Snijders C J 1995a The posterior layer of the thoracolumbar fascia: its function in load transfer from spine to legs. Spine 20:753

Vleeming A, Snijders C J, Stoeckart R, Mens J M A 1995b A new light on low back pain. In: Proceedings from the 2nd interdisciplinary world congress on low back pain. San Diego, California

Vleeming A, Mooney V, Dorman T, Snijders C (eds) 1995c Second interdisciplinary world congress on low back pain: the integrated function of the lumbar spine and sacroiliac joint, parts 1 and 2. San Diego, California

Vleeming A, Pool-Goudzwaard A L, Hammudoghlu D, Stoeckart R, Snijders C J, Mens J M A 1996 The function of the long dorsal sacroiliac ligament: its implication for understanding low back pain. Spine 21(5):556

Vleeming A, Snijders C J, Stoeckart R, Mens J M A 1997 The role of the sacroiliac joints in coupling between spine, pelvis, legs and arms. In: Vleeming A, Mooney V, Dorman T, Snijders C, Stoeckart R (eds) Movement, stability and low back pain. Churchill Livingstone, Edinburgh, p 53

Vleeming A, de Vries H J, Mens J M, van Wingerden J P 2002 Possible role of the long dorsal sacroiliac ligament in women with peripartum pelvic pain. Acta Obstetrica Gynecologica Scandinavica 81(5):430

Waddell G 1998 The back pain revolution. Churchill Livingstone, Edinburgh

Walheim G G, Selvik G 1984 Mobility of the pubic symphysis. Clinical Orthopaedics and Related Research 191:129

Walker J M 1980a Morphological variants in the human fetal hip joint. Journal of Bone and Joint Surgery 62A:1073

Walker J M 1980b Growth characteristics of the fetal ligament of the head of femur: significance in congenital hip disease. Yale Journal of Biology and Medicine 53:307

Walker J M 1981 Histological study of the fetal development of the human acetabulum and labrum: significance in congenital hip disease. Yale Journal of Biology and Medicine 54:255

Walker J M 1984 Age changes in the sacroiliac joint. Proceedings of the 5th International Federation of Orthopaedic Manipulative Therapists. Vancouver, p 250

Walker J M 1986 Age-related differences in the human sacroiliac joint: a histological study; implications for therapy. Journal of Orthopaedic and Sports Physical Therapy 7:325

Watanabe R S 1974 Embryology of the human hip. Clinical Orthopaedics 98:8

Webster D F, Harvey W, Dyson M, Pond J B 1980 The role of ultrasound-induced cavitation in the "in vitro" stimulation of collagen synthesis in human fibroblasts. Ultrasonic 18:33

Weisl H 1954 The articular surfaces of the sacro-iliac joint and their relation to the movements of the sacrum. Acta Anatomica 22:1

Weisl H 1955 The movements of the sacro-iliac joint. Acta Anatomica 23:80

White A A, Panjabi M M 1978 The basic kinematics of the human spine. Spine 3:12

Whittaker J L 2003 Abdominal ultrasound imaging of pelvic floor muscle function in individuals with low back pain. Journal of Manual and Manipulative Therapy (submitted)

Wilder D G, Pope M H, Frymoyer J W 1980 The functional topography of the sacroiliac joint. Spine 5:575

Willard F H 1997 The muscular, ligamentous and neural structure of the low back and its relation to back pain. In: Vleeming A, Mooney V, Dorman T, Snijders C, Stoeckart R (eds) Movement, stability and low back pain. Churchill Livingstone, Edinburgh, p 3

Willard F H, Carreiro J E, Manko W 1998 The long posterior interosseous ligament and the sacrococcygeal plexus. In: Proceedings from the 3rd interdisciplinary world congress on low back and pelvic pain. Vienna, Austria, p 207

Williams P L 1995 Gray's anatomy, 38th edn. Churchill Livingstone, New York

Wroblewski B M 1978 Pain in osteoarthrosis of the hip. Practitioner 1315:140

Wurdinger S, Humbsch K, Reichenback J R, Peiker G, Seewalk H J, Kaiser W A 2002 MRI of the pelvic ring joints postpartum: normal and pathological findings. Journal of Magnetic Resonance Imaging 15(3):324

Wurff P, Hagmeijer R, Meyne W 2000 Clinical tests of the sacroiliac joint. A systematic methodological review: part 1: reliability. Manual Therapy 5(1):30

Wyke B D 1981 The neurology of joints: a review of general principles. Clinics in Rheumatic Diseases 7:223

Wyke B D 1985 Articular neurology and manipulative therapy. In: Glasgow E F, Twomey L T, Scull E R, Kleynhans A M (eds) Aspects of manipulative therapy, 2nd edn. Churchill Livingstone, Melbourne, p 72

Young J 1940 Relaxation of the pelvic joints in pregnancy: pelvic arthropathy of pregnancy. Journal of Obstetrics and Gynecology 47:493

Young J Z 1981 The life of vertebrates, 3rd edn. Clarendon Press, Oxford

Yue G, Cole K J 1992 Strength increase from the motor programme: comparison of training with maximal voluntary and imagined muscle contractions. Journal of Neurophysiology 67(5):1114

Index

Plate section

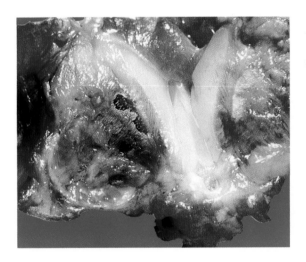

Plate 1 Sacroiliac joint of a fetus at 37 weeks of gestation. Note that the fibrocartilage lining the articular surface of the ilium is bluer than the hyaline cartilage lining the articular surface of the sacrum.

Plate 2 Sacroiliac joint of a male, 3 years of age (the sacral surface is on the right). Note the blue, dull fibrocartilage lining the articular surface of the ilium.

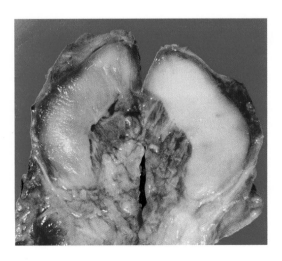

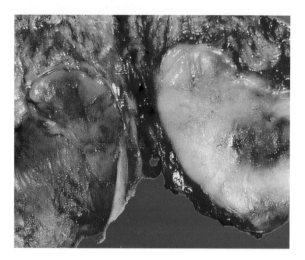

Plate 3 Sacroiliac joint of a male, 17 years of age (the sacral surface is on the right). Note the dull, rough fibrocartilage lining the articular surface of the ilium.

Plate 4 Sacroiliac joint of a male, 40 years of age (the sacral surface is on the right).

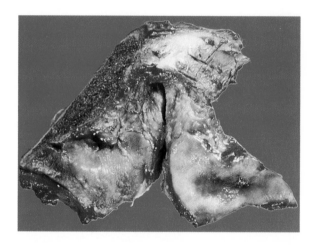

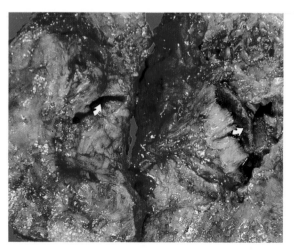

Plate 5 Sacroiliac joint of a female, 72 years of age (the sacral surface is on the left). Note the marked loss of articular cartilage on both sides of the joint as well as the presence of an accessory sacroiliac joint (arrows). (Plates 1–5 are reproduced with permission from Bowen & Cassidy (1981) and the publishers Harper and Rowe.)

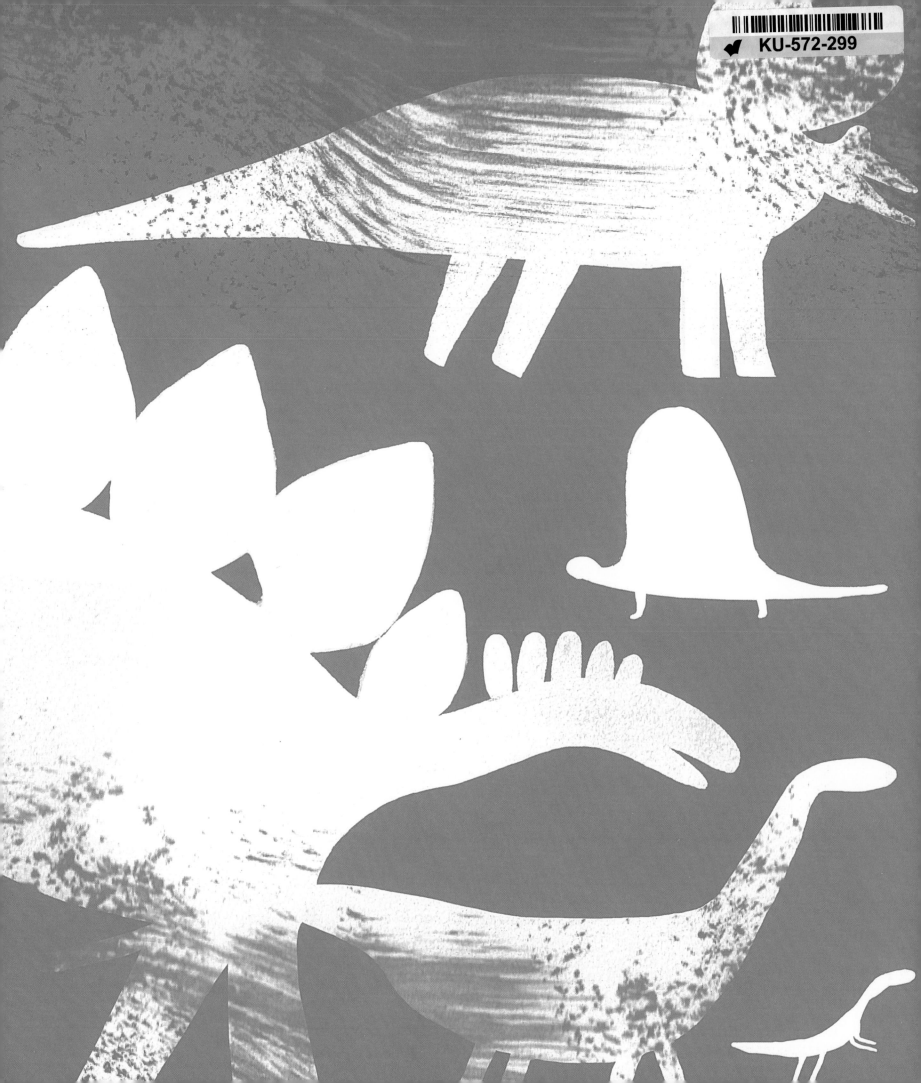

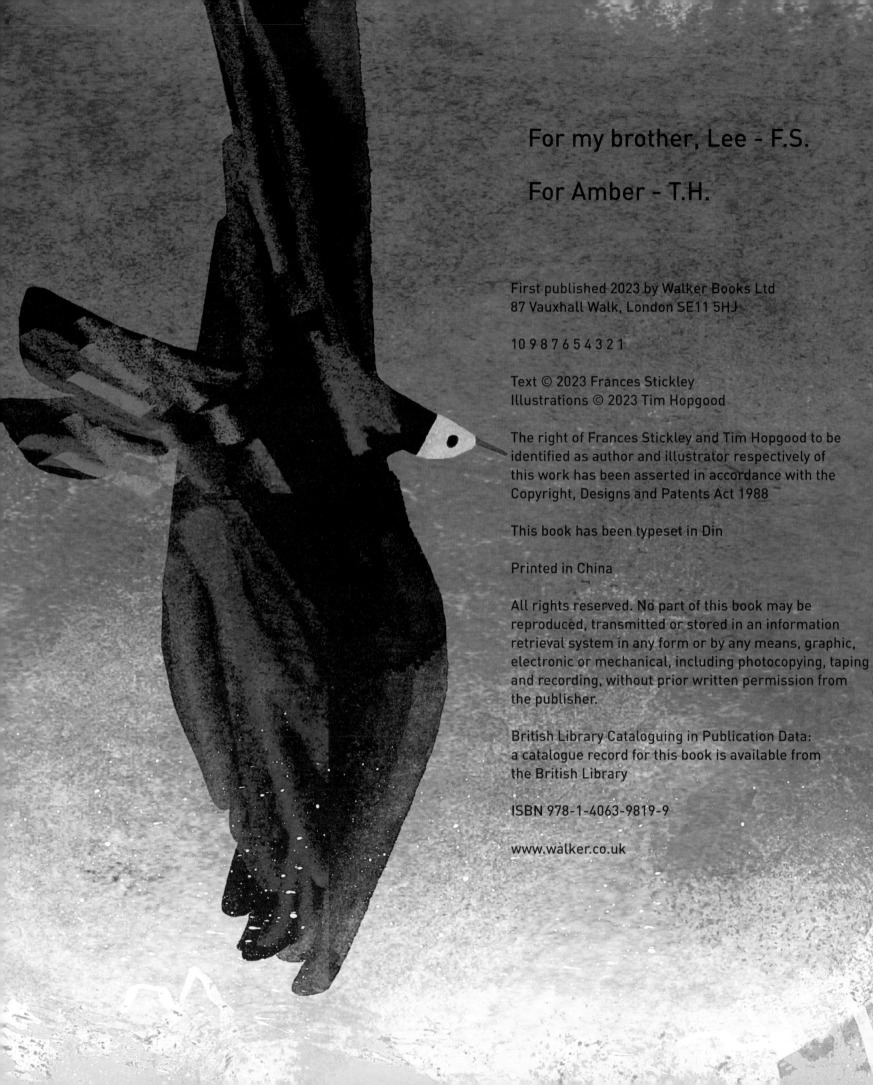

For my brother, Lee - F.S.

For Amber - T.H.

First published 2023 by Walker Books Ltd
87 Vauxhall Walk, London SE11 5HJ

10 9 8 7 6 5 4 3 2 1

Text © 2023 Frances Stickley
Illustrations © 2023 Tim Hopgood

The right of Frances Stickley and Tim Hopgood to be
identified as author and illustrator respectively of
this work has been asserted in accordance with the
Copyright, Designs and Patents Act 1988

This book has been typeset in Din

Printed in China

British Library Cataloguing in Publication Data:
a catalogue record for this book is available from
the British Library

ISBN 978-1-4063-9819-9

www.walker.co.uk

Frances Stickley

LOVE, THE EARTH

ILLUSTRATED BY

Tim Hopgood

WALKER BOOKS
AND SUBSIDIARIES
LONDON • BOSTON • SYDNEY • AUCKLAND

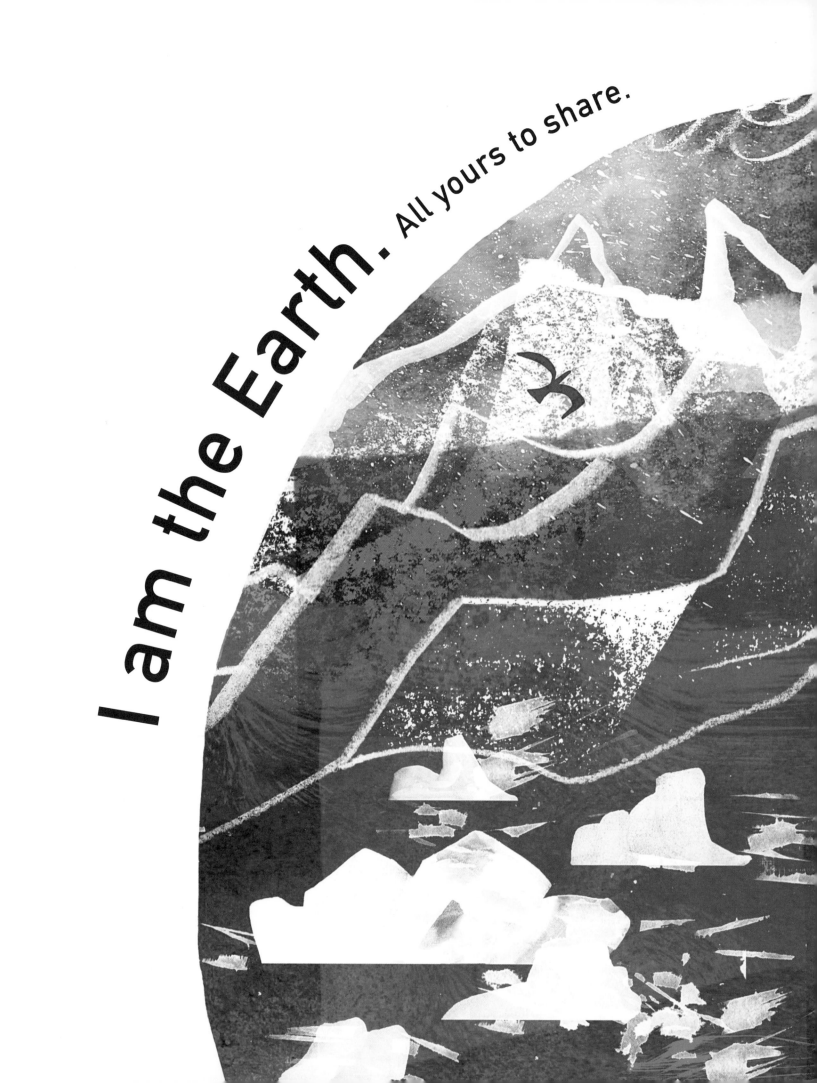

I am the Earth. All yours to share.

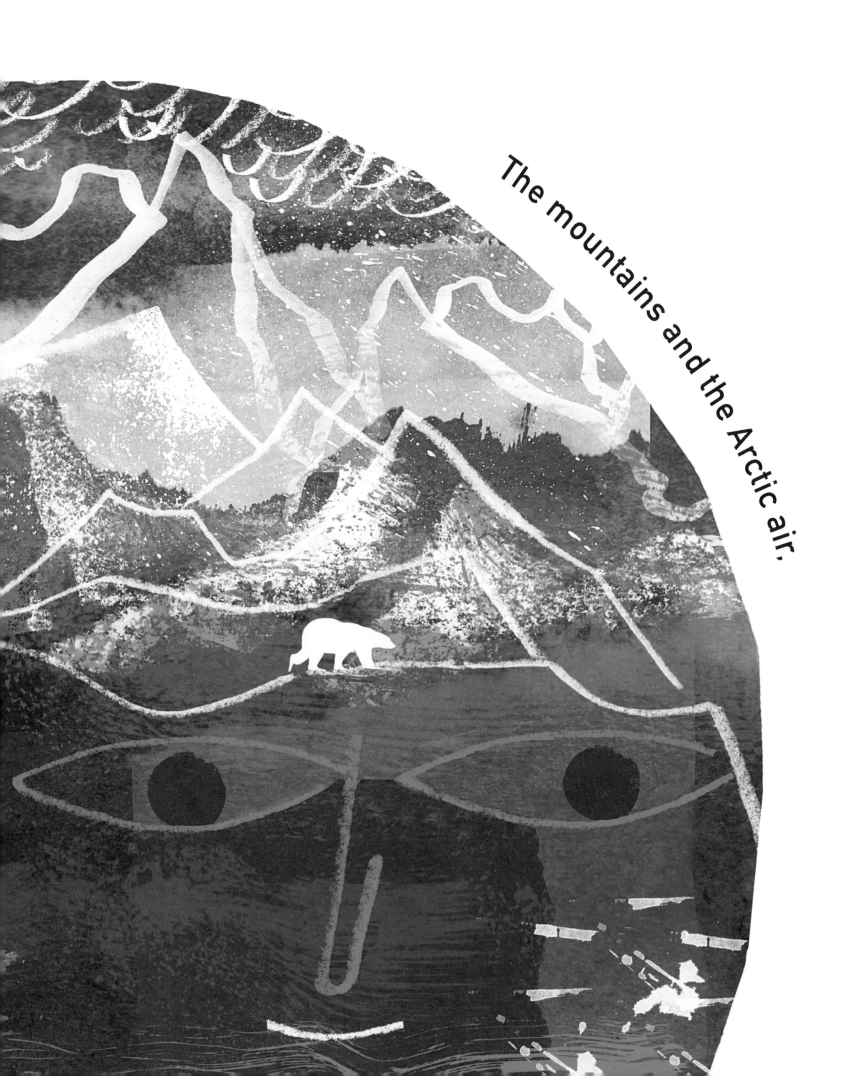

The mountains and the Arctic air.

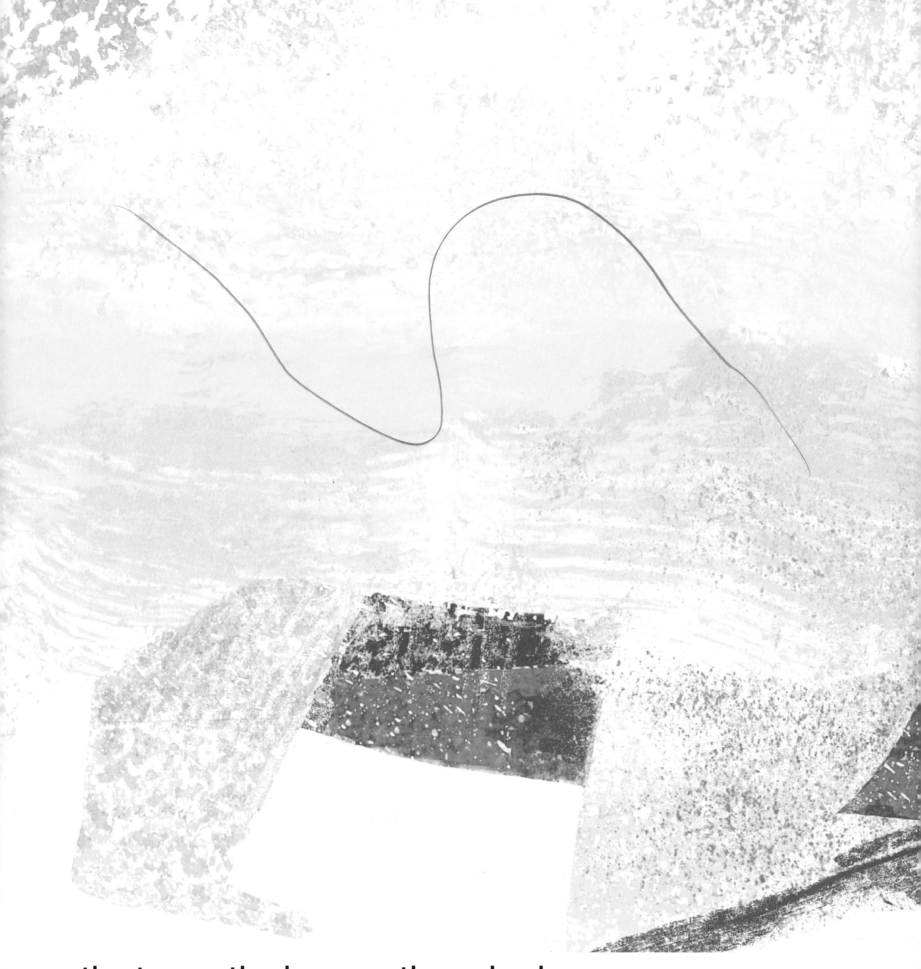

the trees, the breeze, the polar bear,

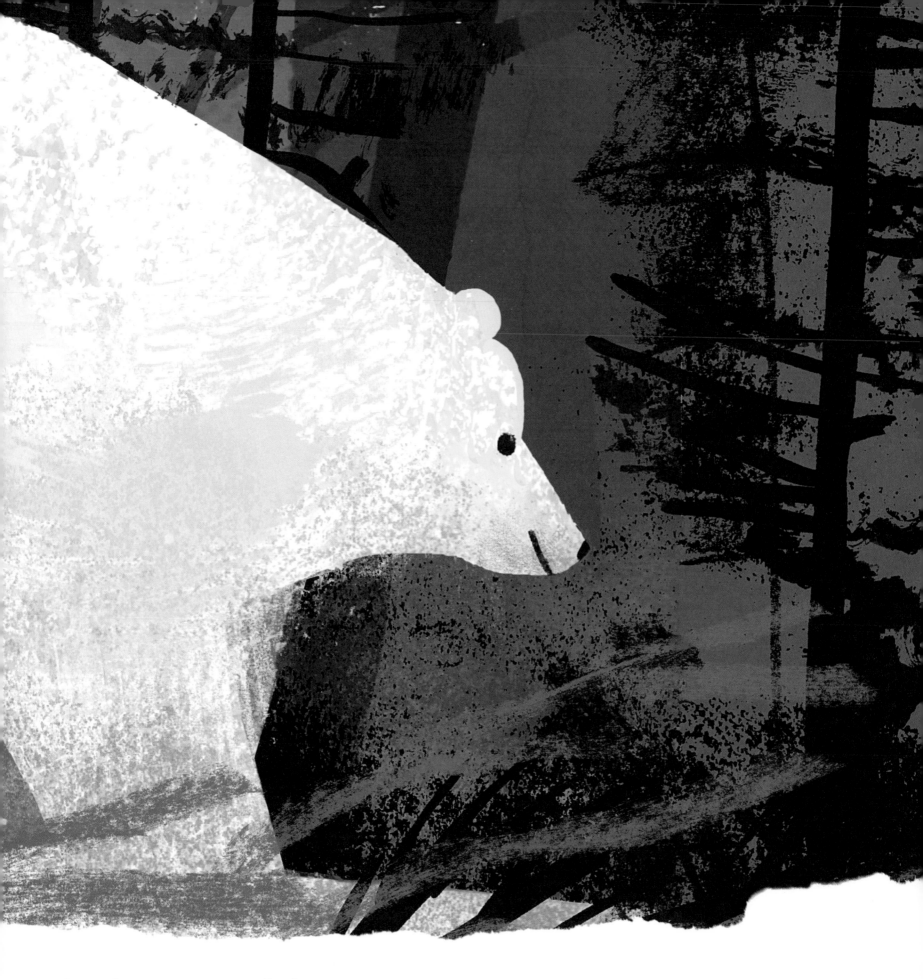

the forests and the sea.

And now you're here, so small and new.

A tiny little dream come true.

Don't worry, I'll take care of you.

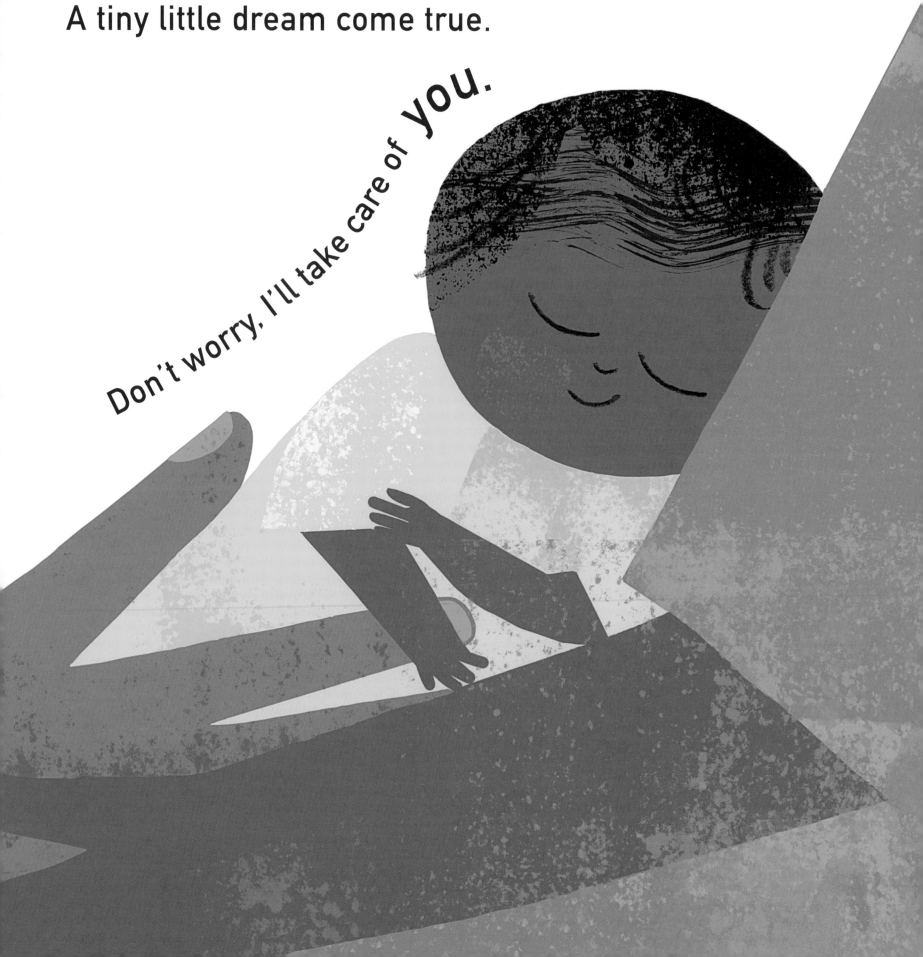

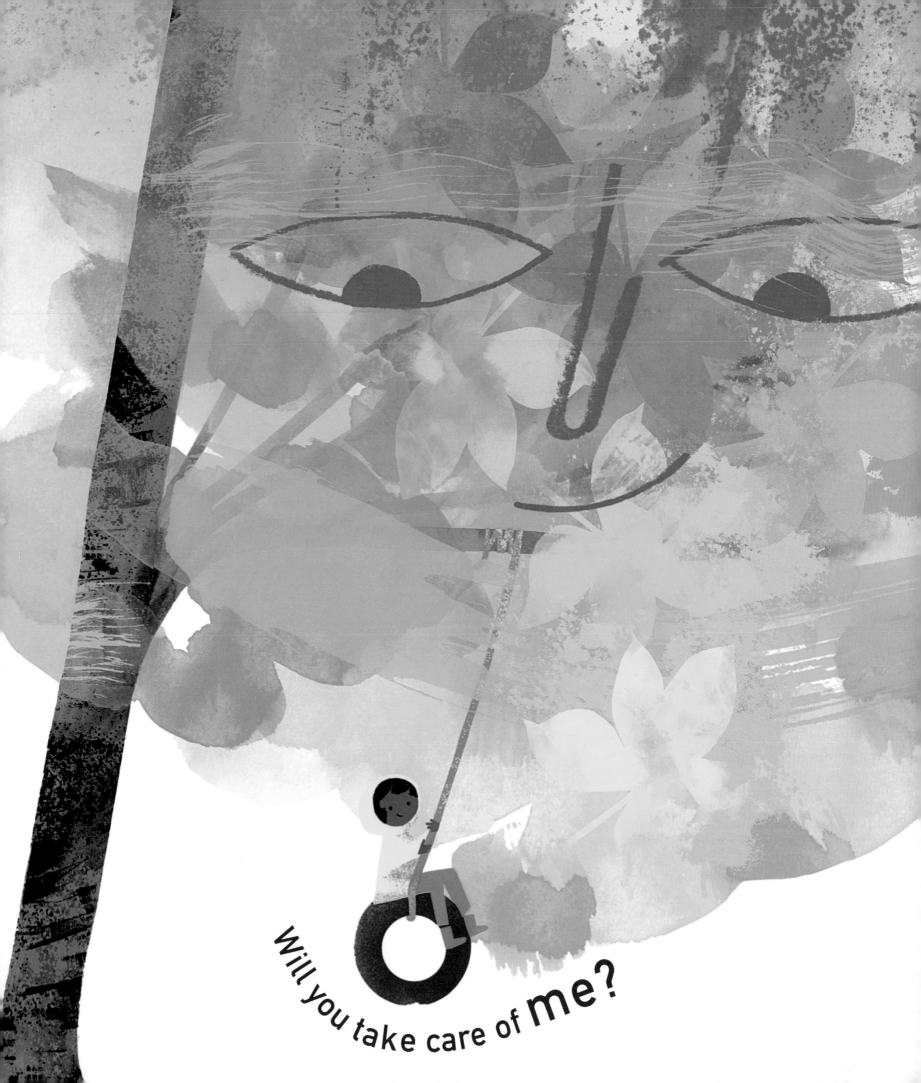

Will you take care of me?

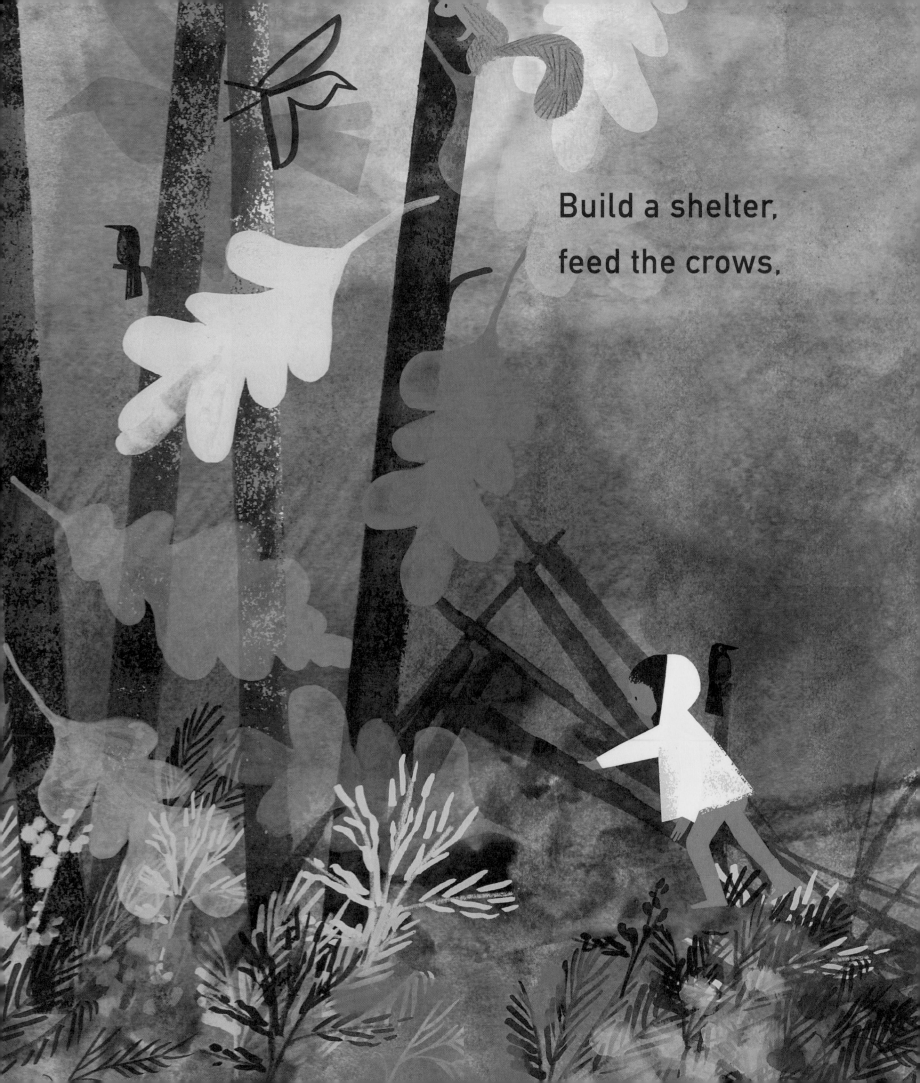

Build a shelter,
feed the crows,

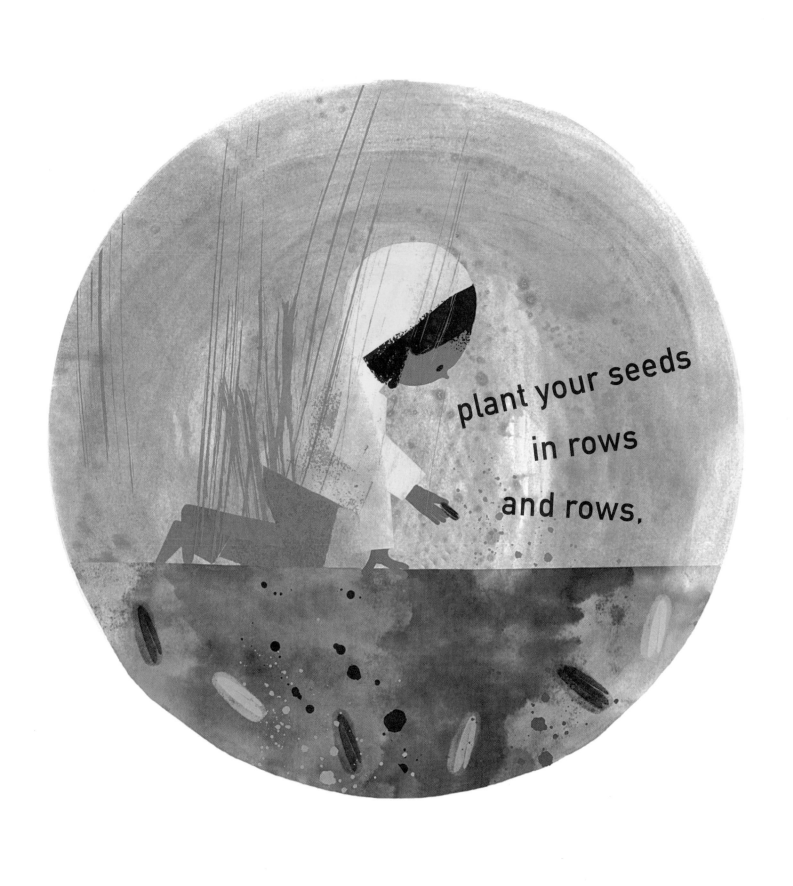

plant your seeds
in rows
and rows,

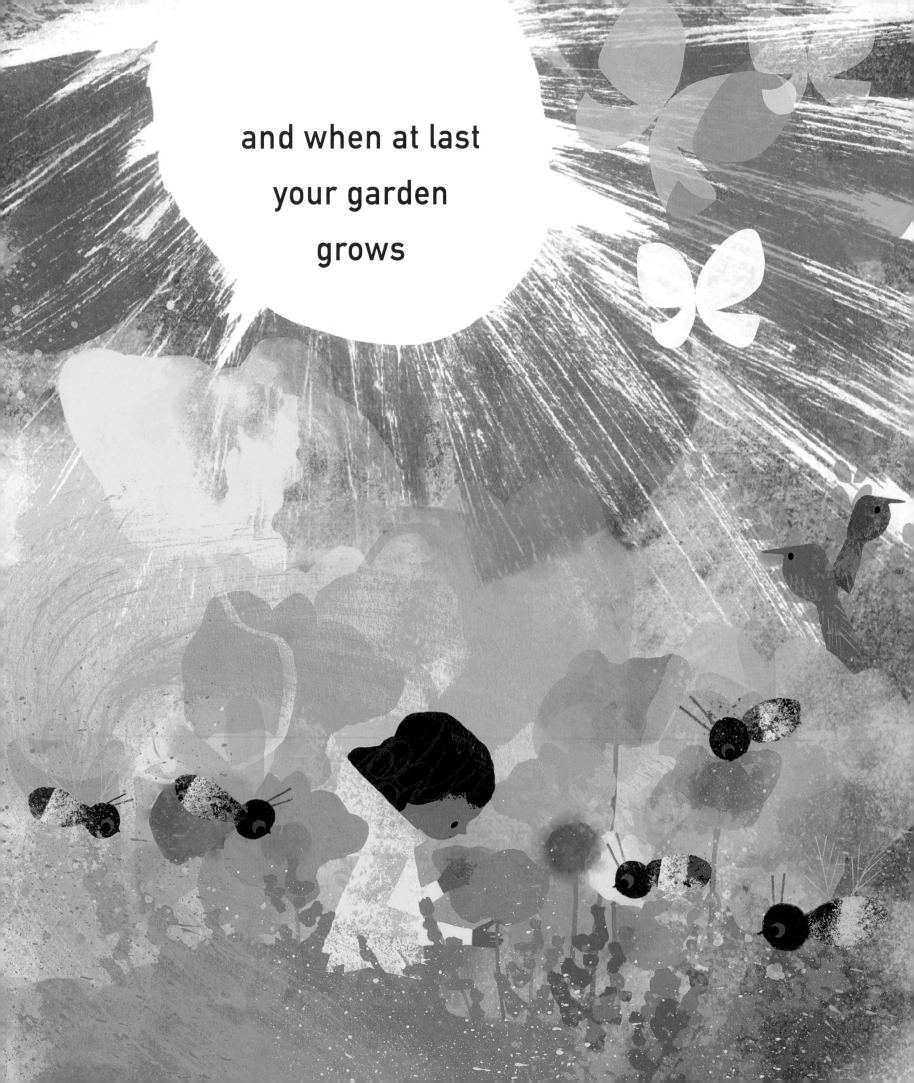

and when at last
your garden
grows

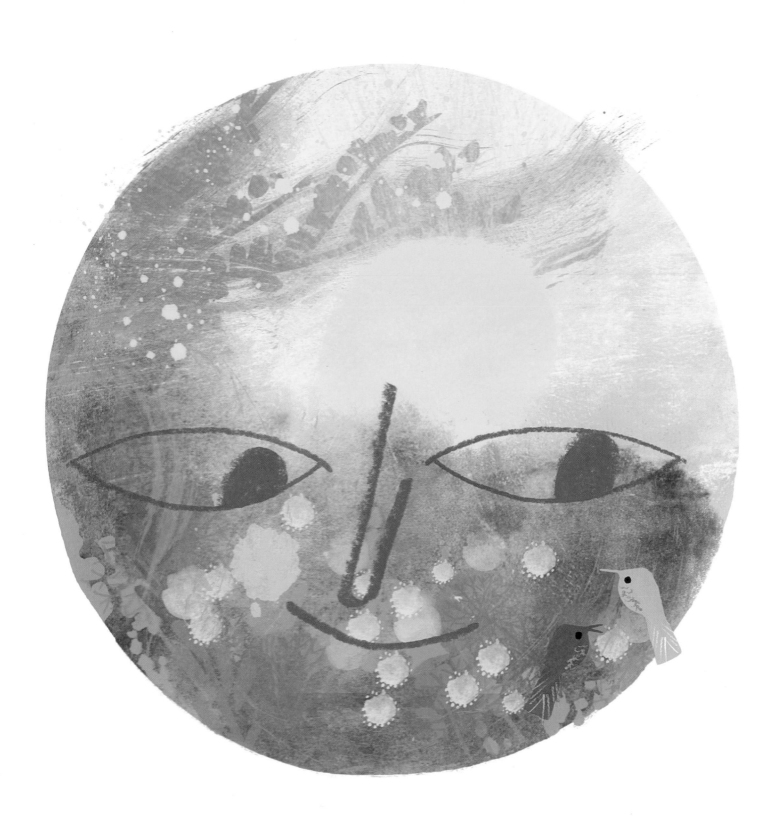

enjoy the bees and birds.

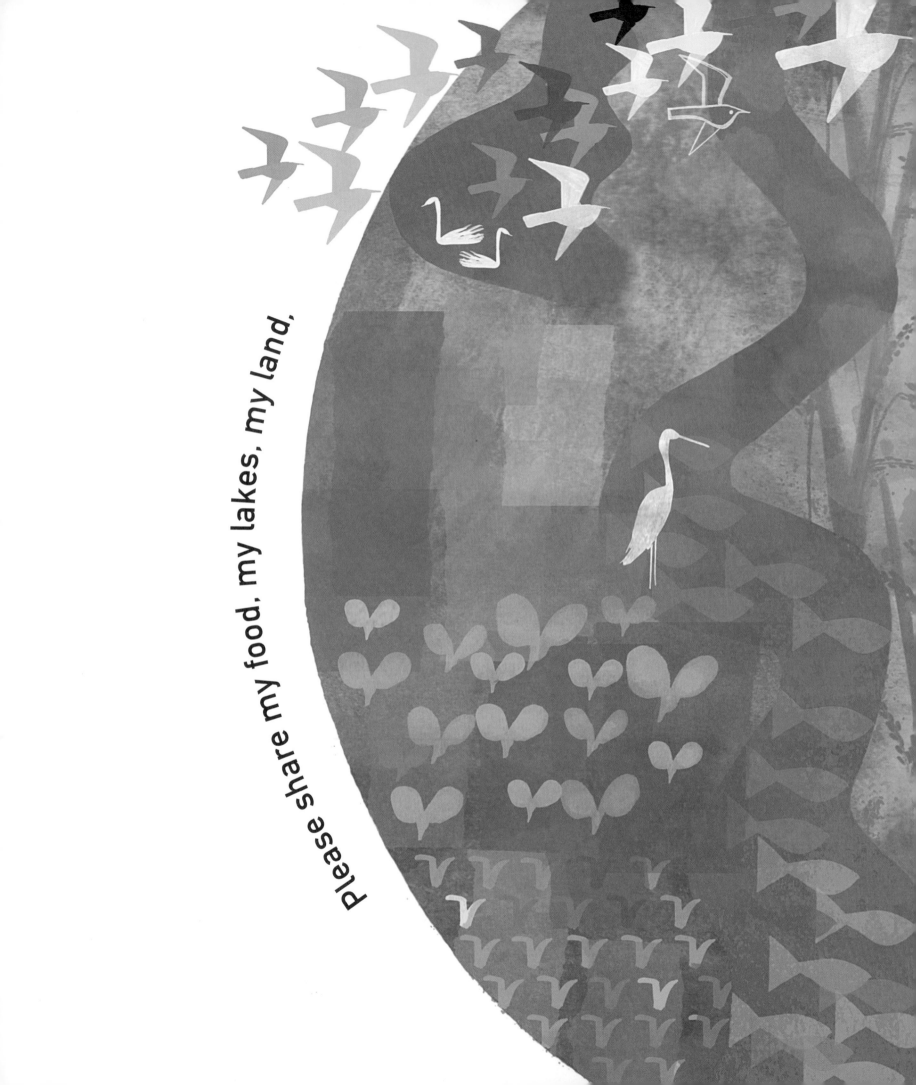

Please share my food, my lakes, my land,

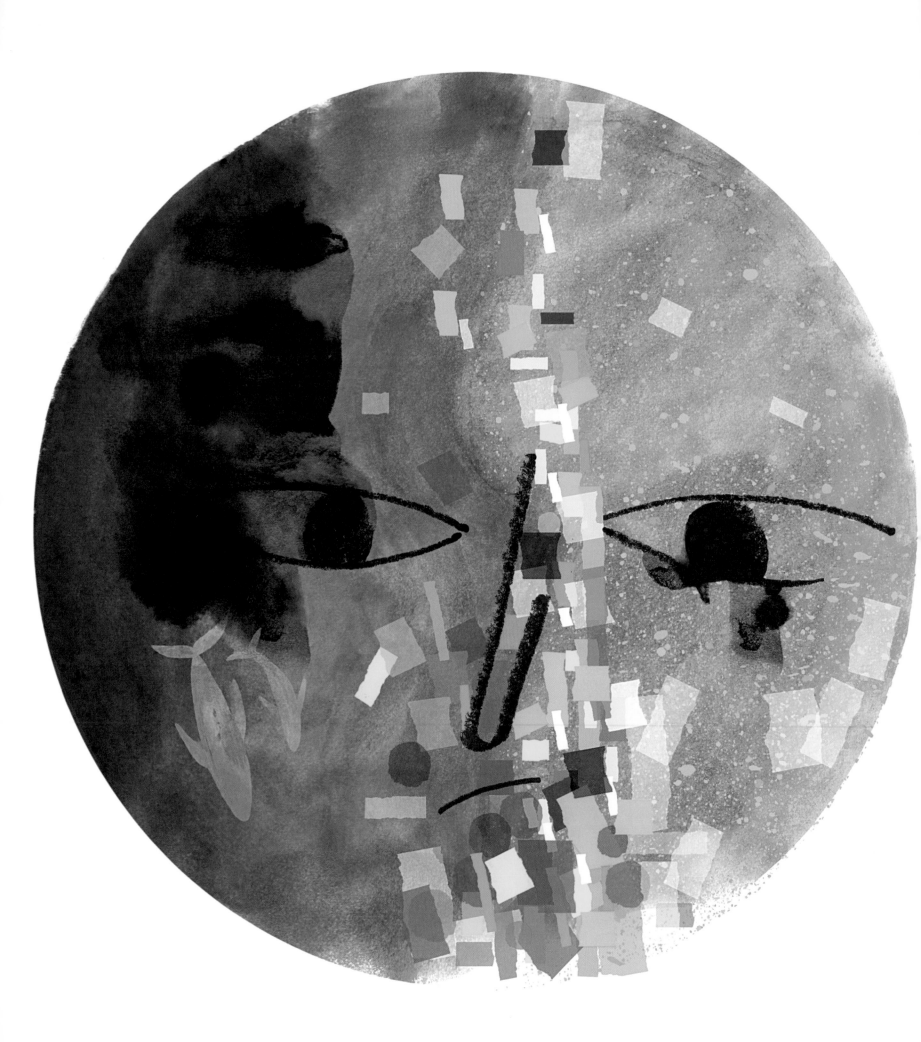

but try to lend
a helping hand.

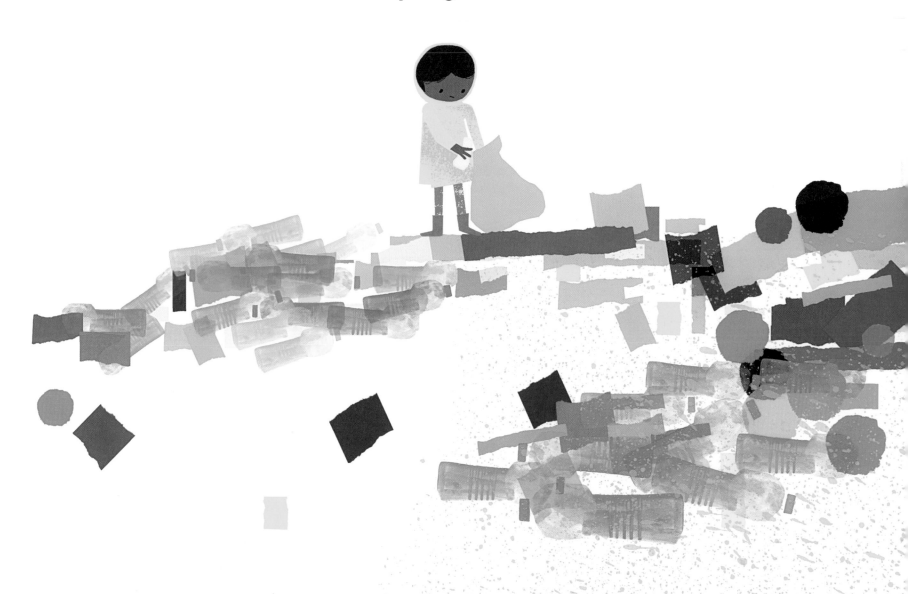

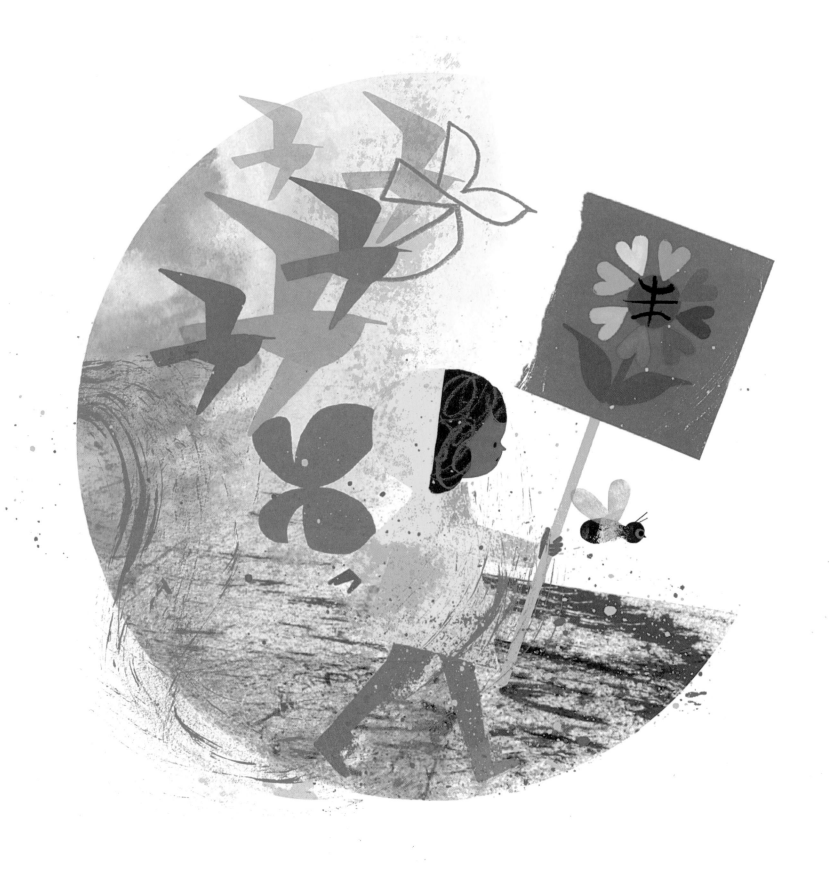

Make your mark and take a stand,

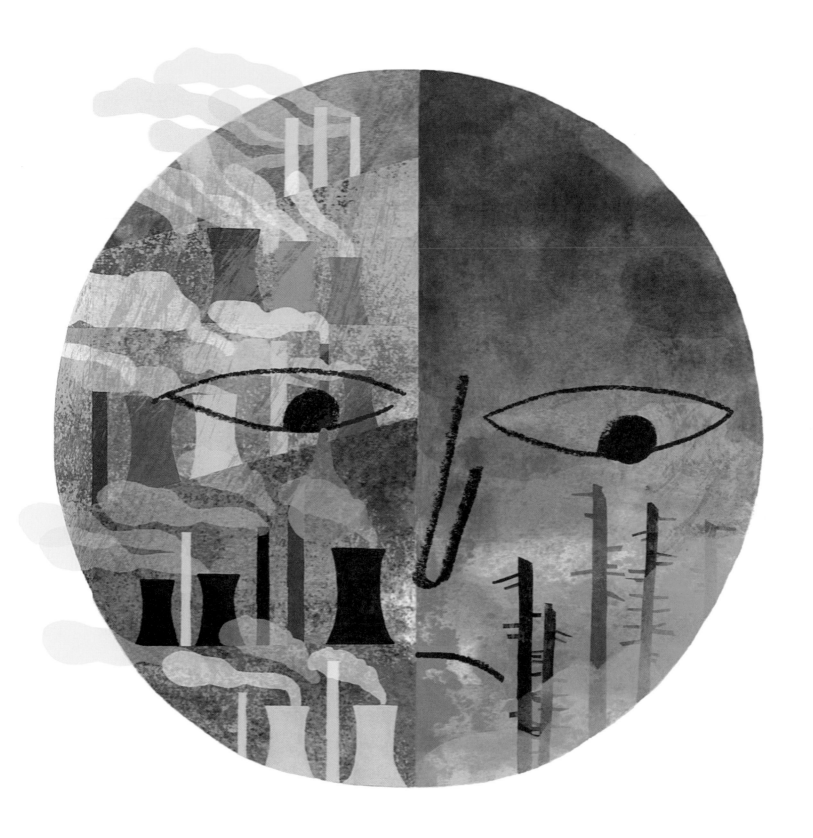

and let your voice

be heard.

I'll keep you safe,
and warm,
and dry.

At night
I'll sing
a lullaby.

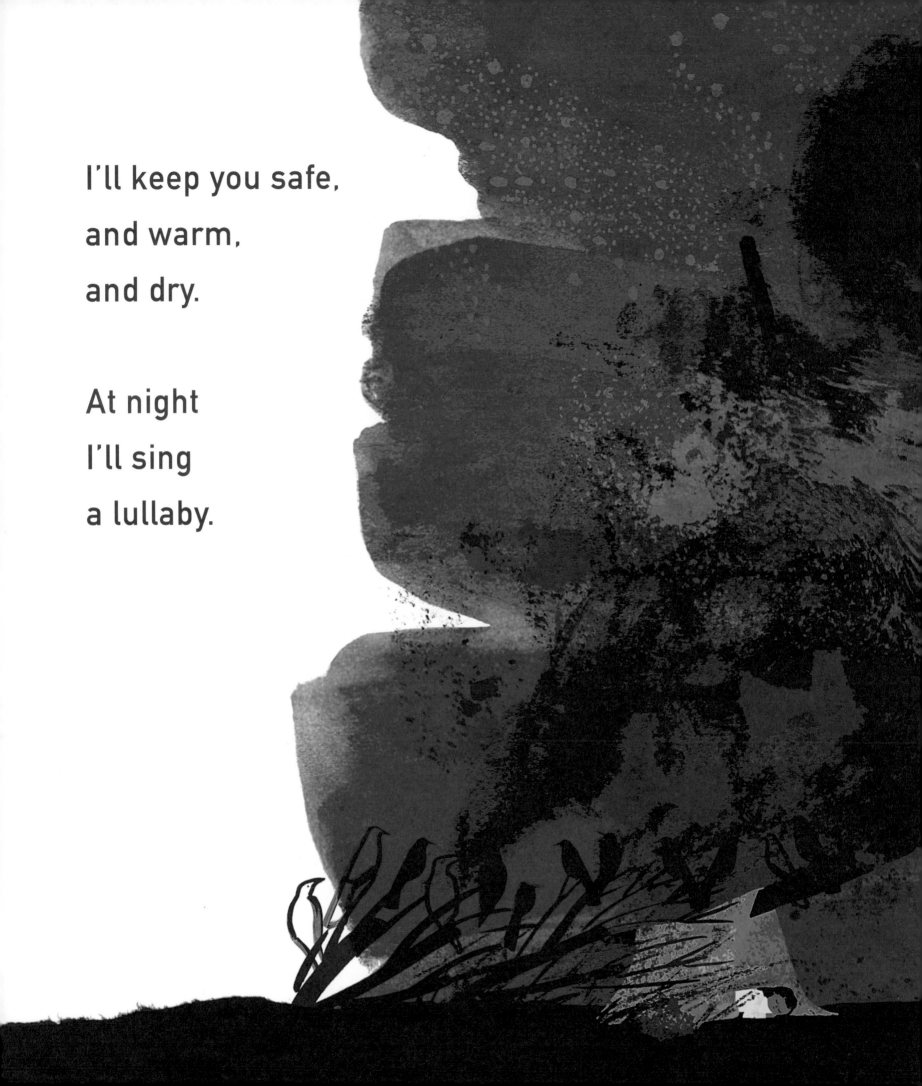

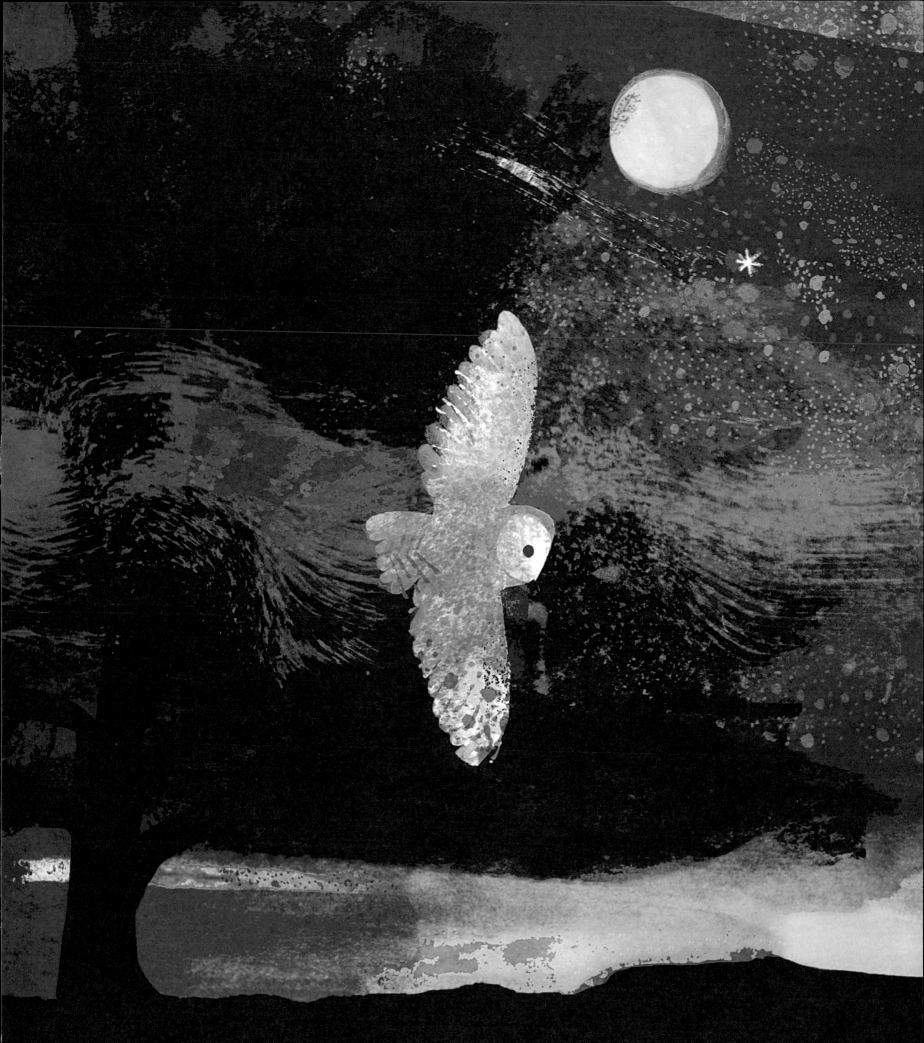

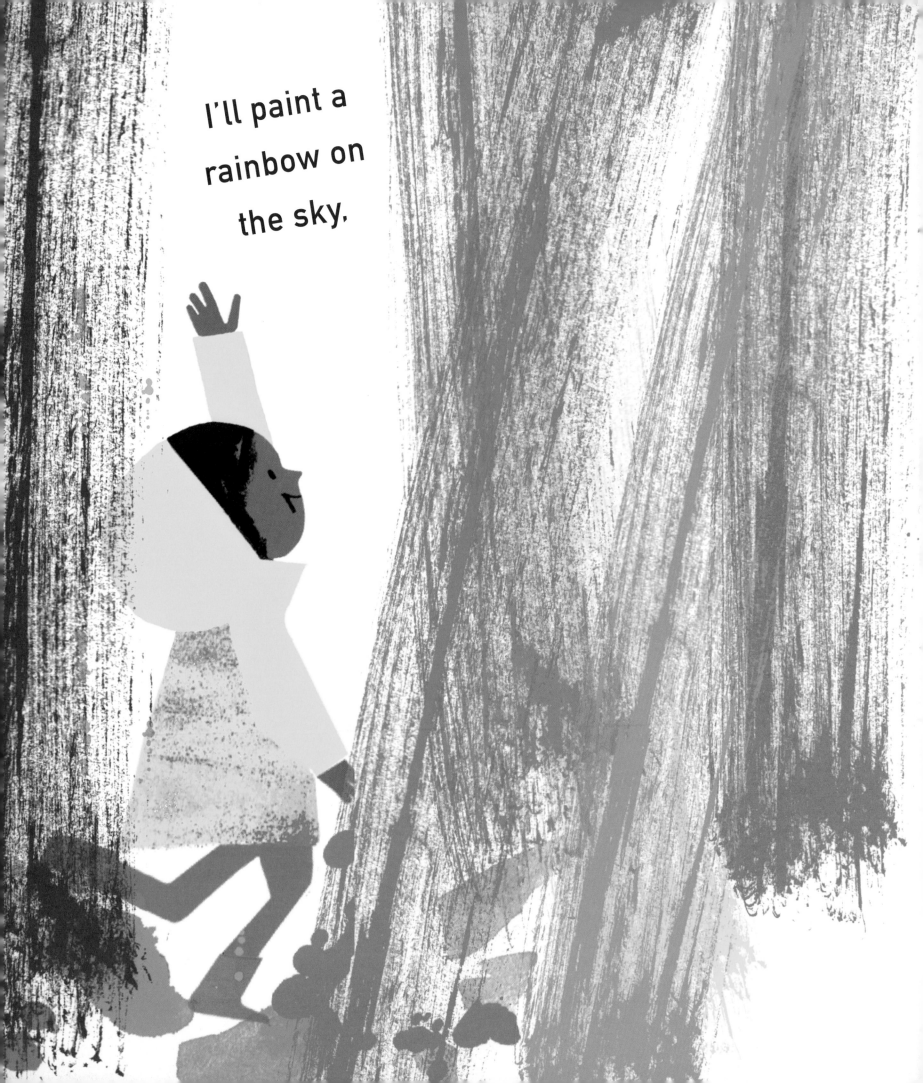

I'll paint a rainbow on the sky,

or cast a stormy spell.

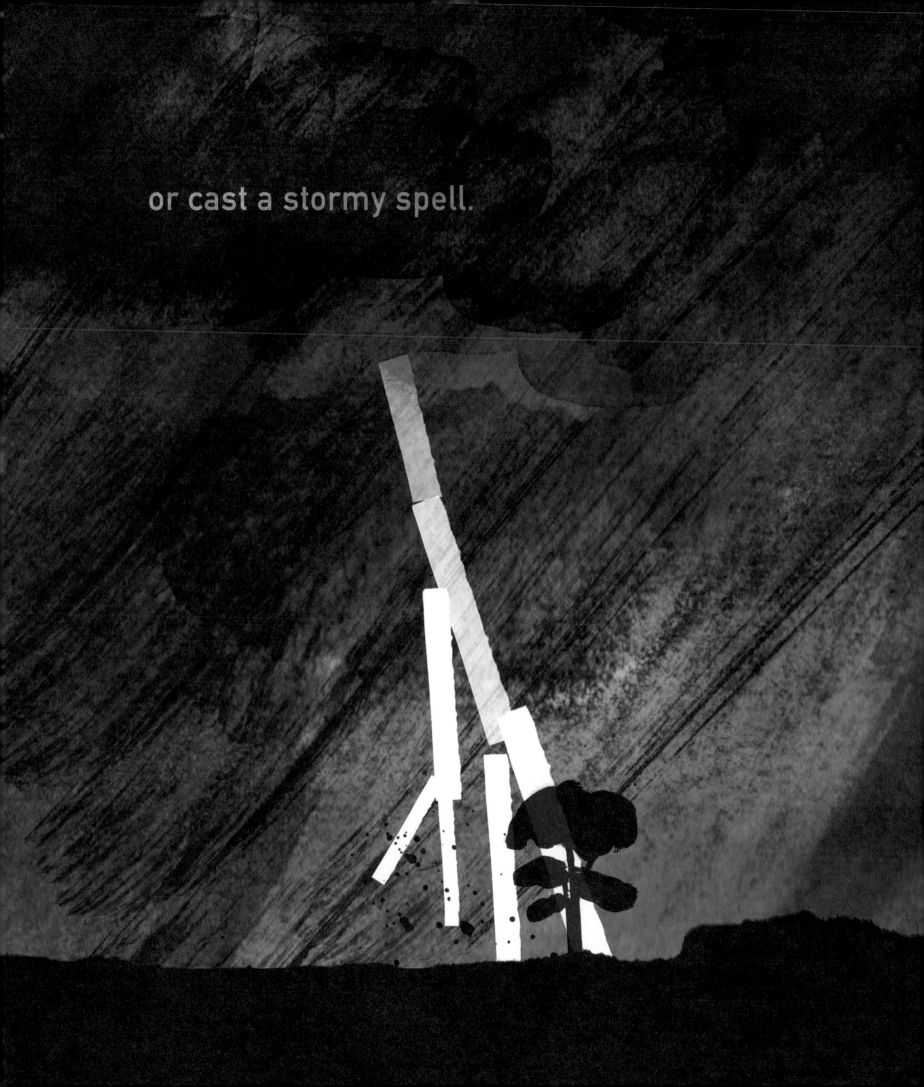

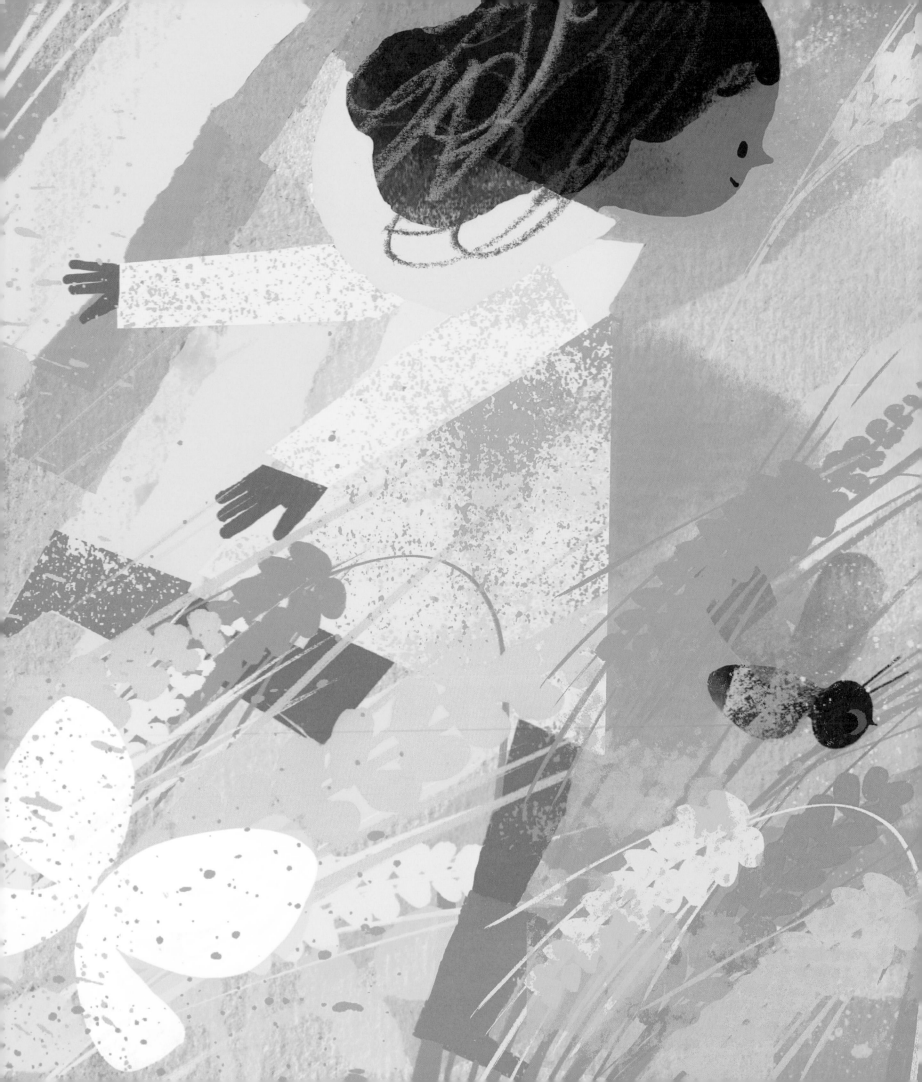

And as you **grow**, and **grow**, and **grow**,

I'll teach you everything I know,

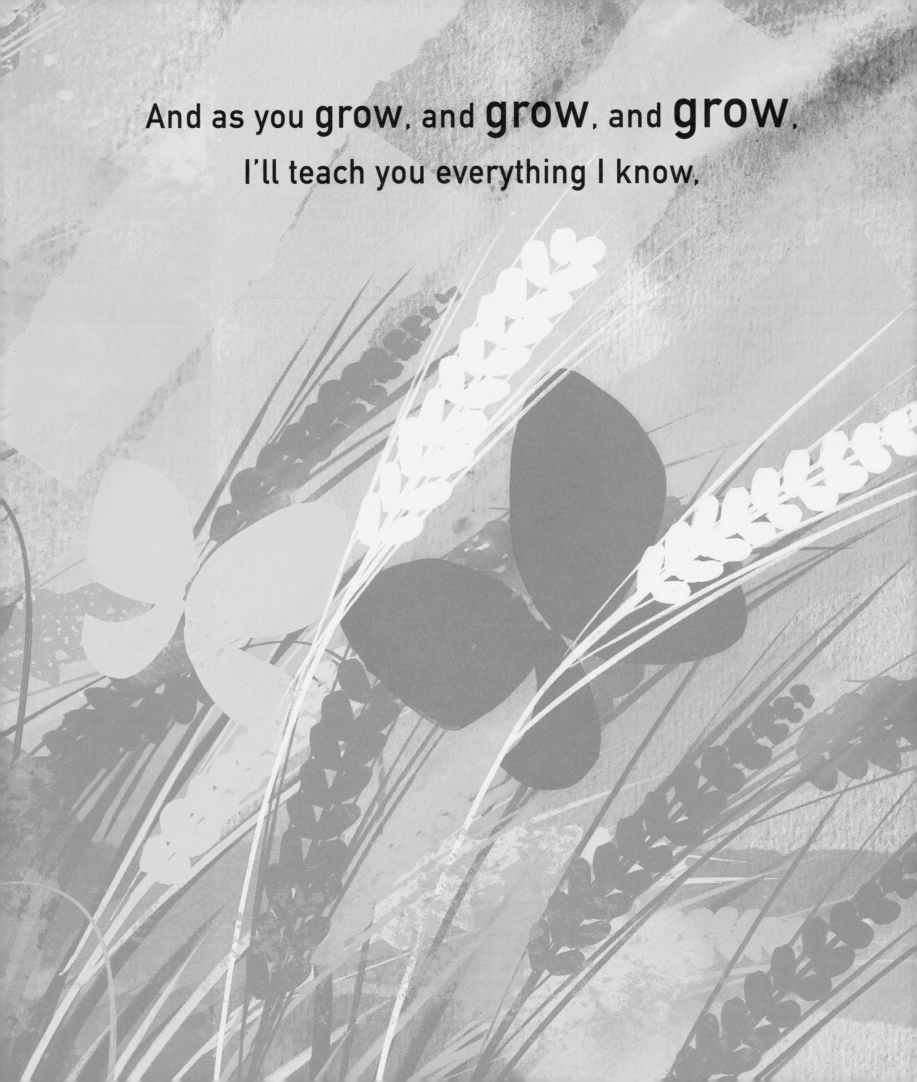

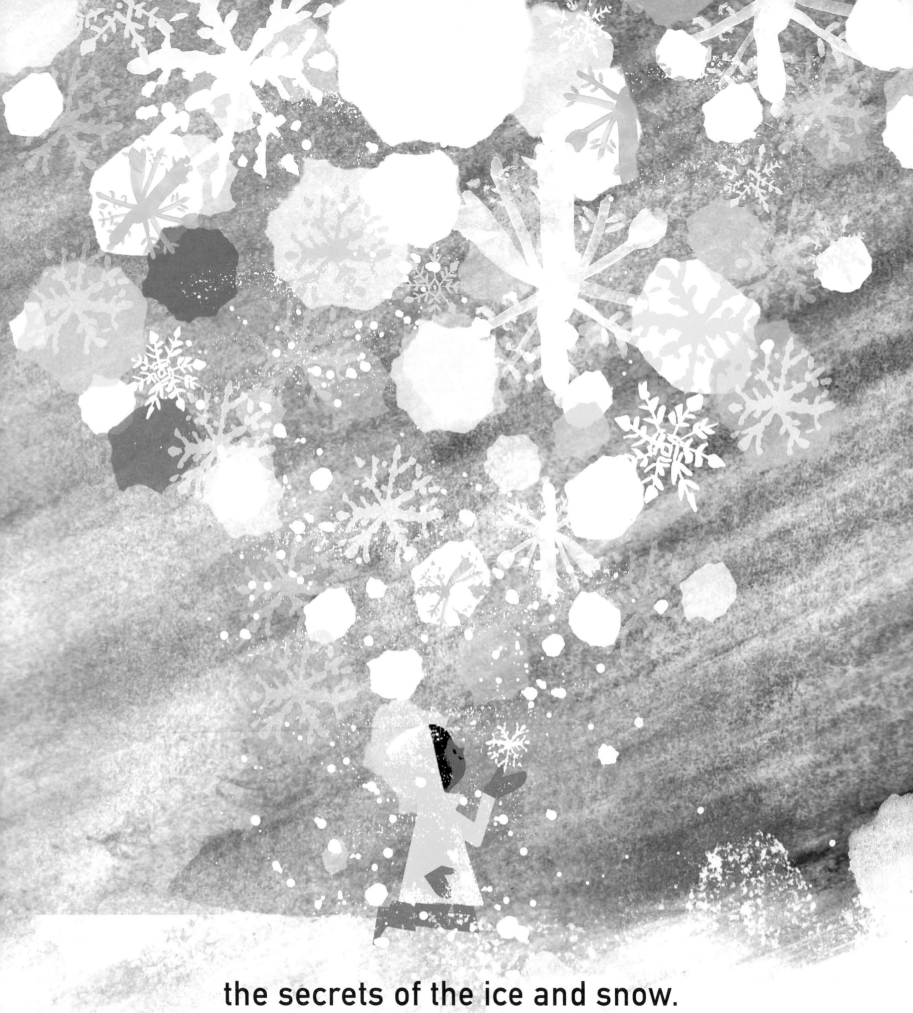

the secrets of the ice and snow.

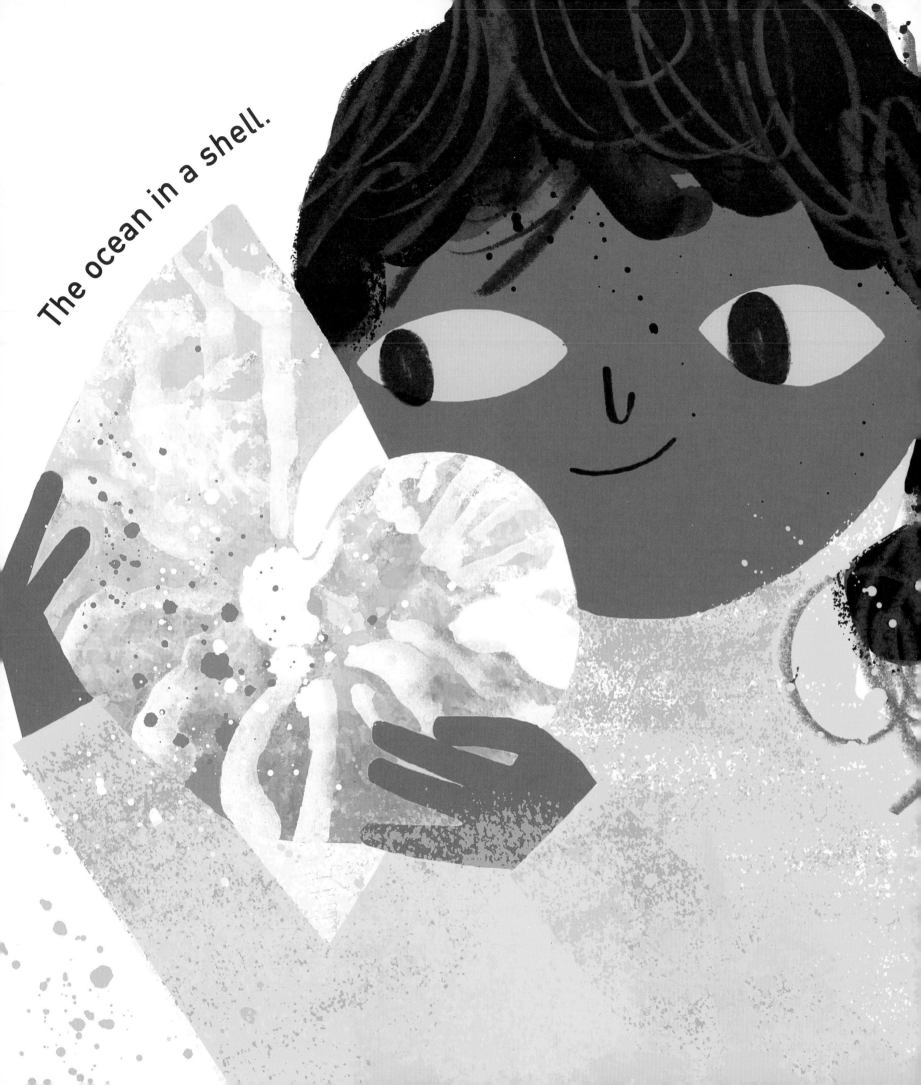

The ocean in a shell.

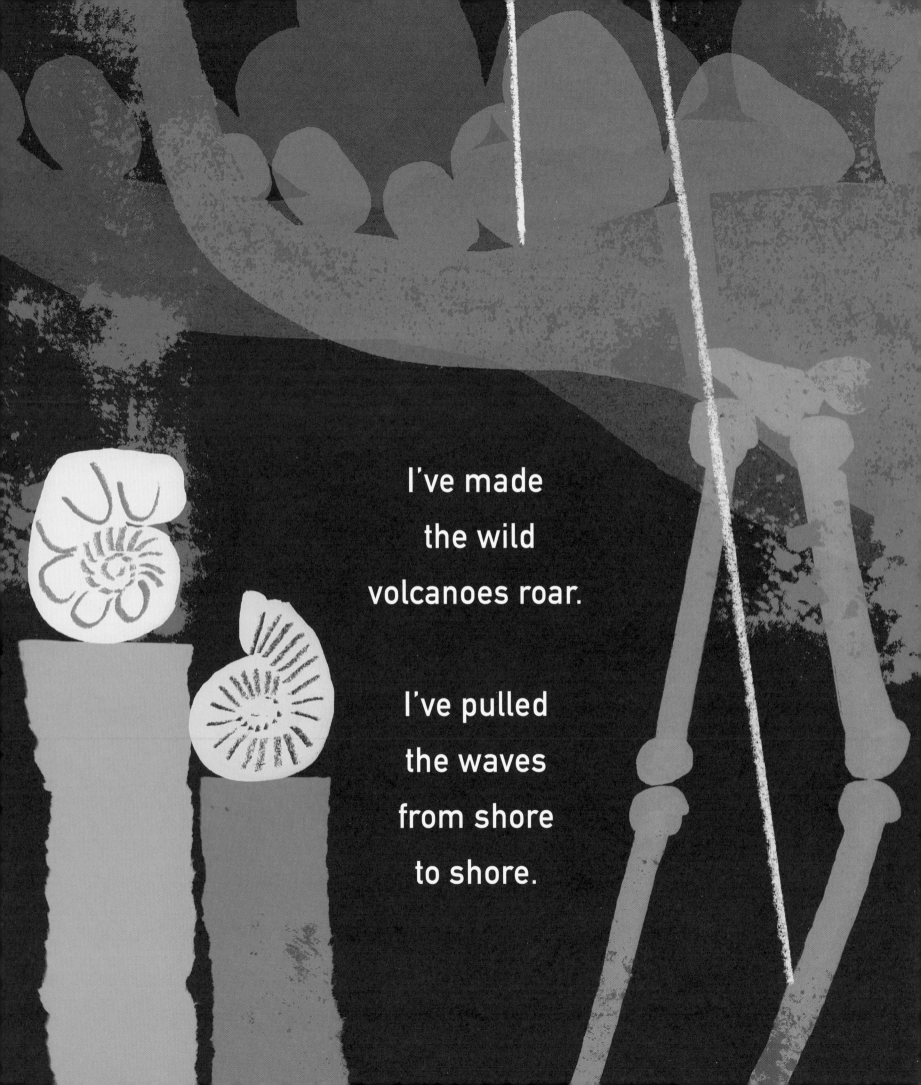

I've made
the wild
volcanoes roar.

I've pulled
the waves
from shore
to shore.

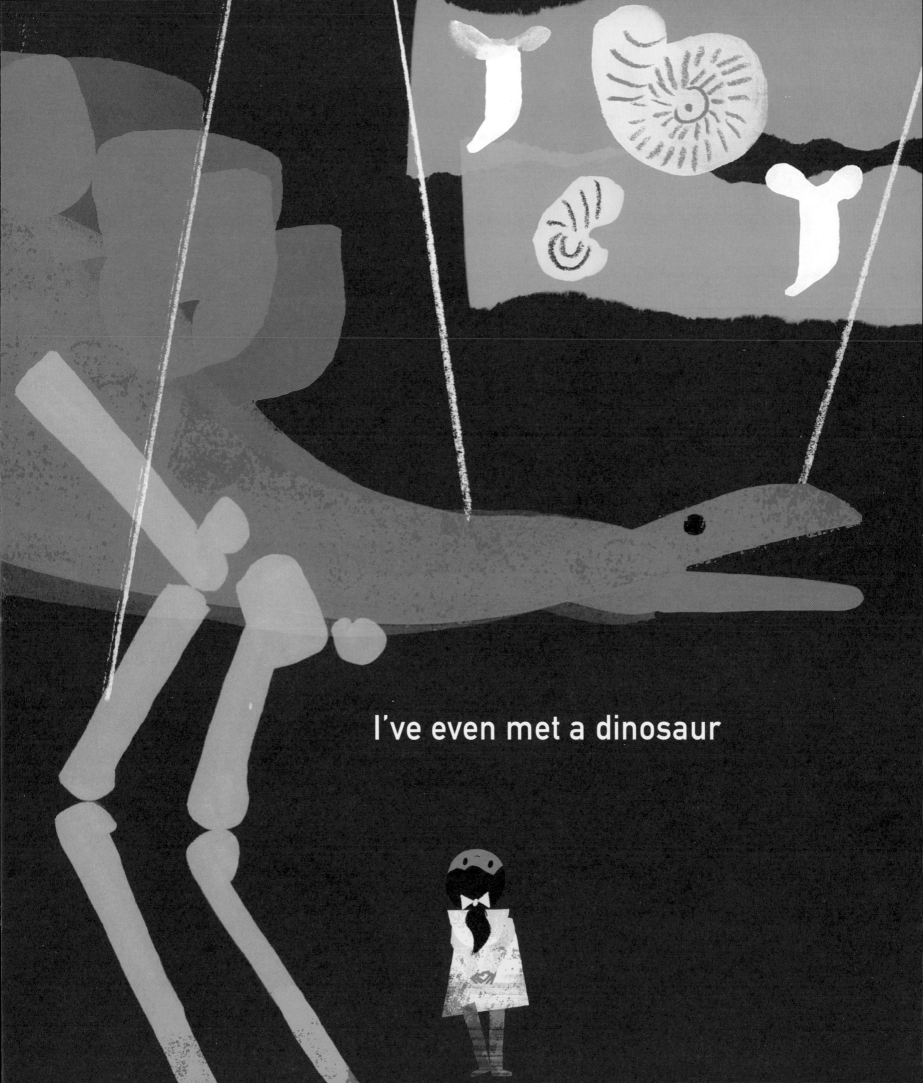

I've even met a dinosaur

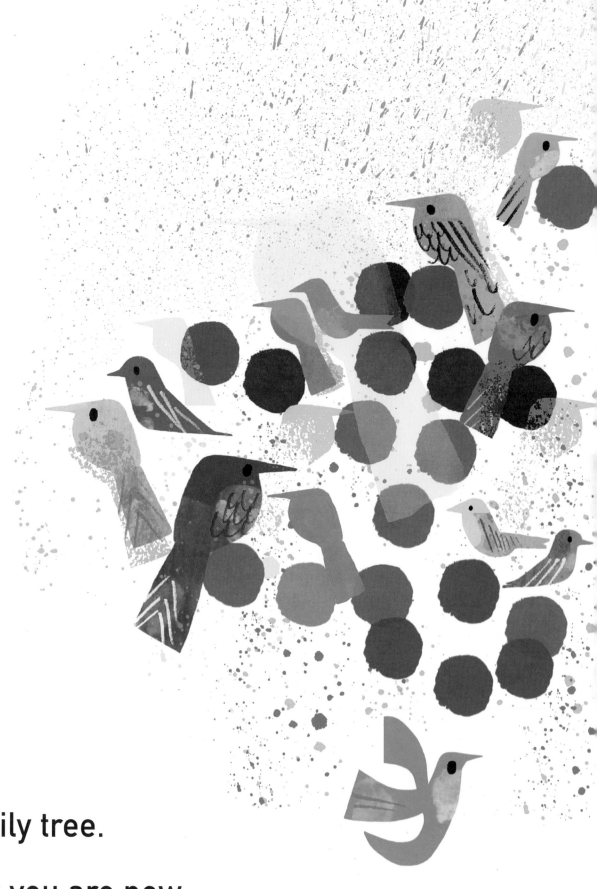

and all your family tree.

For I am old, but you are new.

Just think of all the things *you'll* do.

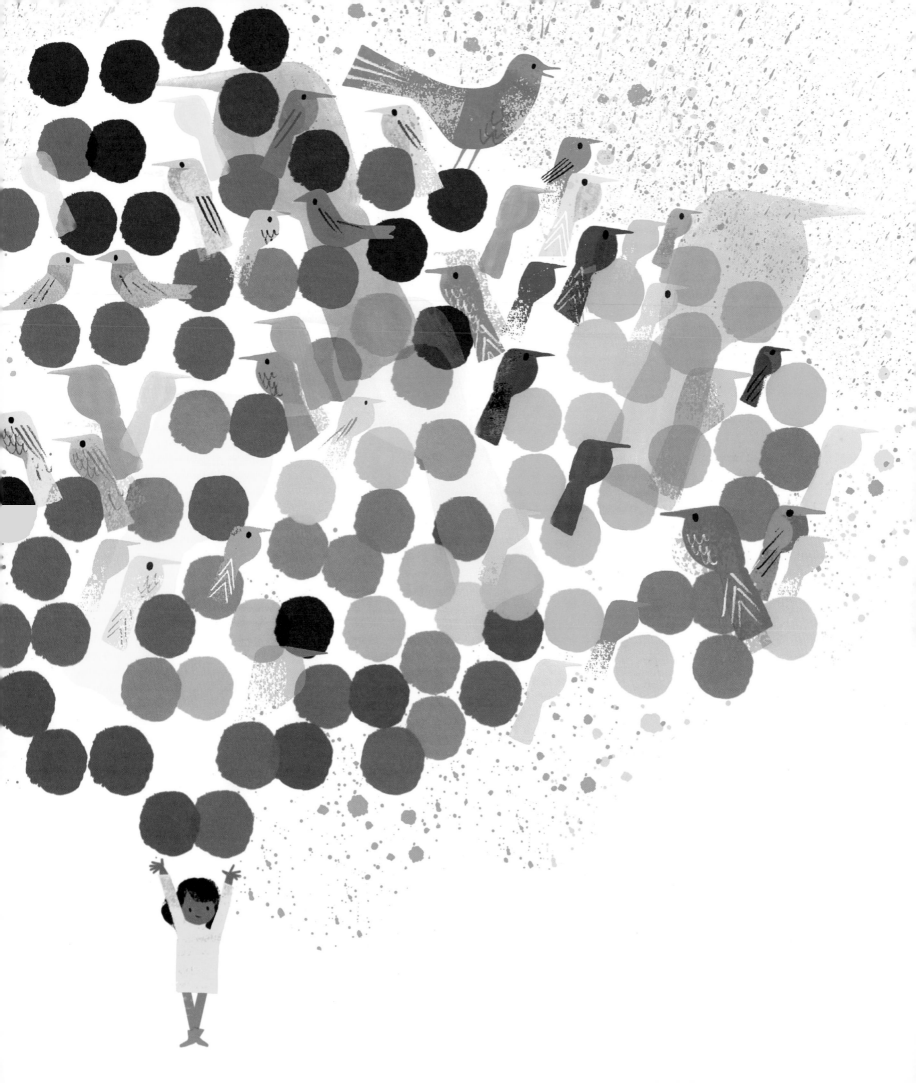

You see, there's only **one** of you,

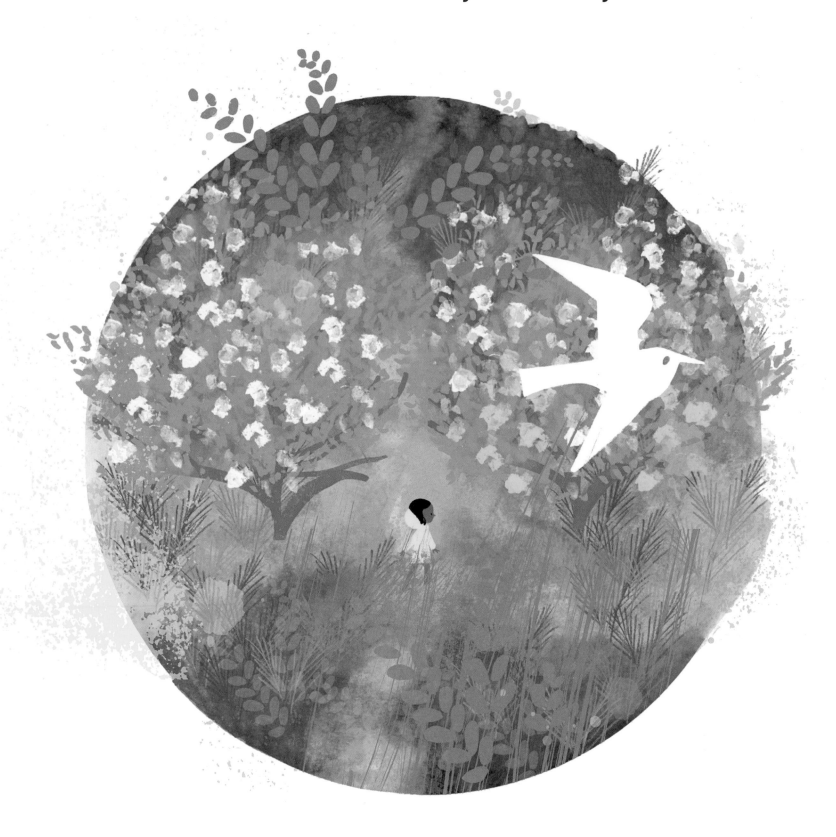

and only **one** of me.

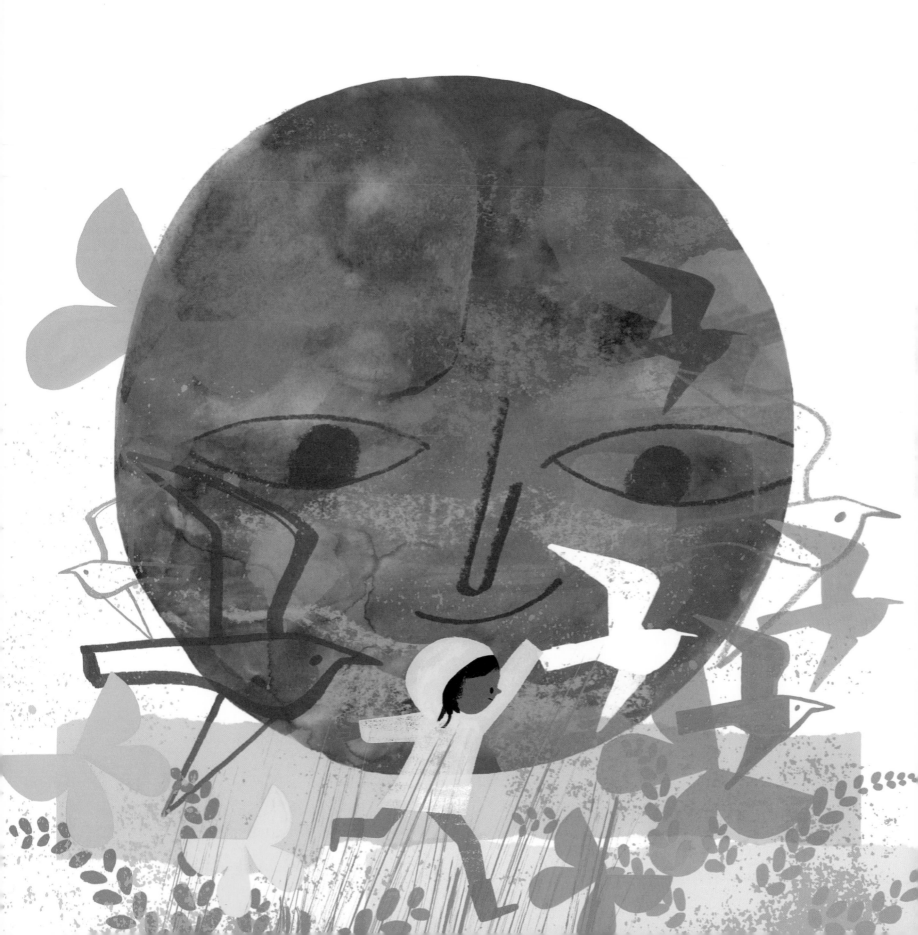

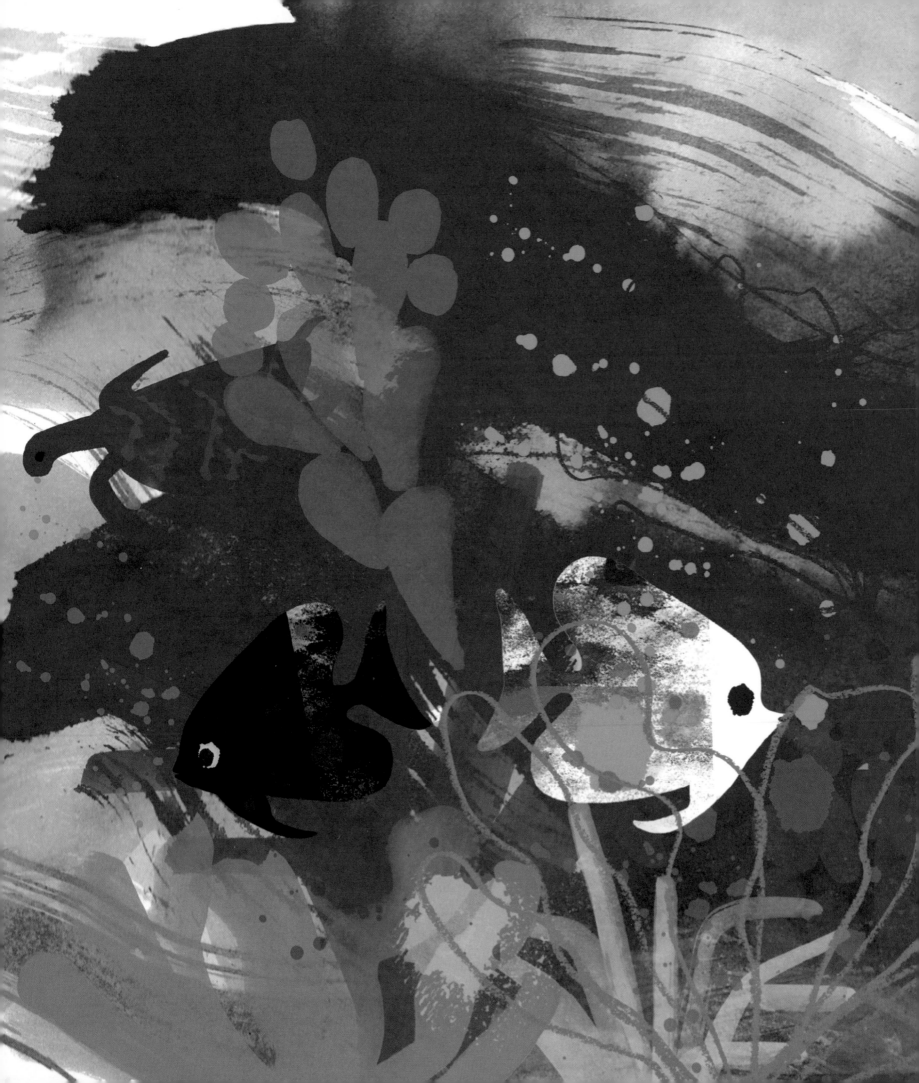

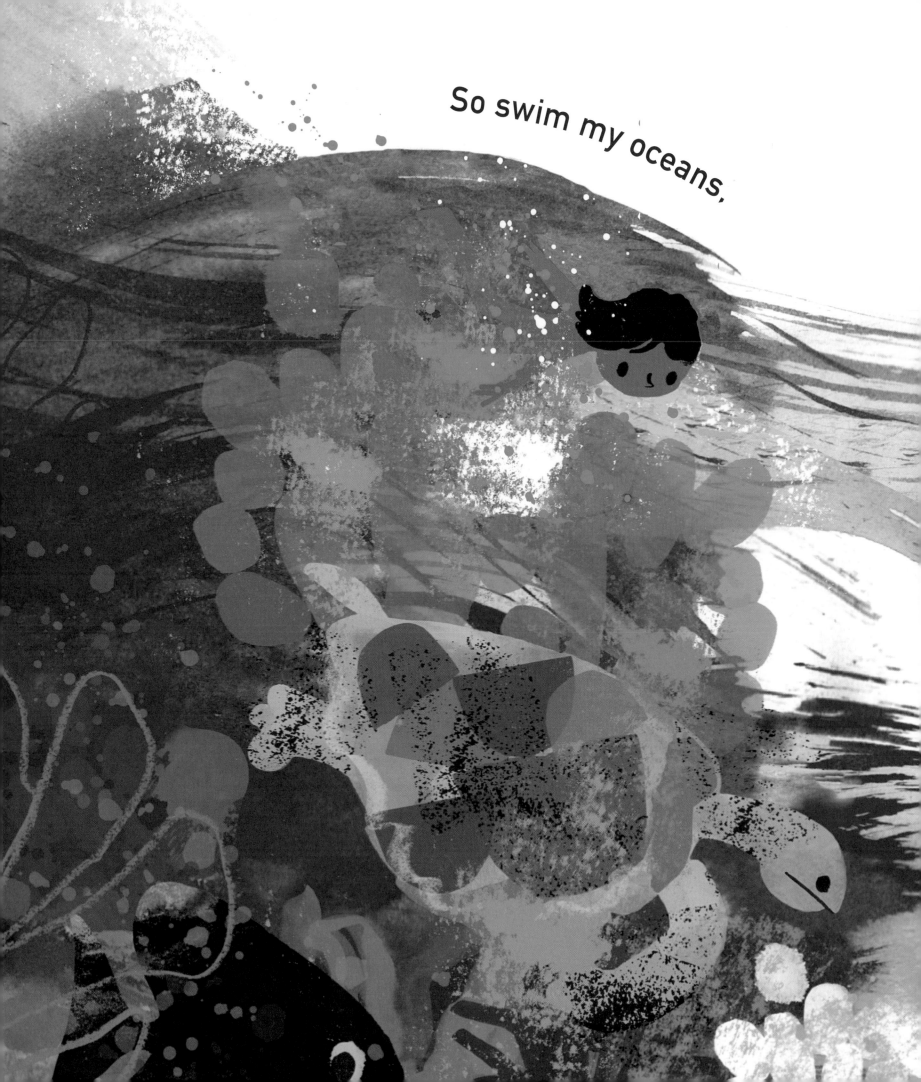

So swim my oceans,

climb my trees.
Kick my leaves into
the breeze.
Marvel at the galaxies
and love with all
your worth.

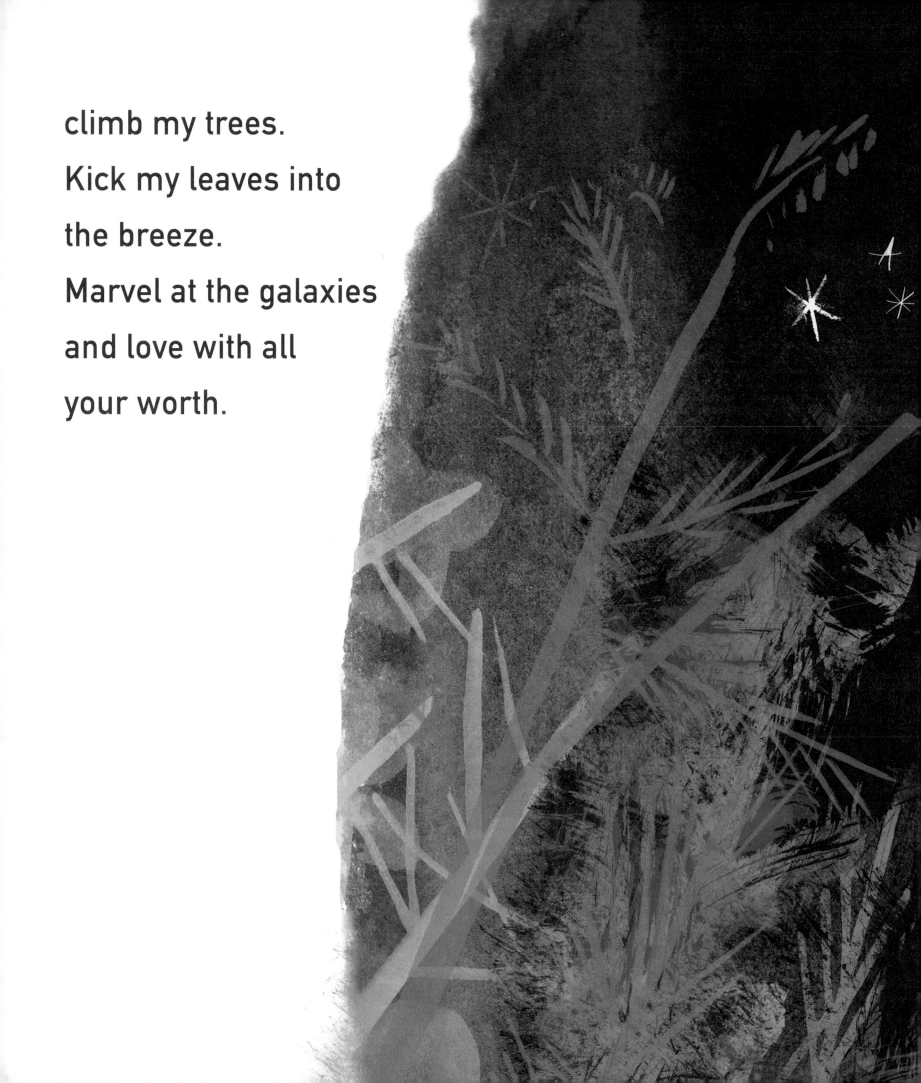

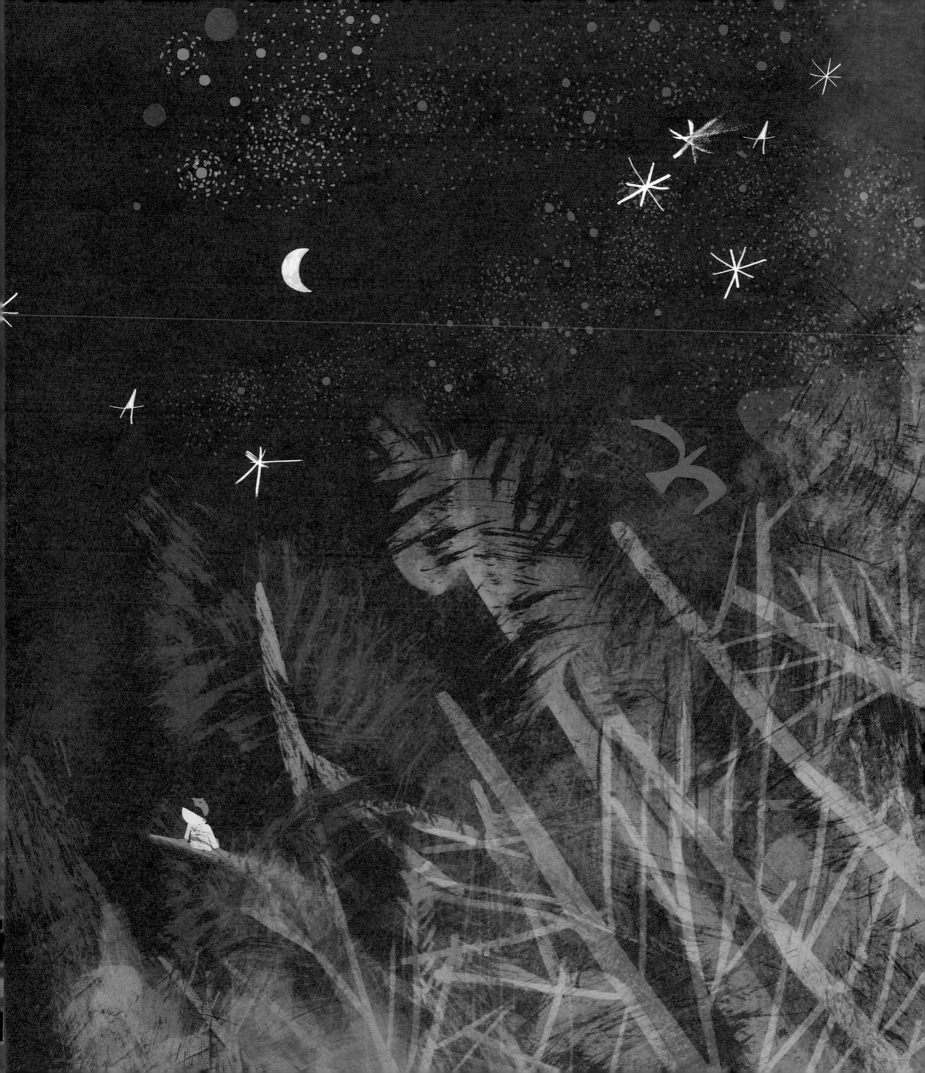

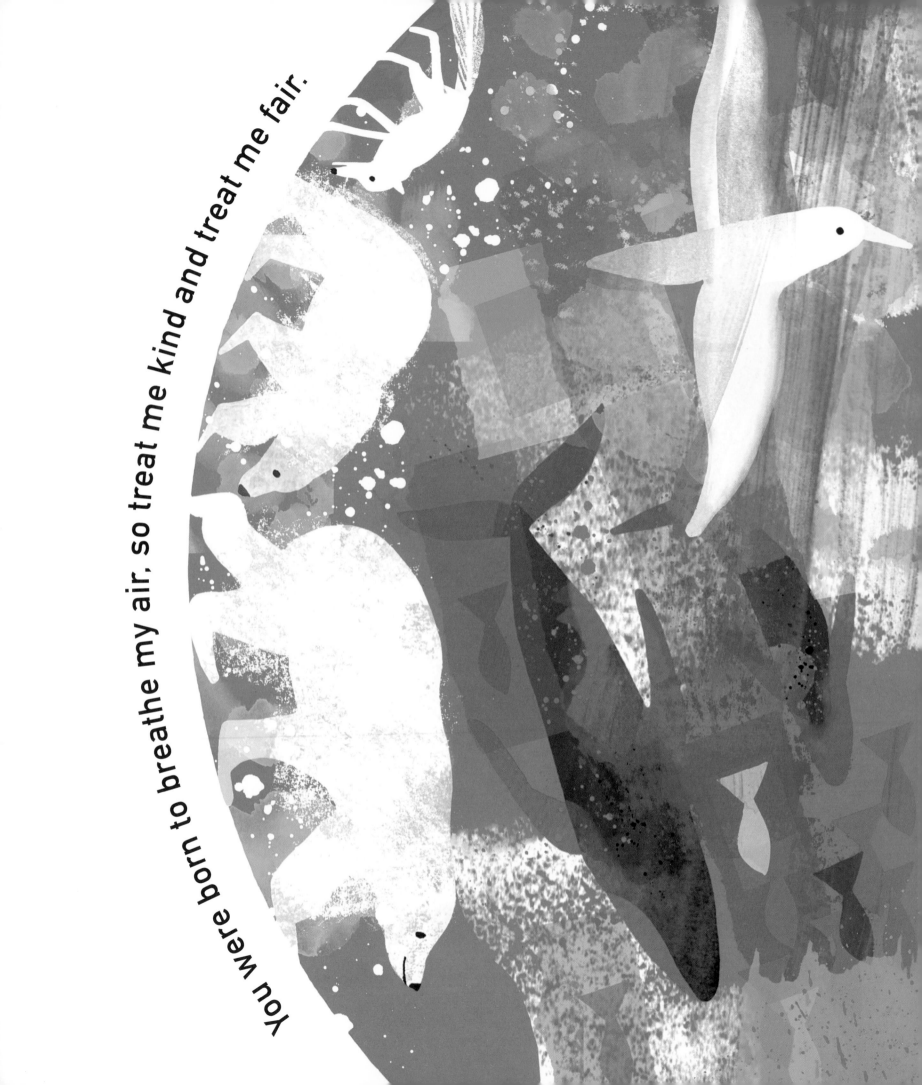

You were born to breathe my air, so treat me kind and treat me fair.

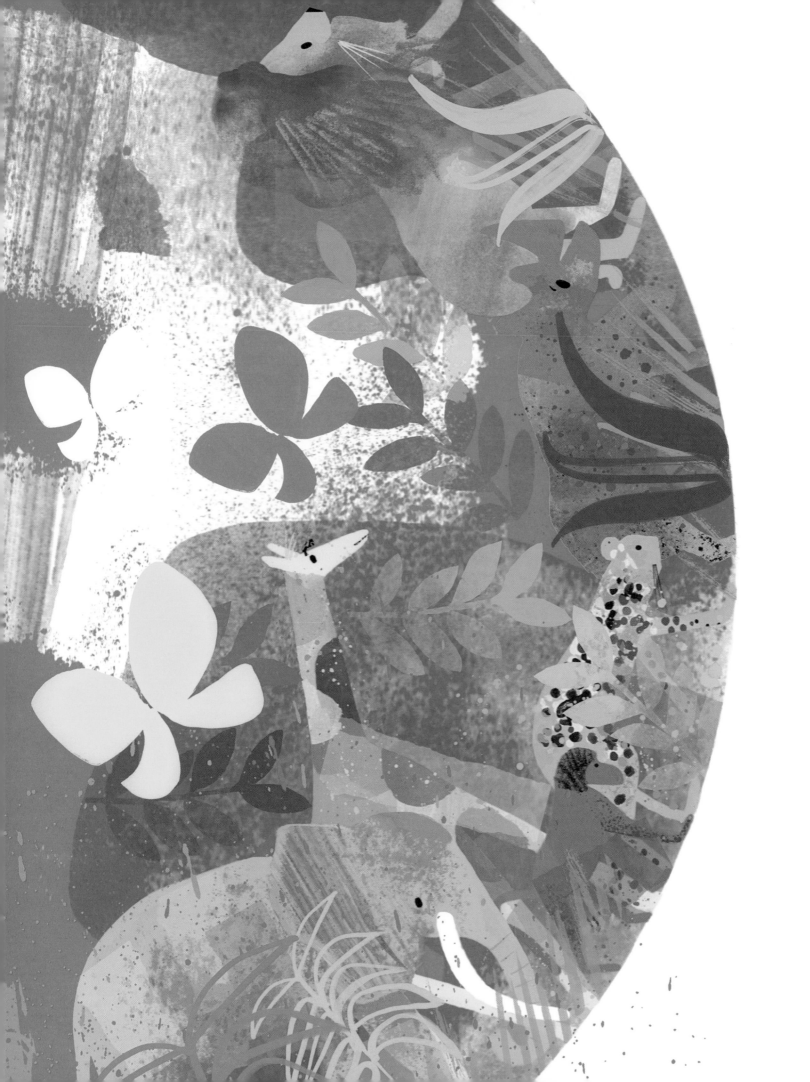

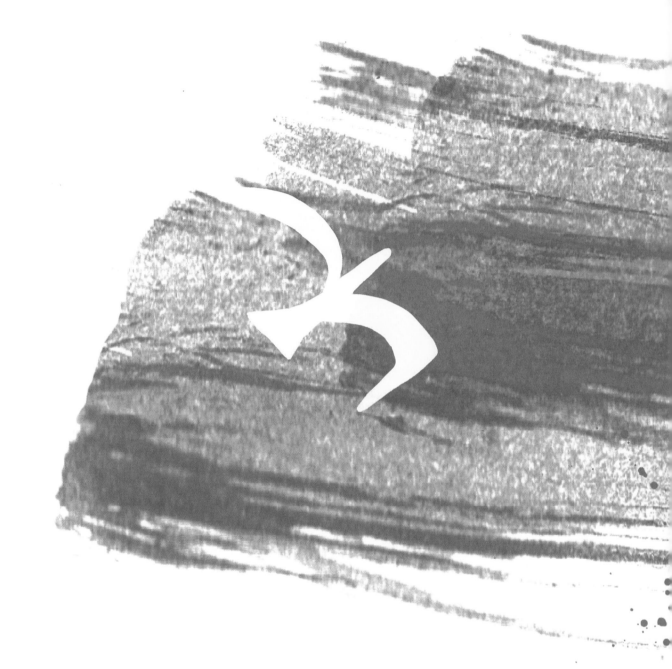

These gifts from me are yours to share.

With all my

Love, the Earth.

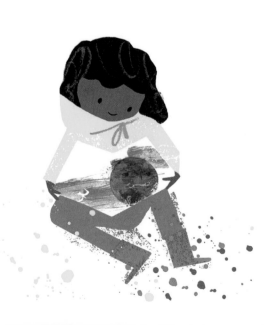

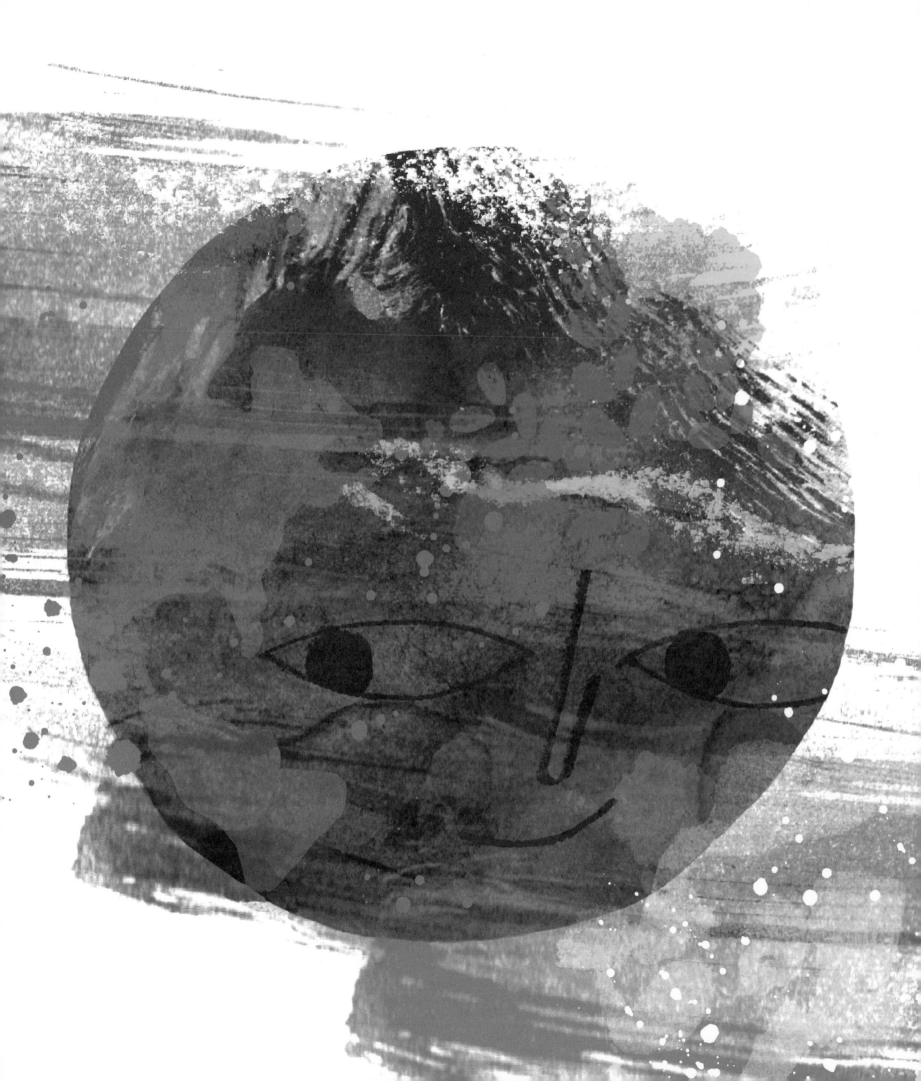

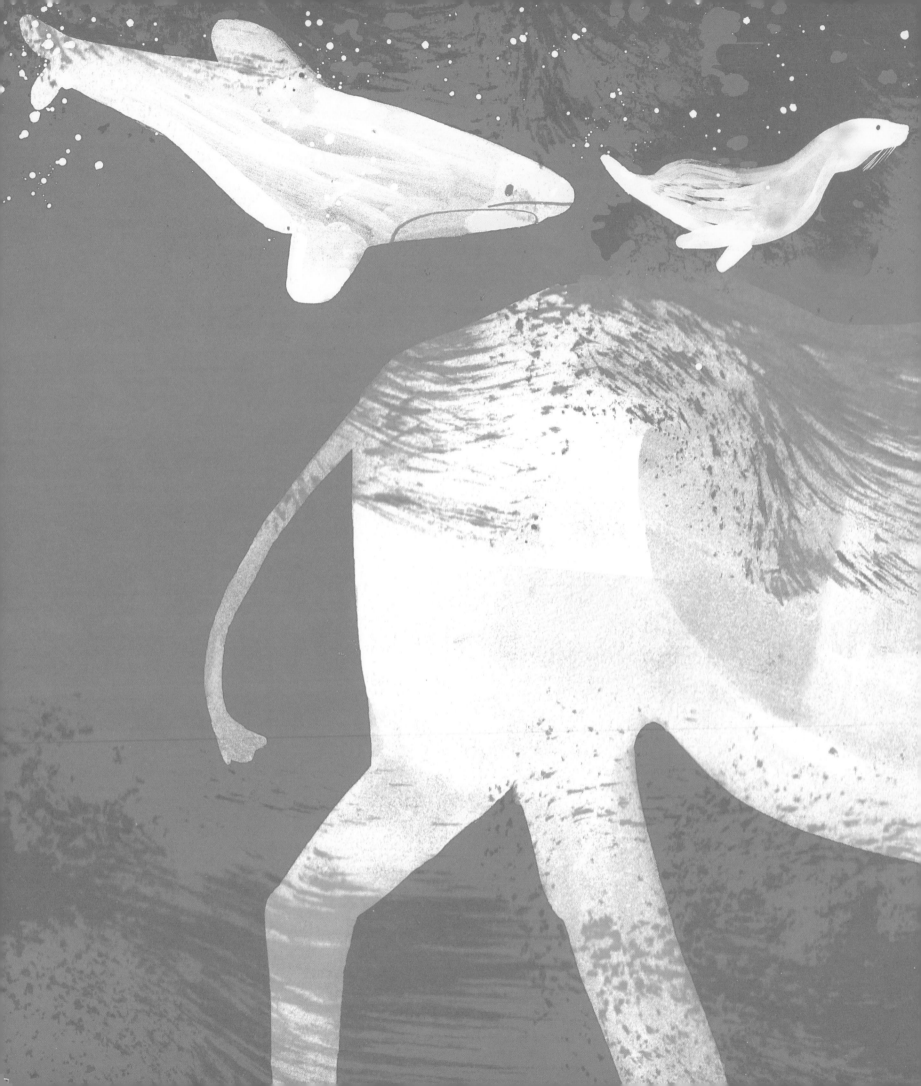